# Renal Disease

# Renal Disease

## *Prevention and treatment*

Edited by

G. Venkat Raman

*Wessex Renal and Transplant Unit*
*St Mary's Hospital*
*Portsmouth*
*UK*

Consulting Editor

T.A. Golper

*Division of Nephrology*
*University of Arkansas for Medical Sciences*
*Little Rock*
*Arkansas*
*USA*

CHAPMAN & HALL MEDICAL

London · Weinheim · New York · Tokyo · Melbourne · Madras

**Published by Chapman & Hall, 2–6 Boundary Row, London SE1 8HN, UK**

Chapman & Hall, 2–6 Boundary Row, London SE1 8HN, UK

Chapman & Hall GmbH, Pappelallee 3, 69469 Weinheim, Germany

Chapman & Hall USA, 115 Fifth Avenue, New York, NY 10003, USA

Chapman & Hall Japan, ITP-Japan, Kyowa Building, 3F, 2-2-1 Hirakawacho, Chiyoda-ku, Tokyo 102, Japan

Chapman & Hall Australia, 102 Dodds Street, South Melbourne, Victoria 3205, Australia

Chapman & Hall India, R. Seshadri, 32 Second Main Road, CIT East, Madras 600 035, India

First edition 1998



Typeset in 10/12pt Palatino by Acorn Bookwork, Salisbury, Wiltshire

Printed in Great Britain by T.J. International, Padstow, Cornwall

ISBN 0 412 45700 8



A catalogue record for this book is available from the British Library

Library of Congress Catalog Card Number: 97-67518

∞ Printed on acid-free text paper, manufactured in accordance with ANSI/NISO Z39.48-1992 (Permanence of Paper).

# Contents

# Contributors

C. Brunton MBChB MRCP
Department of Nephrology and Transplantation
Royal Free Hospital
Pond Street
London
NW3 2QG
UK

K. Erbeck MD
Division of Nephrology
Kidney Disease Program
University of Louisville
615 South Preston Street
Louisville
Kentucky 40202-1718
USA

C.F. George BSc MD FRCP
Professor of Clinical Pharmacology and Dean of the Faculty of Medicine and Biological Sciences
Clinical Pharmacology Group
Medical and Biomedical Sciences Building
Bassett Crescent East
Southampton
SO9 3TU
UK

S. Goldfarb MD PhD
Kidney Disease Program
University of Louisville
615 S Preston
Louisville
Kentucky 40292
USA

T.A. Golper MD FACP
Division of Nephrology
University of Arkansas for Medical Sciences
4301 West Markham
Mail Slot 501
Little Rock
Arkansas 72207 7199
USA

K.P.G. Harris MA MD FRCP
Senior Lecturer in Nephrology
Department of Medicine and Therapeutics
School of Medicine
Leicester General Hospital
Gwendolen Road
Leicester
LE5 4PW
UK

M. Jadoul MD
Department of Nephrology
Cliniques Universitaires St Luc
University of Louvain Medical School
Brussels
Belgium

P. Jungers MD
Professor of Nephrology
University Paris V
Department of Nephrology
Necker Hospital
Paris
France

P.A. Kalra MA MBBChir MRCP MD
Consultant Nephrologist and Honorary Lecturer
Hope Hospital
University of Manchester
Stott Lane
Salford
M6 8HD
UK

H.A. Lee FRCP
Formerly Professor of Renal Medicine
University of Southampton
Consultant Nephrologist
Wessex Renal and Transplant Unit
St Mary's Hospital
Portsmouth
PO3 6AD
UK

R. Maskell DM FRCP
Formerly Associate Specialist
Public Health Laboratory and Wessex Renal Unit
St Mary's Hospital
Portsmouth
PO3 6AD
UK

P.D. Mason BSc PhD FRCP
Consultant Nephrologist
Renal Unit
Churchill Hospital
Headington
Oxford
OX3 7LJ
UK

M.E. McGraw FRCP
Consultant Paediatric Nephrologist
Children's Renal Unit
Southmead Hospital
Bristol
BS10 5NB
UK

J.F. Moorhead FRCP
Professor of Renal Medicine
Department of Nephrology and Transplantation
Royal Free Hospital
Pond Street
London
NW3 2QG
UK

A.R. Noble PhD
Senior Lecturer in Physiology
Department of Physiology and Pharmacology
University of Southampton
Biomedical Sciences Building
Bassett Crescent East
Southampton
SO16 7PX
UK

C.D. Pusey MA MSc FRCP
Renal Unit
Hammersmith Hospital
Du Cane Road
London
W12 0NN
UK

K.M. Shaw MA MD FRCP
Consultant Physician
Queen Alexandra Hospital
Cosham
Portsmouth
PO6 3LY
UK

Z. Varghese PhD FRCPath
Associate Director
Renal Research Unit
Royal Free Hospital
Pond Street
London
NW3 2QG
UK

G.Venkat Raman MBBS MD FRCP
Consultant Renal Physician
Wessex Renal and Transplant Unit
St Mary's Hospital
Portsmouth
PO3 6AD
UK

M. Vennegoor SRD
Senior Renal Dietitian
St Thomas' Hospital Trust
St Thomas' Hospital
Lambeth Palace Road
London
SE1 7EH
UK

D.G. Waller BSc DM MB FRCP
Senior Lecturer in Medicine
Southampton General Hospital
Tremona Road
Southampton SO16 6YD
UK

J. Walls MB ChB FRCP
Professor of Nephrology
School of Medicine
Leicester General Hospital
Gwendolen Road
Leicester
LE5 4PW
UK

G.F. Watts BSc (Hons) DM FRCP
Senior Lecturer in Medicine
University of Western Australia
Consultant Physician
Royal Perth Hospital
Perth (GPO Box X2213)
Western Australia WA 6001

A. Wilkinson MD FRCP
Professor of Medicine
Director, Kidney and Pancreas Transplantation
Medical Specialty Suites
Suite 365
200 UCLA Medical Plaza
Los Angeles
California 90024 1693
USA

# Foreword

*An ounce of prevention is worth a pound of cure*

Everyone knows this ancient saying which, despite its non-metric units, remains as true in medicine as in all areas of human endeavour. Yet how neglected it is in medicine, including nephrology! The glamour and attention is all on what amounts to the *failure* of medicine to avert disasters, to prevent acute and chronic disease. And not only the glamour – also the money. With the annual budget for end-stage renal failure approaching $10 billion each year in both the USA and Japan, and even in Britain perhaps half a billion dollars, and a patient in acute renal failure costing $2000 per day, we have financial as well as humanitarian reasons to ask ourselves why we do not spend more time thinking about and working on prevention rather than crisis intervention or end-stage palliation.

Imagine a country where the rate of end-stage renal failure exceeds 1000 per million inhabitants per year. In fact you do not have to imagine such a country, because numerous countries in the developing world remain in exactly this situation. You can look also at what has been achieved by prevention in so-called developed countries. In the year that Queen Victoria ascended the throne of Britain in 1837, 600 deaths per million each year were attributed to nephritis alone, and Richard Bright was able to speak of ten or twenty nephrotics lying in the wards of any hospital in London. Life expectancy at birth was slightly less than 40 years. In recent years, the figure for ESRD from nephritis is about one-twentieth of this, and a life expectancy of twice that in 1837 is available to citizens of this fortunate country. How was this achieved? Not by any organized plan, or by medical intervention at all, but by improvements in housing, diet and hygiene which permitted the control of what we now regard as 'tropical' diseases such as malaria, streptococcal pyoderma, leprosy, cholera and bladder stones.

Of course, prevention has been evidently possible in many areas of nephrology for some time, obstructive uropathy is an example, yet still elderly men present to renal units with acute or chronic renal failure as a result of benign prostatic enlargement. Their 'successful' treatment by dialysis represents a complete failure of preventative medicine. The removal of medicinal toxins such as some analgesics and some industrial poisons such as lead from the environment has helped, but is not yet complete.

However, the list of preventable conditions leading to renal failure has extended steadily. Even ten years ago, diabetes would have been listed as a disease in which nothing can be done to avert the appearance or progression of the diabetic nephropathy. Now we know from prospective controlled trials that not only can the progress be slowed by ACE inhibitors, but that better control of glycaemia can reduce the proportion of type I diabetics developing nephropathy at all: this has fallen from about half to about a quarter during the past half century.

Control of disease progression has not yet, in general, arisen from a better understanding of the mechanisms leading to cirrhosis of the kidney. Limitation of protein intake, recommended as long ago as 1838, remains contentious and lowering of serum lipids has yet to be demonstrated in humans to slow progression. However, control of hypertension became possible during the 1950s at a terrible price in side-effects of the drugs used. Now it can be achieved in almost all patients, provided that enough effort is spent in teaching the patient to manage his or her lifetime commitment to therapy. Many failures result from the blood pressure not being taken or the pills not being taken. How much money do we spend on staff and programmes to treat hypertension in the community compared with that spent on end-stage renal disease?

This book is a timely reminder and a detailed consideration of our need to shift the emphasis of our thinking in nephrology away from the superficially exciting areas of crisis medicine to the much more cost-effective areas of prevention and slowing progression. Not only cost-effective in terms of cash, but also in terms of human suffering. If some readers are persuaded to change their thinking in this direction, its goal will have been achieved.

J. Stewart Cameron
Emeritus Professor of Renal Medicine
Guy's Campus, UMDS, London

# Introduction

Renal disease is an expensive high-intensity subspecialty of medicine. The major complication of a variety of diseases is the development of end stage renal failure, owing to the propensity for kidneys to lock in to an 'autoself destruct' mode. Where this used to be uniformly lethal, the last 30 years have seen dramatic developments in dialysis and transplantation, to the extent that at least in developed countries, patients do not die of renal failure any more (unless allowed to do so).

The euphoria that has accompanied these enormous strides has been tempered recently by the realization of the costs to society. With increasing availability of renal replacement therapies, and public awareness and expectations, the 'incidence' of end stage renal failure treatment is steadily increasing across the world. In Western Europe and USA the incidence of new patients varies from 70 to 120 patients per million population. The chronic shortage of cadaveric organs has led to an ever-increasing waiting list for transplantation. Furthermore a substantial proportion of patients coming onto dialysis are elderly, many of whom will not be physically fit to be considered for transplantation. Thus dialysis requirements are progressively rising and stretching the resources available.

The need for treating renal disease early, with a view to preventing the progression to end stage, is now well appreciated, for all the reasons mentioned above. A great deal of research has gone into identifying mechanisms of progression, as well as the factors contributing to it. The result has been an explosion of knowledge in all aspects of nephrology. Textbooks have been progressively increasing in size and there are a number of reference-style large texts in this field. However, there is a singular lack of a concise and up-to-date handbook, which is easy to read and transport. That was the reason for my decision to create such an entity. Furthermore, with the rising trend for a team approach towards the management of patients with renal disease, there is a need to educate paraclinical staff including nurses, dietitians, and pharmacists. Again, for this reason I felt that a book that was relatively concise would have a wide appeal. Lastly, a lot of emphasis has been placed on renal replacement therapy, and not enough has been said and done about preventative aspects. By the term prevention, I refer not only to the prevention of progression of renal disease, but also the prevention of other serious systemic disease, cardiovascular in particular, in patients with renal disease. This book combines all the points mentioned thus far, and hopefully will serve as a ready and useful guide for a wide spectrum of healthcare professionals, in particular nephrologists, both trained and in training.

I would like to acknowledge the considerable editorial help offered by my co-editor Tom Golper. I would like to express my sincere gratitude to my ever cheerful and uncomplaining secretary, Linda Rogers. Last but not least, I thank my family for their patience and understanding.

G. Venkat Raman

# 1

# Renal physiology

*A.R. Noble*

The fundamental processes of urine formation, filtration at the glomerulus followed by selective reabsorption and secretion by tubular epithelial cells, are well established. In the past, studies concerned with the regulation of these processes have mainly concentrated on endocrine control by aldosterone, antidiuretic hormone (ADH), angiotensin II (Ang II) and atrial natriuretic peptide (ANP), together with neural control mediated by the sympathetic nervous system. It is now recognized that local hormones exerting paracrine effects on cell populations which include vascular smooth muscle, the mesangial cells of the glomerulus and tubular epithelial cells are also of primary importance in the overall regulation of kidney function. In this chapter both endocrine and paracrine control mechanisms will be considered. In general the references quoted are to major review articles rather than specific research papers.

## 1.1 GLOMERULAR FILTRATION AND RENAL BLOOD FLOW

Textbooks of physiology are written about male subjects, weighing 70 kg and aged 20–25 years, who have no pathology. In such a subject, under resting conditions the kidneys receive approximately 20–25% of cardiac output, a blood flow of about 1.25 l/min or, assuming a haematocrit of 45%, a renal plasma flow of around 700 ml/min. Together, the kidneys have 2–3 million nephrons in which the glomeruli produce an ultrafiltrate of plasma at a rate of about 125 ml/min or 170 l/day. The filtration fraction (FF), glomerular filtration rate (GFR) expressed as a percentage of renal plasma flow (RPF) is therefore about 20%. Most of

*Renal Disease.* Edited by G. Venkat Raman. Published in 1998 by Chapman & Hall, London. ISBN 0 412 45700 8.

the water and the solutes in the filtrate are reabsorbed into the peritubular capillaries during passage down the nephron. For obvious reasons, in clinical practice, GFR should be expressed as a function of body surface area (standardized to $1.73\,m^2$). For any given individual, every aspect of these basic statistics of kidney function is conditional upon age, gender, body weight and pathological changes both inside and outside the kidney. Age-related changes in renal function have recently been reviewed [1].

### 1.1.1 The glomerular filter

In moving from the plasma into the lumen of Bowman's capsule the filtrate must pass through three layers, all of which contribute to the functional characteristics of the glomerulus (reviewed in refs 2 and 3). Selectivity of the filter is determined both by the molecular size of solutes and by the presence of a net negative electrical charge carried on glomerular structures. The three layers of the filter are as follows.

1. **The blood capillary endothelial cell layer**. The hydraulic conductivity of this layer, which has very large fenestrae, is high. It is about 100 times more permeable than any other capillary bed and 100 000 times as permeable as the cerebral vasculature, which has no fenestrae. On the basis of size, the glomerular endothelial cell layer is only an effective permeability barrier to blood cells. However, a strongly anionic glycocalyx contributes to the charge-selectivity of the glomerular filter. The negative charge probably helps to reduce penetration by small proteins, such as albumin.
2. **The glomerular basement membrane (GBM)**. This non-cellular layer is approximately twice the thickness of basement membranes found outside capillary endothelia elsewhere in the body. The GBM is composed of glycoproteins, particularly type IV collagen, non-collagenous sialoglycoproteins, such as laminin and fibronectin, and proteoglycans, including heparan sulphate. These constituents of the GBM are produced by the podocytes and, to a lesser extent, during development by the capillary endothelial cells. Functionally, the GBM is the primary filter in the glomerulus [4, 5]. Under electron microscopy, three layers have been identified in the GBM, the lamina interna next to the endothelial cells, a middle layer called the lamina densa and the lamina externa to which the podocytes are attached. It is thought that the lamina densa, and particularly the type IV collagen component, is the most effective part of the filter on the basis of size. The lamina interna and lamina externa primarily provide an electrostatic anionic barrier (reviewed in ref. 6).

   The thickness of the GBM is variable and this may be associated with changes in hydraulic conductivity. The podocyte responds to increased physical stress or to cytokines, such as interleukin-1 (IL-1) and transforming growth factor-beta (TGF-$\beta$), with increased extracellular matrix production. The epithelial cells, endothelial cells and mesangium of the glomerulus, together with plasma enzymes, also produce matrix degrading proteins which can reduce the thickness of the GBM (reviewed in ref. 7).

3. **The visceral epithelial cells or podocytes**. These are structurally the most complex component of the filter. The cell body lies in the urinary space but the cells have a series of primary processes which form multiple secondary and tertiary processes called pedicels or foot processes. These are attached to the GBM. Retention of the structural integrity of the glomerulus is the result of both cell-to-cell and cell-to-GBM adhesion. Several types of molecule are involved including proteins of the $\beta_1$-integrin subfamily, immunoglobins and other cell adhesion molecules (reviewed in ref. 8).

   The complex arrangement of the podocytes produces a series of slit pores through which the filtrate must pass and which cover between 3 and 10% of the total GBM area. The foot processes have a contractile apparatus [9] which may function to vary the slit width and thus contribute to the overall permeability of the glomerular filter [10].

   In addition to synthesizing the constituents of the GBM, the podocytes also express the sialoglycoprotein podocalyxin. This protein provides a highly anionic coating to the podocytes which contributes to the charge selectivity of the glomerulus. Additionally, podocalyxin is important in maintaining the architecture of the glomerulus [11]. The precise role of the podocytes in determining $K_c$, the filtration coefficient per unit area of the glomerular endothelium, still requires considerable clarification.

In a normal kidney the permeability characteristics for the glomerular filter can be summarized as follows. Substances with a molecular radius less than 1.8 nm, and which do not carry an electrical charge, are filtered freely. For example, an uncharged polysaccharide dextran molecule with a relative molecular mass of 5500 and a molecular radius of 1.5 nm is freely filtered. Neutral dextrans above 4.0 nm in radius are almost completely excluded from the filter. For dextrans with radii between 1.5 and 4.0 nm there is a size-related partial filtration. If a molecule carries a negative charge it is filtered less easily than a neutral molecule and if it carries a net positive charge it will be filtered more easily. Experimentally, neutralizing the negative charge on the wall of the glomerulus causes the filter to operate entirely on a size basis.

Human plasma albumin (relative molecular mass 69 kD) has a molecular radius of 3.55 nm and is polyanionic. About 70 000 g of albumin pass through the vasculature of the kidneys in a day but only about 7 g/day appears in the filtrate, 0.01% of the total. Normally all the filtered albumin is reabsorbed in the proximal tubule and so none appears in the urine. Although possessing a very low permeability to proteins, the glomerular filter nevertheless maintains a very high permeability to water.

The remaining structural component of the glomerulus is the mesangium. This consists of cells and extracellular matrix occupying the centrilobular region of the glomerular tuft and thus appearing to be connective tissue-like. Two main cell types have been identified as the mesangial cells, which in some ways are similar to smooth muscle cells, and the bone marrow-derived phagocytic cells. The cells of the mesangium are surrounded by a matrix, major components of which include collagens IV and V, fibronectin, laminin, entactin/nidogen and proteoglycans such as chondroitin sulphate and heparan sulphate. There has been much recent interest in the role played by the mesangium in the regulation of glomerular function (referred to below) and in immunologically mediated mechanisms of renal disease (reviewed in refs 12–14).

### 1.1.2 Forces driving filtration

The Starling forces which determine GFR represent a balance between the hydrostatic pressure gradient and a colloid osmotic pressure gradient. These forces can be summarized mathematically as follows:

$$\mathrm{GFR} = K_f[P_{\mathrm{CAPILL}} - P_{\mathrm{TUB}}) - (\pi_{\mathrm{CAPILL}} - \pi_{\mathrm{FILT}})]$$

where $K_f$ is the filtration coefficient, i.e. the permeability of the filter for the whole kidney(s). This parameter is returned to later in this chapter.

This Starling equation can be adapted to apply to single nephron glomerular filtration rate (SNGFR) by replacing $K_f$ with $K_g$, a filtration coefficient appropriate to a single glomerulus.

$P_{\mathrm{CAPILL}}$ is the glomerular capillary blood pressure, the primary force driving filtration. Typical normal figures at the afferent end of the glomerular capillary would be 45 mm Hg and at the efferent end 44 mm Hg. The regulation of glomerular capillary blood pressure is discussed below.

$P_{\mathrm{TUB}}$ is the tubular fluid pressure, typically about 10 mm Hg uniformly along the interface with the capillary. Tubular pressure opposes filtration and if it rises markedly, as in the case of urinary outflow obstruction, filtration will cease.

$\pi_{\mathrm{CAPILL}}$ is the colloid osmotic pressure exerted by the proteins in plasma. This component of the Starling forces opposes filtration. Most of the total osmotic pressure of blood plasma (about 5000 mm Hg) is attributable to the small molecules, particularly sodium and chloride ions. The concentrations of these substances in the plasma and the filtrate are effectively identical and so there is no osmotic gradient produced by them. Only about 0.5% of the total osmotic pressure of plasma is generated by the large non-filterable molecules (colloids). A typical value for $\pi_{CAPILL}$ at the afferent arteriolar end of the glomular capillary is 25 mm Hg. Movement of water across the filter means that protein left in the glomerular capillary becomes more concentrated and so $\pi_{CAPILL}$ rises to about 34 mm Hg at the efferent arteriolar end of the capillary.

$\pi_{FILT}$ is the colloid osmotic pressure of the tubular fluid. As the protein content of the filtrate is normally very small, about 0.01% of $\pi_{CAPILL}$, the numerical value for $\pi_{FILT}$ is effectively zero. This will not of course be true if significant amounts of albumin permeate the glomerular filter as a result of a pathological process.

Using the normal values quoted above for the component Starling forces we can calculate that the net filtration pressure at the afferent arteriolar end of the glomerular capillaries is approximately 10 mm Hg and at the efferent arteriolar end it is close to zero.

## 1.2 REGULATION OF GLOMERULAR CAPILLARY BLOOD PRESSURE

Much of the experimental work which provided direct measurements of glomerular capillary pressure was carried out in the Munich–Wistar rat, a strain in which the glomeruli persist on the surface of the kidney into adulthood. The glomeruli are accessible for investigations using direct micropuncture techniques [15].

Glomerular capillary pressure is determined fundamentally by the perfusion pressure in the renal artery (arterial blood pressure) and locally by the balance between the afferent and efferent arteriolar resistances. Potentially, an increase in afferent or a decrease in efferent arteriolar tone will lead to a fall in glomerular capillary blood pressure and therefore to a decrease in GFR. Conversely, a decrease in afferent or an increase in efferent arteriolar tone will increase both glomerular capillary pressure and GFR. In practice, in the normal kidney, both renal blood flow (RBF) and GFR are maintained at a relatively constant level over a wide range of arterial blood pressures, the phenomenon of autoregulation. This is achieved by adjustment of pre and post glomerular vascular resistances (reviewed in ref. 16). All of the blood vessels from the arcuate artery through to the glomerular efferent arteriole are involved. Many factors have been identified which modulate the tone of these vessels and these are now discussed individually.

### 1.2.1 Sympathetic nervous system

The kidney has a rich sympathetic adrenergic innervation particularly to the glomerular afferent and efferent arterioles and to the mesangial cells. Stimulation of the renal nerves leads to a rise in renal vascular resistance and hence to a reduction in RBF and GFR. This is primarily mediated through post-junctional $\alpha_1$-adrenoceptors and it is thought that a more intense vasoconstriction occurs in the afferent, rather than efferent, arterioles [17]. In addition, almost all segments of the nephron and the renin-secreting juxtaglomerular (JG) cells are to some degree under the control of an adrenergic innervation. Studies carried out mainly in the rat have shown that the proximal tubule has a particularly rich population of $\alpha_1$- and $\alpha_2$-receptors. $\beta_1$-Adrenoceptors have also been located on the cortical thick ascending limb of the loop of Henle, the distal convoluted tubule and the cortical collecting duct [17]. This complicates any interpretation of the role of the renal sympathetic nerves in the overall regulation of kidney function.

Of the many actions of the renal sympathetic nerves, increases in renin secretion are experimentally the most sensitive to nerve stimulation followed by changes in tubular sodium and water reabsorption. The least sensitive are the changes in renal blood flow and GFR (reviewed in ref. 18). It is therefore quite possible to alter renin secretion rate by electrically stimulating the renal nerves without any concurrent alteration in sodium excretion or renal haemodynamics. The increase in renin secretion in this circumstance is mediated through $\beta_1$-adrenoceptors. More intense nerve stimulation leads to changes in renin secretion rate which are the net result of direct effects on JG cells plus indirect renal baroreceptor-detected changes in arterial blood pressure and altered tubular sodium handling detected at the macula densa [19].

### 1.2.2 Renin–angiotensin system (RAS)

The simplistic view that renin is an endocrine agent produced by the juxtaglomerular cells in the afferent arteriole of the glomerulus still holds true. It must, however, be modified to encompass renin and angiotensins produced by other cell types as paracrine agents. Actions of angiotensin II (Ang II) on the renal vasculature and on GFR have been reviewed in detail [20–22].

Ang II, generated by renin from the $\alpha_2$-globulin angiotensinogen (renin substrate), is a powerful vasoconstrictor. Blockade of the RAS with angiotensin-converting enzyme (ACE) inhibitors [23] or with angiotensin receptor antagonists [24], reduces renal vascular resistance and increases renal blood flow. This suggests that Ang II is tonically effective as a renal vasoconstrictor under normal conditions. In situations where renin secretion is increased, for instance by sodium depletion, renal artery stenosis or heart failure, pharmacological blockade of the RAS markedly reduces renal vascular resistance.

Although the effectiveness of Ang II as an intrarenal vasoconstrictor is unquestioned, the site of action within the renal vasculature is more contentious. It has been suggested that Ang II can act on almost all vascular sites within the kidney but it appears to differentially constrict the efferent arteriole rather than the afferent arteriole. Indeed, some authors suggest that Ang II has little or no action on preglomerular vessels. The consequence of the effects on the efferent arteriole is a rise in glomerular capillary pressure and an increase in GFR. The RAS therefore helps to maintain GFR in the face of a fall in renal perfusion pressure.

Ang II has other effects within the kidney which potentially alter GFR by reducing the filtration surface area and $K_f$. These effects include contraction of the mesangial cells and a mitogenic action leading to mesangial cell proliferation. Ang II-induced contraction of the vasa recta in the renal medulla would reduce blood flow in this region of the kidney and may contribute to sodium retention.

Many of the actions of Ang II within the kidney are opposed by endogenous physiological antagonists. These include atrial natriuretic peptide (ANP), nitric oxide and renal prostaglandins. Thus, prostaglandin synthetase inhibitor drugs may potentiate Ang II-induced renal vasoconstriction. Intra-renal production of adenosine increases the constrictor actions of Ang II on the renal vasculature.

Ang II may have a paracrine role in many tissues in addition to its endocrine functions. Local paracrine effects may well contribute to the pharmacological effects of drugs acting on the RAS. Of particular interest is local generation of Ang II in the heart and blood vessels. This contributes to the process of vascular and cardiac remodelling which occurs in many cardiovascular disease states. Remodelling is characterized by cellular hypertrophy and hyperplasia and also by changes in extracellular matrix production, deposition and degradation [25]. Some of these changes may be reversed by treatment with converting enzyme inhibitors.

### 1.2.3 Endothelins

The first member of the endothelin (ET) family was discovered in 1988 by Yanigisawa. Actions of these peptides within the kidney have been the subject of several recent reviews [26–29]. The ET peptides seem to act primarily as paracrine or autocrine agents but under some circumstances circulating ET may have endocrine effects. The ET family of three 21-amino acid peptides, designated ET-1, ET-2 and ET-3, each have two disulphide Cys–Cys bonds in their structure. The peptides have an interesting structural homology with the sarafotoxin family of vasoconstrictor peptides found in the venom of a snake, the Israeli burrowing asp (*Atractaspis engaddensis*). All three ET peptides are expressed in humans although ET-2 may be mainly produced in the intestine. ET-3 is produced within the kidney but in much smaller amounts than ET-1. It is assumed that ET-1 is responsible for most of the physiological actions of the ET family.

The ET-1 molecule is synthesized first as a pre-propeptide which is then subjected to post-translational modification to a propeptide (big-ET) and then to the mature peptide. The final peptide does not appear to be stored in vesicles and so regulation of the secretion of these peptides is likely to be primarily at the level of transcription and translation.

Every cell type within the glomerulus expresses ET-1 and production is regulated by a host of vasoactive agents, cytokines and other proteins such as erythropoietin and thrombin [29]. In general terms, factors which have a mainly vasoconstrictive or cell proliferative effect such as Ang I, vasopressin, interleukin-1 and transforming growth factor-beta, increase ET-1 production. Vasodilator agents including ANP, brain natriuretic peptide (BNP) and nitric oxide (NO) inhibit ET-1 release from glomerular cell populations. The ET peptides evoke both short-term responses, such as smooth muscle contraction, and long-term responses such as mesangial cell mitogenesis within the kidney.

ET-1 is a very potent renal vasoconstrictor although, in response to acute infusion, this may be preceded by a transient prostaglandin-mediated vasodilation. The dominant effect, vasoconstriction, affects both afferent and efferent glomerular arterioles, although constriction is greater in the efferent than the afferent arteriole, leading to a net increase in the intraglomerular pressure. Other blood vessels within the kidney, such as the arcuate artery, are also constricted by ET peptides. A characteristic of ET-induced vasoconstriction is a very prolonged response which typically lasts 30 to 60 min following a single exposure to the peptide. The effects described above would appear to suggest that ET peptides should cause an increase in SNGFR. This, however, is complicated by concurrent effects on the mesangium.

### 1.2.4 Atrial natriuretic peptide (ANP)

ANP is secreted from cardiac atrial myocytes. The product of gene transcription is a pre-proANP which has between 149 and 153 amino acids depending on the species. A signal peptide at the amino-terminal end of the molecule is cleaved prior to storage in granules as a 126 amino acid proANP. In response to hormone release stimuli, a 28-amino acid active ANP peptide is cleaved from the carboxy-terminal end of the pro-ANP molecule. The active peptide has one Cys–Cys disulphide bridge which is essential for biological activity. Aspects of ANP synthesis and release have been reviewed in ref. 30.

A large number of factors are known to modulate ANP gene expression including stretch in the atrial and ventricular walls, glucocorticoids, thyroid hormones, endothelin, $\alpha_1$-adrenergic agonists, growth factors and prostaglandins. Similarly, a long list of factors, of which atrial stretch is probably the most important, are proposed to regulate the release of stored hormone [30]. A further influence on circulating ANP levels is enzymic inactivation, a potential site for pharmacological manipulation. Inactivation of a circulating small peptide, such as ANP, is likely to involve a number of non-specific, as well as relatively specific, pathways. Clearance receptors for ANP are widely distributed in many tissues but are particularly numerous in the renal cortex, vascular endothelium and smooth muscle cells [31].

ANP markedly increases GFR by raising glomerular capillary blood pressure. This is achieved by virtue of afferent arteriolar dilation together with ANP-induced efferent arteriolar constriction. In many experimental studies, because of these opposing effects, total renal vascular resistance is relatively unchanged in response to ANP infusion. Dilator actions of ANP on the renal vasculature have been linked through receptors to particulate guanylate cyclase activation and production of cyclic GMP (reviewed in refs 31–34). However, not all the experimental data fits comfortably with this hypothesis and increasingly the vasodilator actions of ANP are being linked to a cyclic GMP-independent mechanism (reviewed in ref. 35). The ANP-induced vasoconstriction of the efferent arteriole may be linked to an inhibition of adenylate cyclase and reduced cyclic AMP formation.

Other natriuretic peptides identified include brain natriuretic peptide (reviewed in ref. 36) and C-type natriuretic peptide (CNP), both initially isolated from brain tissue, and the peptide urodilatin (reviewed in ref. 37). Together with ANP, these peptides share considerable structural homology, each with a 17-amino acid ring formed by a disulphide bond. Precise definition of their physiological roles remains to be established.

### 1.2.5 Nitric oxide pathway

Nitric oxide is produced by many cell types but most notably by vascular endothelial cells, macrophages and nerve cells. L-Arginine is the substrate for both a constitutive and an inducible form of the enzyme nitric oxide synthase (NOS). Expression of the inducible NOS depends on the presence of certain cytokine agents. This inducible enzyme is not present under normal conditions but, once expressed, releases nitric oxide for prolonged periods. The constitutive enzyme is cytosolic and is $Ca^{2+}$/calmodulin dependent. Release of NO synthesized via the constitutive pathway occurs for relatively short periods, after receptor activation by agonists such as acetylcholine or bradykinin, or in response to physical stimulation of the cells. The NO produced in this way acts as a transduction mechanism in a wide range of physiological responses.

Progress in clarifying the physiological roles of NO has been aided by the development of arginine analogues which act as competitive inhibitors of both constitutive and inducible NOS. These include $N^G$-monomethyl-L-arginine (L-NMMA) and $N^G$-nitro L-arginine methyl ester (L-NAME). These and similar compounds inhibit the production of NO by endothelial cells. Several reviews of fundamental studies on nitric oxide are available [38].

Acetylcholine (ACh) and bradykinin (BK) have long been identified as potent renal vasodilators which do not significantly alter GFR or SNGFR. These effects are assumed to be secondary to receptor-linked NO production by vascular endothelial cells and a subsequent paracrine action on underlying smooth muscle. However, more recent studies also point to complex interactions with prostaglandins (PGs) [39]. Prostaglandins $E_1$, $E_2$ and $I_2$ (prostacyclin) are all potent renal vasodilators which also do not significantly alter GFR or SNGFR. In relation to ACh-induced renal vasodilation it is proposed that, whenever either NO or PG synthesis is inhibited by drugs, the overall vasodilator response in the kidney is not compromised as the missing dilation is compensated for by the alternative vasodilator mechanism [40].

Finally, in relation to the interpretation of data concerning the effects of NO and PGs on GFR, the concurrent effects of these agents on the mesangial cells on $K_f$ must be borne in mind. These aspects of renal function are dealt with later in this chapter.

### 1.2.6 Other renal vasoactive agents

Many other vasoactive substances exist, including histamine and glucocorticoids which are both renal vasodilators. The effects of these compounds are often secondary to modulation of the production of cyclic AMP, prostaglandins or another endothelium-derived vasoactive agent.

## 1.3 TUBULOGLOMERULAR FEEDBACK

Thus far in this chapter we have concentrated on the forces which determine GFR and the control mechanisms which can potentially alter it. If GFR did vary widely it would be necessary to regulate tubular reabsorptive mechanisms over an equally wide range in order to avoid acute volume depletion or fluid overload.

The concept of tubuloglomerular feedback (TGF) is that a change in the tubular function or environment is detected downstream in the nephron and the information transmitted back to the glomerulus. The result is a local change in vascular resistance, and a consequent alteration in GFR, which opposes the initial disturbance. This therefore creates a classical negative feedback loop which tends to optimize GFR. As all the components of the feedback loop exist within each nephron, the TGF mechanism is essentially stabilizing SNGFR in all the nephrons in parallel. Evidence concerning the mechanisms involved has mainly been derived from micropuncture studies on individual nephrons (reviewed in refs 41–44).

The detection site within the nephron is believed to be the macula densa cells at the start of the distal tubule. The signal detected is a flow-dependent change in the composition of the tubular fluid. An increase in the fluid flow rate in the ascending limb of the loop of Henle will mean more $Na^+$ and $Cl^-$ presented to the macula densa. Changes in each of these ions have been variously proposed to provide the trigger for the TGF response but some studies suggest that total solute concentration is detected. Given the composition of plasma, and therefore of the glomerular filtrate, the $Na^+$ and $Cl^-$ contents will necessarily be the largest components of total tubular solute concentration. The response is inhibition of renin secretion and Ang II production, leading to a fall in the GFR – the converse occurs when the intratubular delivery of $Na^+$ and $Cl^-$ drops. The other component of this response consists of afferent arteriolar constriction.

The chemical mediator which transmits vasoconstriction-generating information from the macula densa to the adjacent preglomerular arterioles is unclear. Candidates include adenosine, ATP and products of arachidonic acid metabolism through the lipoxygenase or cyclooxygenase pathways. The resulting vasoconstriction in the afferent arterioles involves a calcium entry step which can be blocked with calcium channel-blocking drugs. Among the agents which are postulated to modulate the functional characteristics of the TGF loop are Ang II, ANP, prostaglandins and NO.

The TGF mechanism appears to be important in adjusting GFR to a level appropriate to volume homeostasis across a wide range of physiological and pathological conditions.

### 1.3.1 Filtration coefficient ($K_f$)

The movement of filtrate across the glomerulus is equal to the product of the net driving pressure for filtration and the ultrafiltration coefficient

($K_f$). The value of $K_f$, in turn, is the product of the intrinsic permeability of the glomerular structures and the surface area available for filtration. It is thought that the mesangial cells influence both $K_f$ and renal haemodynamics. They respond to vasoactive hormones, such as Ang II and ET peptides, with a contractile response and a reduction in $K_f$.

The mesangial cells also synthesize NO and this may be triggered by a variety of cytokines including IL-1$\beta$ and tumour necrosis factor-alpha (TNF-$\alpha$). However, the NOS enzymes in the endothelial cell and in the mesangial cells are somewhat different. The endothelial cell enzyme is a constitutive, $Ca^{2+}$/calmodulin-dependent enzyme which responds immediately to increased intracellular [$Ca^{2+}$], with increased NO production. The mesangial cell NOS is similar to the macrophage enzyme and is apparently $Ca^{2+}$/calmodulin independent. More recent studies have shown that calmodulin is tightly bound in inducible NOS enzymes and effectively forms an enzyme subunit. As cytokines act by increasing NOS gene expression at the transcriptional level there is significant delay before NO release is increased. Complex interactions occur between a number of signalling pathways leading to mesangial cell NOS induction [45]. Biochemical aspects of NO production [46] and actions of NO on the glomerulus [47] have been reviewed.

The macrophage-type NOS enzyme in mesangial cells may well have functions in addition to the regulation of renal haemodynamics and $K_f$. These could include a cytotoxic role similar to the macrophage, particularly in relation to inflammatory reactions. It is known that some mesangial cells can phagocytose immune complexes and large molecules. This activity would be helpful in keeping the glomerular filter clear of debris.

## 1.4 THE RENAL TUBULE: CELLULAR MECHANISMS AND CONTROL

Epithelia in all parts of the nephron consist of a single layer of cells. These cells, like transporting epithelia in the gut, have a very distinct polarity and the plasma membrane surface can be divided into a luminal (apical) surface in contact with the filtrate and a basolateral surface bathed by the interstitial fluid. The sodium pump (Na/K ATPase), which provides the drive for much of the reabsorptive functions of the nephron, is limited to the basolateral membrane. Studies on the Na/K ATPase have been reviewed [48]. Tight junctions between cells separate the luminal and basolateral membranes. The determination of polarity in a cell is provided by elements of the cytoskeleton [49].

Movement of solutes and water across epithelia can follow one of two distinct routes, the trans-cellular route or the paracellular route through tight junctions between adjacent cells. Movement of substances via the paracellular route is entirely passive and the selectivity of what may pass by this route is primarily determined by the tight junctions. The limiting steps for the transport of substances via the trans-cellular route are the movement across the luminal and the basolateral membranes of the cells. All active, ATP-consuming, transport processes utilize the trans-cellular route.

### 1.4.1 The proximal tubule

The proximal tubule is not a homogeneous segment of the nephron. It can be divided into an extensively convoluted part (pars convoluta) which is entirely within the cortex of the kidney and a straight part (pars recta) which extends into the outer stripe of the outer medulla. Bicarbonate, glucose and amino acid reabsorption takes place in the early part of the pars convoluta linked to $Na^+$ reabsorption. Sodium and chloride-linked reabsorption predominates in the second part of the pars convoluta and in the pars recta.

In the proximal tubule, the paracellular pathway contributes less than 1% of the total surface area of the epithelium. Nevertheless, this is the major route for passive diffusion of ions across the epithelium. In the second half of the proximal tubule, a significant amount of $Na^+$ and $Cl^-$ reabsorption takes place by the paracellular route and this accounts for about one-third of the total NaCl reabsorption in the proximal tubule. The remaining NaCl reabsorption utilizes the trans-cellular route. In the proximal tubule, 50–70% of the filtered $Na^+$, $Cl^-$ and water is reabsorbed. The trans-cellular component of this process is aided by the electrical potential of $-50$ to $-70\,mV$ across the luminal side of the epithelial cell (inside of cell has net negative charge). This potential is generated by the combination of passive diffusion of $K^+$ out of the cell and active $Na^+$ extrusion at the basolateral side using the Na/K ATPase.

Water movement in the proximal tubule is the passive consequence of active solute transport. This osmotically driven water movement occurs mainly via the trans-cellular pathway [50]. The actual osmotic gradients generated across the epithelium are quantitatively small but, because of the high water conductivity, bulk flow of water is enormous. In the proximal tubule, the Na/K ATPase, located in the basolateral membrane of the epithelial cells, is the main generator of an osmotic gradient. Intracellular $[Na^+]$ is maintained at a low level by expulsion of $Na^+$ against a concentration gradient across the basolateral membrane. Entry of $Na^+$ at the luminal membrane can therefore occur passively down a concentration gradient. The role played by mechanisms which couple transepithelial $Na^+$ transport and the basolateral $K^+$ conductance has been recently reviewed [51].

Most of the other active transport processes in the proximal tubule operate in a manner secondary to the movement of sodium ions across the luminal membrane down an electrochemical gradient. A range of sodium-coupled co-transporters on the luminal side of the cell move organic and inorganic solutes into the cell. These solutes include glucose, amino acids, mono and di-carboxylic acids, phosphate and sulphate. The properties of these proximal tubule transporters have been reviewed [52].

Of the order of 90% of filtered $HCO_3^-$ and nearly 100% of filtered glucose and other organic solutes is reabsorbed in the proximal tubule. Glucose uptake is limited by the numerical availability of sodium/glucose co-transport carrier molecules, thus giving rise to the concept of 'tubular maximum' ($T_m$) for glucose. If excessive amounts of glucose are filtered, due to a high plasma [glucose], then the maximum capacity of the carrier molecules to reabsorb glucose is exceeded. As the glucose carriers effectively only exist in the proximal tubule epithelial cells, glucose cannot be reabsorbed further down the nephron and glycosuria will result.

The role of hormones in the regulation of proximal tubular function has been a matter of some controversy. Ang II stimulates proximal tubule $Na^+$ reabsorption at low ($10^{-13}$ to $10^{-10}$M) dose ranges whilst at higher concentrations ($10^{-9}$M and above) it inhibits reabsorption [53]. Ang II acts through an electoneutral $Na^+/H^+$ exchange mechanism. The source of Ang II for these actions is of interest. Locally generated Ang II, as well as hormone provided through the blood supply, is available to the proximal tubule. Local concentrations of Ang II could therefore be high enough to cause inhibition of $Na^+$ transport. Ang II is filtered freely at the glomerulus and so can reach the luminal membrane of the proximal tubule cells. Ang II receptors are present on both the brush border and basolateral sides of the epithelial cells and are coupled through several parallel signal transduction pathways. The receptors are present in the highest number in the first part of the proximal tubule. The stimulatory effects of Ang II on the basolateral side are inhibited by ANP and by parathyroid hormone (PTH) [53].

In addition to the effects mediated through epithelial receptors, Ang II also constricts afferent and efferent arterioles. Changes in renal tubular hydrostatic and colloid osmotic pressures as a consequence of this lead to increased $Na^+$ and water reabsorption in the proximal tubule.

In summary, the proximal tubule is the site for reabsorption of 60–70% of filtered water and solutes in the nephron. Reabsorption is isosmotic, the fluid reaching the end of the proximal tubule having the same osmotic strength as the fluid entering this segment of the nephron as the glomerular filtrate.

### 1.4.2 The loop of Henle

The prime function of the loop of Henle (LOH) is to establish a gradient of osmolality in the renal interstitium and therefore in the tubular fluid. Thus, in the cortex of the kidney interstitial osmolality is the same as blood plasma, about 275–290 mosmol/kg. In the tip of the medulla, interstitial osmolality is of the order of 600 mosmol/kg under conditions where a dilute urine is produced and up to 1200 mosmol/kg under conditions of maximum water retention. This provides an osmotic gradient between tubular fluid in the collecting duct (CD) and the interstitial fluid which drives water reabsorption in the terminal segment of the nephron. The potential therefore exists to excrete urine with up to four times the osmolality of plasma although, in practice, this is rarely required under normal lifestyle conditions. The LOH also has a role in acid–base balance which is discussed in a later section.

In the LOH, approximately 20% of the filtered load of ions, including $Na^+$, $Cl^-$, $K^+$, $Mg^{2+}$ and $Ca^{2+}$ and $HCO_3^-$ is reabsorbed. These events take place almost entirely within the thick ascending limb of the LOH (ALH). As with the proximal tubule, reabsorption of most solutes is driven by the Na/K ATPase located in the basolateral membrane of the epithelial cells.

Movement of $Na^+$ across the luminal brush border membrane of the ALH is mediated by a symport mechanism which couples movement of one $Na^+$, one $K^+$ and two $Cl^-$ ions. The $Na^+$ ions move down their concentration gradient into the cell and are expelled actively at the basolateral side, thus maintaining a low intracellular [$Na^+$]. Although this provides a $Na^+$-linked drive to move $K^+$ into the cell against a concentration gradient, once released inside the cell $K^+$ tends to diffuse back out into the tubular lumen.

Chloride movement into the cell at the luminal side of the epithelial cell is also linked to $Na^+$ flux via the $Na^+/2Cl^-/K^+$ co-transport mechanism. In this case, $Cl^-$ is moving against both a concentration and an electrical gradient as intracellular [$Cl^-$] is relatively high and the inside of the cell has a net negative charge. At the basolateral side of the cell, $Cl^-$ leaves the cell passively. The balance of charged ions moving across the epithelial cell (effectively one $Na^+$ and two $Cl^-$) means that the lumen of the thick ALH becomes progressively more positively charged. This has the effect of driving more $Na^+$ out of the lumen via the paracellular route. The tight junctions between the epithelial cells are cation selective and $K^+$, $Mg^{2+}$ and $Ca^{2+}$ also cross from the tubular fluid by the paracellular route.

Reabsorption of NaCl in the ALH is blocked by 'loop-diuretic' drugs. Frusemide and its derivatives piretanide and bumetanide are secreted into the tubular fluid in the proximal tubule and block the $Na^+/2Cl^-/K^+$ co-transporter from the luminal side. The loop diuretic ethacrynic acid acts by a mechanism which is independent of this co-transport system.

In summary, under normal conditions, $Na^+$ reabsorption in the ALH can proceed either via a trans-cellular route or a paracellular route. Quantitatively, these two pathways are roughly equivalent. The thick ALH is impermeable to water and so the fluid leaving this segment of the nephron has an osmolality of less than 150 mosmol/kg, approximately half the osmotic strength of blood plasma. Solute reabsorbed in the ALH can enter the descending limb of the LOH which is freely permeable to water and solutes. The tubular fluid effectively equilibrates with the surrounding interstitial fluid and becomes progressively more concentrated going down the LOH and less concentrated going up the ALH. In this way, the osmotic gradient between cortex and medulla is maintained.

### 1.4.3 The distal tubule

The term 'distal tubule' is not an entirely satisfactory one from either the structural or the functional viewpoint. Morphologically, the distal tubule consists of an initial straight part, referred to as the cortical thick ascending limb (CTAL) and a distal convoluted tubule (DCT) which starts shortly after the macula densa and is distinguished by an abrupt increase in epithelial cell height.

From a functional viewpoint, the CTAL behaves in similar fashion to the ALH and the term 'early diluting segment' is sometimes used to refer to this part of the nephron. The DCT can be functionally grouped with the subsequent cortical connecting tubule (CCT) and cortical collecting duct (CCD) even though there are morphological differences between these segments of the tubule. The term 'late diluting segment' is used to functionally identify this part of the nephron. The late diluting segment is relatively impermeable to both water and urea. These aspects of tubular function are considered in Section 1.4.4. Tubular fluid enters the CTAL as a hypotonic fluid and becomes even more hypotonic as a result of further $Na^+$ and $Cl^-$ reabsorption. The late diluting segment of the distal nephron is a site for the regulation of $Na^+$ excretion by aldosterone and ANP and for urine acidification.

The epithelia in the later part of the DCT have two cell types, principal cells and intercalated cells. Principal cells reabsorb $Na^+$ and water and secrete $K^+$ whereas the intercalated cells secrete $H^+$. The latter function is discussed in Section 1.7.

The drive for $Na^+$ reabsorption in the principal cells of the late diluting segment is again provided primarily by the Na/K ATPase on the basolateral side of the epithelial cell. This maintains a low intracellular $[Na^+]$ and low intracellular electronegativity. Entry of $Na^+$ at the luminal side of the cells is thought to occur passively through water-filled ion channels and is not linked to the movement of any other solute.

Potassium ions are secreted into the lumen of the tubule in two steps. They initially enter the epithelial cell against a concentration gradient through the basolateral membrane, because of the activity of the Na/K ATPase and the negative charge on the inside of the cell. Intracellular $[K^+]$, at about 140 mM, is much higher than luminal $[K^+]$, which is of the order of 10 mM. $K^+$ can therefore diffuse across the luminal membrane through an ion selective channel into the tubule. This movement will of course be opposed by the negative charge on the inside of the cell. The movement of $Na^+$ and $K^+$ in opposite directions across the luminal membrane would tend to maintain the electrical neutrality of the tubular fluid. However, as $K^+$ can also leave the principal cells through channels in the basolateral membrane there is a tendency to develop an electrical potential gradient across the epithelial cells in this segment of the tubule with the lumen negative relative to the basolateral side. This provides an electrical gradient for the reabsorption of $Cl^-$ via the paracellular route. The luminal membrane of the principal cells is relatively impermeable to $Cl^-$ but the basolateral membrane appears permeable [54].

$Na^+$ reabsorption and $K^+$ excretion in the principal cells is regulated by aldosterone. For many years it was assumed that this simply followed increased Na/K ATPase activity. Our understanding of the actions of aldosterone has now become more sophisticated [55, 56]. Current models of aldosterone action still include the classical steroid hormone-type I nuclear or cytosolic receptor-linked, gene transcription-mediated, component. This response, which would have a latency of the order of two to eight hours, is relatively non-specific as the receptor has an equivalent affinity for aldosterone and the mineralocorticoids cortisol and corticosterone. The genomic response to aldosterone results in *de novo* synthesis of additional Na/K ATPase molecules and also other aldosterone-induced proteins. The number of $Na^+$ and $K^+$ channels in the luminal membrane is also increased by aldosterone, resulting in enhanced $Na^+$ entry into epithelial cells and increased $K^+$ extrusion. Other aspects of the action of aldosterone, which have a more rapid response, cannot be explained in this way.

The second component of aldosterone action on $Na^+$ reabsorption is mediated through a plasma membrane receptor which is coupled through protein kinase C and the inositol phosphate pathway. Aldosterone measurably increases inositol trisphosphate ($IP_3$) production within 60 s. This leads to increased $Na^+/H^+$ antiporter activity resulting in an increase in intracellular [$Na^+$]. As the rate at which the Na/K ATPase functions is rate limited by intracellular [$Na^+$] this immediately leads to increased $Na^+/K^+$ exchange across the basolateral membrane. The plasma membrane receptor does not accept cortisol, corticosterone or dexamethasone as ligands and is therefore specific for aldosterone [57].

Pharmacologically, the genomic actions of aldosterone can be blocked by the competitive inhibitor spironolactone. The $Na^+$ channel blockers amiloride and triamterene have a similar overall action to spironolactone but act by a different mechanism. As amiloride reduces $Na^+$ influx into the epithelial cell, this means that the lumen-negative trans-epithelial potential difference is reduced in the presence of this diuretic. This change in potential difference will reduce the tendency for $K^+$ to diffuse into the lumen and so amiloride is referred to as a potassium-sparing diuretic. Amiloride, predictably, does not block the plasma membrane receptor-mediated events [57] although this component of the aldosterone response is blocked by spironolactone.

Physiologically, aldosterone secretion is inhibited by ANP. Increased levels of Ang II, ACTH and $K^+$ all increase aldosterone synthesis and ANP blocks the response to all these agents. The cellular mechanisms involved have been reviewed [58].

### 1.4.4 The collecting duct

This segment contains the confluence of many nephrons into cortical and medullary sections of the collecting duct. The cortical collecting duct functions in a similar way to the DCT and has already been dealt with. The medullary collecting duct is frequently further subdivided on a functional basis although there is no very obvious morphological transition. This division comprises firstly, the outer and inner stripes of the outer medullary collecting duct (OMCD) and secondly, the inner medullary collecting duct (IMCD). The IMCD is the final arbiter of urinary $Na^+$ and water excretion and is the site therefore of complex endocrine and paracrine hormone-mediated events [59, 60]. Two main epithelial cell types exist. The principal cells are primarily involved in $Na^+$ and $Cl^-$ reabsorption and antidiuretic hormone-stimulated water reabsorption. The intercalated cells are involved in $HCO_3^-$ and $H^+$ transport and are referred to later in the section on acid–base balance.

The principal cells of both the OMCD and IMCD have many similarities to those already described in the DCT. Reabsorption of $Na^+$ and $Cl^-$ is again driven by the basolateral membrane Na/K ATPase. Entry of $Na^+$ down both a concentration and electrical gradient across the luminal membrane is through water-filled, amiloride-sensitive channels. The number of $Na^+$ channels open appears to be the rate-limiting step in this process. ADH increases $Na^+$ transport in the collecting duct and this is thought to be linked to an increased density of open $Na^+$ channels in the luminal membrane (reviewed in ref. 61).

The Na/K ATPase in the basolateral membrane of the IMCD epithelial cells is sensitive to aldosterone, which stimulates transport, but the inner medulla also has high local concentrations of prostaglandin $E_2$ ($PGE_2$) which inhibits the ATPase. Several mediators, including members of the ANP family, IL-1 and ET peptides inhibit $Na^+$ transport in this segment by stimulating $PGE_2$ synthesis [59].

Tubular reabsorption of $Na^+$ in the medulla is known to be affected by changes in renal medullary haemodynamics. Precise evaluation of this has in the past been limited by the methods available to study medullary blood flow but several new methods have now been developed [62]. Only 10–15% of total renal blood flow enters the medulla. Changes in flow rate alter the renal interstitial pressure and the osmotic potential of the medullary interstitium. Evidence is emerging of multiple endocrine and paracrine influences on medullary blood flow which lead to changes in renal sodium excretion [63].

The osmotic gradient created in the tubular and interstitial fluid between the cortex and medulla is generated by the tubular mechanisms in the loop of Henle (see the previous section). All nephrons contribute to the osmotic environment of the cortex and outer medulla but only those nephrons with long loops of Henle, the juxtamedullary nephrons which form 15% of the total nephron population, are able to influence the environment in the inner medulla. The importance of the osmotic gradient is that it exposes the basolateral side of the collecting duct cells to a hypertonic environment in the medulla. If the collecting duct is impermeable to water the hypotonic fluid entering from the distal tubule will pass through and be excreted relatively unchanged. If the collecting duct is made permeable to water by the actions of the antidiuretic hormone (ADH; vasopressin) then osmotic equilibrium occurs with water moving out of the collecting duct and the urine inside the tubule can potentially reach an osmolality of 1200 mosmol/kg, about four times plasma osmolality. The details of the functioning of the countercurrent mechanism are outside the scope of this chapter but have been reviewed elsewhere [64–66].

The characteristics of the actions of ADH on urine flow are a fast onset and fast termination. This is partly associated with the short physiological half-life of the hormone, a few minutes. Many aspects of the action of ADH remain to be elucidated but the fundamentals can be summarized as follows.

ADH binds to specific V2 receptors activating an array of signal transduction mechanisms which include activation of adenylate cyclase and cyclic AMP formation. The speed of the subsequent physiological responses suggests effects on existing membrane structures rather than a protein synthesis-linked event. It is proposed that vesicles containing large numbers of water channels (aggrephores) are moved from the cytoplasm to the luminal membrane. Insertion of the water channels into the membrane increases water permeability, an event which can be quickly reversed by the removal of ADH. The intracellular mechanisms which accompany these events have been reviewed [67–70]. The actions of ADH on collecting duct epithelial cells may be attenuated physiologically by agonists for $\alpha_2$-adrenoceptors [70] and by $PGE_2$ [71]. Pharmacologically, lithium ions inhibit adenylate cyclase and hence reduce the physiological effects of ADH.

Urea is freely filtered at the glomerulus with a typical normal filtrate concentration of 4 mmol/l. Some reabsorption of urea takes place in the proximal tubule and some urea may diffuse back into the tubule in the thin limbs of the loop of Henle. However, the ALH, distal tubule and cortical and outer medullary collecting duct are impermeable to urea. The consequence is that the urea concentration in the fluid entering the inner medullary collecting duct in a normal kidney will be of the order of 120 mmol/l. This provides a substantial gradient for urea to diffuse out into the interstitial fluid in the medulla. The inner medullary collecting duct is permeable to urea and fast movement out of the tubular fluid can occur due to specific urea transporter proteins in both the luminal and basolateral membranes. Permeability to urea is regulated by ADH which acts by increasing the number of functional transporters in the luminal membrane [72].

Recycling of urea from the inner medullary collecting duct into the interstitial fluid contributes significantly to the development of the osmotic gradient between cortex and the medullary papilla. In the presence of high levels of ADH more urea will be reabsorbed and contribute to the interstitial osmolality [72]. There will therefore be a greater osmotic gradient for reabsorption of water from the tubule into the interstitium and urine with a high osmolality can be produced. Reduced production of urea, when a low-protein diet is consumed, impairs the ability of the kidney to produce a highly concentrated urine.

## 1.5 THE ROLE OF THE KIDNEY IN SODIUM HOMEOSTASIS

Typical $Na^+$ intake in the Western world is of the order of 100–200 mmol/day. There are wide variations outside this range depending on personal dietary preference and ethnic/geographical factors. In order to stay in balance, sodium intake must be balanced by sodium loss from the body. Non-renal losses in sweat and faeces are variable but typically account for about 10% of overall $Na^+$ intake. Sodium balance is finely regulated by the kidneys.

The daily amount of $Na^+$ filtered at the glomerulus of a normal kidney is the product of filtrate [$Na^+$] – 140 mmol/l and the GFR – 170 l/day. This comes to 23 800 mmol of $Na^+$ filtered per day, vastly more than daily intake. Looked at a different way, the kidney would only need to have a GFR of about 1 l/day to filter the load of $Na^+$ to be excreted into the tubular fluid. The kidney then has no problem filtering enough $Na^+$ to provide for excretion, and renal function is all about retaining appropriate amounts of $Na^+$ from the filtrate. The concept of fractional excretion (F.E.) of a substance is sometimes useful in such circumstances:

$$\text{F.E.} = \frac{\text{Amount of substance excreted per unit time}}{\text{Amount of substance filtered per unit time}}$$

In the case of $Na^+$, F.E. is of the order of 0.5%

A daily intake of $Na^+$ of 150–200 mmol is a significant proportion of total body sodium content. The typical 70 kg person contains about 4000 mmoles of $Na^+$ mainly held in the extracellular fluid (ECF). An ECF volume of 19 l with [$Na^+$] = 140 mmol/l accounts for 2660 mmoles of $Na^+$ content. Disturbances of $Na^+$ excretion will lead to changes in the osmolality and/or volume of the ECF. The normal range for the osmolality of blood plasma is 275–290 mosmol/kg. As plasma [$Na^+$] is about 140 mmol/l and plasma [$Cl^-$] is about 105 mmoles/l, these two ions account for about 80% of the osmotic potential of plasma. The plasma proteins, in contrast, account for less than 1%.

An alternative way of looking at these figures is that, assuming plasma [$Na^+$] remains unchanged, failure to excrete one day's average intake of salt would lead to the retention of an extra litre of water. The kidneys of a normal person can regulate $Na^+$ excretion to stay in balance over a range of intake from less than 10 mmoles/day to over 500 mmoles/day. The major sites of regulation and control mechanisms which have been dealt with earlier in this chapter are as follows.

1. Glomerulus – regulation of GFR by Ang II and ANP helps to determine the amount of $Na^+$ entering the nephron.
2. Proximal tubule – site for reabsorption of 60–70% of filtered $Na^+$. Ang II has a dose-dependent biphasic effect in this segment of the nephron.
3. Loop of Henle – site for the reabsorption of about 20% of filtered $Na^+$ but the most important role of this segment of the nephron is to generate an osmotic gradient allowing the kidney to produce urine with either a high or low osmolality as appropriate.

4. Distal tubule – site of further $Na^+$ reabsorption regulated by the action of aldosterone. Synthesis of aldosterone in the zona glomerulosa of the adrenal cortex is stimulated by Ang II and inhibited by ANP.
5. Inner medullary collecting duct – final site for the regulation of $Na^+$ and water excretion by aldosterone, ADH and multiple paracrine influences.

Many other chemical mediators are involved in modulating renal sodium handling, often by actions on the basolateral Na/K ATPase; these are reviewed elsewhere [73]. Of intriguing interest over many years, but still unresolved, are the reports of an endogenous inhibitor of Na/K ATPase, a digoxin-like natriuretic hormone, which is thought to originate in the hypothalamus [74, 75].

## 1.6 THE ROLE OF THE KIDNEY IN POTASSIUM HOMEOSTASIS

A typical dietary intake of potassium in the Western world is about 100 mmoles per day. Distribution within the body fluid compartments is quite different from sodium: about 98% of total body $K^+$ is located within cells and the extracellular fluid only contains 2%. The resting membrane potential of excitable cells, about −70 mV, is primarily a potassium diffusion potential and therefore approaches the potassium equilibrium potential $E_K$ (normally about −90 mV). Because the resting potential is primarily determined by the ratio of $[K^+]$ inside and outside the cell, even small changes in the extracellular fluid $[K^+]$ will result in significant changes in membrane potential. When $[K^+]$ exceeds 5.5 mmol/l, it will tend to depolarize cells and result in increased excitability of nerves and muscles. If $[K^+]$ rises to levels in excess of 7 mmoles/l, there is a severe risk of cardiac arrest. In contrast, hypokalaemia, a plasma $[K^+]$ less than 3.5 mmoles/l, will tend to hyperpolarize cells and reduce nerve and muscle excitability, sometimes leading to muscle weakness.

The response to ingestion and absorption of a $K^+$ load will initially be to deposit the extra $K^+$ inside cells under the control of insulin and adrenaline, followed by excretion of the $K^+$ mainly (92%) via the kidneys under the regulation of aldosterone. The remaining 8% of dietary $K^+$ is excreted in the faeces. These mechanisms can normally cope with a daily $K^+$ intake which is up to about 20 times normal without any significant increase in plasma $[K^+]$.

When the glomerular filtration rate is compromised, entry of $K^+$ into the tubular fluid by filtration is reduced, although this is a relatively minor component of renal $K^+$ handling. On the basis of GFR = 170 l/day and plasma $[K^+]$ = 4 mmoles/l, filtered $K^+$ is 680 mmoles/day. If

GFR is only 10% of normal, although this is still sufficient to keep the patient alive, filtered $K^+$ is now less than the normal daily intake. This is quite different from the way the kidney regulates $Na^+$ excretion.

In the nephron, approximately 70% of filtered $K^+$ is reabsorbed in the proximal tubule and a further 20% in the ALH. The main site for regulation of $K^+$ excretion is, however, secretion into the urine in the connecting tubule of the distal tubule and the collecting duct. This process is under the control of aldosterone. Inhibition of the action of aldosterone, either directly by drugs, such as spironolactone, or indirectly by blockade of the formation of the major stimulatory hormone for aldosterone synthesis, Ang II, may therefore lead to hyperkalaemia.

Increased flow rate down the nephron, as in diuretic therapy, also stimulates $K^+$ secretion. A rise in plasma $[K^+]$ has the same effect. It is suggested that the increase in tubular pressure during diuresis may activate stretch-sensitive potassium channels in the luminal membrane of the intercalated cells. This increases the passage of $K^+$ into the tubule lumen down its electrochemical gradient [76].

Acidosis is associated with increased plasma $[K^+]$ as $K^+$ ions leave the cells. The filtered load of $K^+$ will therefore increase. However, acidosis also reduces $K^+$ secretion in the nephron by inhibiting the Na/K ATPase. As uptake of $K^+$ at the basolateral side is reduced, the $K^+$ extrusion at the luminal side of the epithelial cell is also reduced. ADH, by increasing water permeability in the luminal membrane of the collecting duct, also increases permeability to $K^+$. The result is an increase in the diffusion of $K^+$ back into the tubule lumen. It is suggested that this may prevent excessive potassium retention during periods of antidiuresis [77].

## 1.7 THE ROLE OF THE KIDNEY IN ACID–BASE BALANCE

The role of the kidney in acid–base balance is not merely confined to excretion of $H^+$. Adequate buffering of $H^+$ during transport in the blood between the site of production and the site of excretion is essential if an acceptably narrow range of $[H^+]$ is to be maintained in the body fluids. The bicarbonate buffer is of major importance not only because of its considerable buffer capacity but also because, as part of compensation mechanisms, the $[HCO_3^-]$ can be adjusted by altered generation of bicarbonate. The roles of the tubular mechanisms in acid–base homeostasis may therefore be summarized as:

1. reabsorption of filtered $HCO_3^-$;
2. *de novo* generation of $HCO_3^-$;
3. excretion of $H^+$.

The first of these roles is quantitatively the most onerous task and has been reviewed [78]. In a normal person with a GFR of 170 l/day and a plasma [$HCO_3^-$] of 24 mmoles/l the filtered load of $HCO_3^-$ is 4080 mmol/day. About 90% of this load is reabsorbed in the proximal tubule. Dissociation of carbonic acid within the epithelial cells yields an $H^+$ ion which can enter the filtrate via a $Na^+/H^+$ antiporter mechanism in the luminal membrane. Together with $HCO_3^-$ in the filtrate, the $H^+$ reforms $CO_2$ and water. The $CO_2$ produced becomes part of the dissolved pool of $CO_2$ in the body fluids which have equilibrated with alveolar air. Inside the proximal tubule cell, having dealt with the fate of the $H^+$ ion produced from carbonic acid there remains an $HCO_3^-$. This can leave the cell across the basolateral membrane either through a $3Na^+/1\ HCO_3^-$ symport mechanism or in exchange for $Cl^-$ entering the cell via a basolateral membrane antiport mechanism. These events in the proximal tubule reabsorb filtered $HCO_3^-$ but do not acidify the urine.

A further portion of the filtered load of $HCO_3^-$ is reabsorbed in the loop of Henle, mainly by the thick ascending limb, using a mechanism similar to that in the proximal tubule. In both these segments of the nephron, because reabsorption across the luminal membrane involves a $Na^+/H^+$ antiporter, factors which alter [$Na^+$] within the proximal tubule or the loop of Henle will have a secondary effect on $HCO_3^-$ reabsorption.

The remaining 5% or so of filtered $HCO_3^-$ which has escaped the proximal tubule and loop of Henle segments of the nephron is reabsorbed in the intercalated cells of the distal tubule and collecting duct. The mechanism in the collecting duct is independent of $Na^+$ ions as the protons are actively pumped across the luminal membrane by an $H^+$ ATPase. Active pumping of $H^+$ into the tubular fluid leads to the reabsorption of the remaining filtered $HCO_3^-$ and starts the process of urine acidification. The roles played by the collecting duct intercalated cells in the acidification of urine have been reviewed [79, 80].

The $H^+$ extruded by cells in the distal segments of the nephron is derived from the dissociation of carbonic acid into $H^+$ and $HCO_3^-$. Several mechanisms by which $HCO_3^-$ can cross either the basolateral membrane or luminal membrane have been identified [79, 80]. Bicarbonate entering the interstitial fluid after all the filtered $HCO_3^-$ has been reabsorbed represents an addition to the buffer capacity of the body. One $HCO_3^-$ will be formed for each $H^+$ actively extruded into the tubular fluid. A typical load of $H^+$ excreted in this way would be about 100 mmol/day, mainly derived from the oxidative metabolism of amino acids. The amount of new $HCO_3^-$ generated is therefore also 100 mmol/day.

The maximum [$H^+$] concentration of urine is about $30 \times 10^{-6}$ mol/l (pH 4.5). The $H^+$ daily load to be excreted is about 100 mmol/day. If all the acid was excreted as free $H^+$ this would require a daily urine volume of over 3000 l. This illustrates very simply the need for buffers in urine. The important mechanisms include (i) excreting $H^+$ bound to ammonia, mainly generated by the deamination of glutamine, as ammonium ($NH^+_4$) ion and (ii) generation of dihydrogen phosphate.

Several hormones have been shown to affect renal acid–base mechanisms. Aldosterone appears to promote $HCO_3^-$ reabsorption in the distal nephron. In the proximal tubule PTH inhibits reabsorption of both $HCO_3^-$ and phosphate [81] but it is considered to increase the absorption of $HCO_3^-$ in the loop of Henle and the other distal parts of the nephron [80]. In the thick ascending limb of the loop of Henle both ADH and glucagon inhibit $HCO_3^-$ reabsorption but in the distal tubule and cortical collecting duct ADH stimulates $HCO_3^-$ reabsorption while glucagon promotes $HCO_3^-$ secretion [81].

## REFERENCES


1. Lindeman, R.D. (1993) Renal physiology and pathophysiology of aging. *Contrib. Nephrol.*, **105**, 1–12.
2. Abrahamson, D.R. (1987) Structure and development of the glomerular capillary wall and basement membrane. *Am. J. Physiol.*, **253**, F783–F794.
3. Kanwar, Y.S. and Venkatachalam, M.A. (1992) Ultrastructure of glomerulus and juxtaglomerular apparatus, in *Handbook of Physiology*, section 8, Renal Physiology (ed. E.E. Windhager), American Physiological Society, New York and Oxford University Press, Oxford, pp. 3–40.
4. Caulfield, J.P. and Farquhar, N.G. (1974) The permeability of glomerular capillaries to graded dextrans. *J. Cell. Biol.*, **63**, 883–903.
5. Kanwar, Y.S., Liu, Z.Z., Kashihara, N. and Wallner, E.I. (1991) Current status of the structural and functional basis of glomerular filtration and proteinuria. *Semin. Nephrol.*, **11**, 390–413.
6. Remuzzi, A. and Remuzzi, G. (1994) Glomerular perm-selective function. *Kidney Int.*, **45**, 398–402.
7. Baricos, W.H. and Shah, S.V. (1991) Proteolytic enzymes as mediators of glomerular injury. *Kidney Int.*, **40**, 161–73.
8. Goligorsky, M.S., Lieberthal, W., Racusen, L. and Simon, E.E. (1993) Integrin receptors in renal tubular epithelium: new insights into pathophysiology of acute renal failure. *Am. J. Physiol*, **264**, F1–F8.
9. Drenckhahn, D. and Franke, R.-P. (1988) Ultrastructural organisation of contractile and cytoskeletal proteins in glomerular podocytes of chicken, rat, and man. *Lab. Invest.*, **59**, 673–82.
10. Ronco, P.M., Ardaillou, N., Verroust, P. and Lelongt, B. (1994) Pathophysiology of the podocyte: a target and a major player in glomerulonephritis. *Adv. Nephrol. Necker Hosp.*, **23**, 91–131.
11. Kriz, W., Hackenthal, E., Nobiling, R. *et al.* (1994) A role for podocytes to counteract capillary wall distension. *Kidney Int.*, **45**, 69–76.
12. Kashgarian, M. and Sterzel, R.B. (1992) The pathobiology of the mesangium. *Kidney Int.*, **41**, 524–9.

13. Veis, J.A. (1993) An overview of mesangial cell biology. *Contrib. Nephrol.*, **104**, 115–26.
14. Davies, M. (1994) The mesangial cell: a tissue culture view. *Kidney Int.*, **45**, 320–7.
15. Brenner, B.M., Troy, J.L. and Daugharty, T.M. (1971) The dynamics of glomerular ultrafiltration in the rat. *J. Clin. Invest.*, **50**, 1776–80.
16. Holstein-Rathlou, N.-H. and Marsh, D.J. (1994) Renal blood flow regulation and arterial pressure fluctuations: a case study in nonlinear dynamics. *Physiol. Rev.*, **74**, 637–81.
17. Barajas, L. and Powers, K. (1990) Monoaminergic innervation of the rat kidney: a quantitative study. *Am. J. Physiol.*, **259**, F503–F511.
18. DiBona, G.F. (1982) The functions of the renal nerves. *Rev. Physiol. Biochem. Pharmacol.*, **94**, 76–181.
19. DiBona, G.F. (1992) Sympathetic neural control of the kidney in hypertension. *Hypertension*, **19**, suppl. I, I-28 – I-35.
20. Navar, L.G. and Rosivall, L. (1984) Contribution of the renin–angiotensin system to the control of intrarenal haemodynamics. *Kidney Int.*, **25**, 857–68.
21. Hall, J.E. (1986) Regulation of glomerular filtration rate and sodium excretion by angiotensin II. *Fed. Proc.*, **45**, 1431–7.
22. Johnson, C.I., Fabris, B. and Jandeleit, K. (1993) Intrarenal renin–angiotensin system in renal physiology and pathophysiology. *Kidney Int.*, **44**, suppl. 42, S-59 – S-63.
23. Macfadyen, R.J., Lees, K.R. and Reid, J.L. (1991) Tissue and plasma angiotension converting enzyme and the response to ACE inhibitor drugs. *Br. J. Clin. Pharmacol.*, **31**, 1–13.
24. Timmermans, P.B.M.W.M., Wong, P.C., Chiu, A.T. *et al.* (1993) Angiotensin II receptors and angiotensin II receptor antagonists. *Pharmacol. Rev.*, **45**, 205–51.
25. Struijker-Boudier, H.A.J., Smits, J.F.M. and De May, J.G.R. (1995) Pharmacology of cardiac and vascular remodelling. *Ann. Rev. Pharmacol. Toxicol.*, **35**, 509–39.
26. Simonson, M.S. (1993) Endothelins: multifunctional renal peptides. *Physiol. Rev.*, **73**, 375–411.
27. Simonson, M.S. and Dunn, M.J. (1993) Endothelin peptides and the kidney. *Ann. Rev. Physiol.*, **55**, 249–65.
28. Marsen, T.A., Schramek, H. and Dunn, M.J. (1994) Renal actions of endothelin: linking cellular signaling pathways to kidney disease. *Kidney Int.*, **45**, 336–44.
29. Kohan, D.E. (1993) Endothelins in the kidney: physiology and pathophysiology. *Am. J. Kidney Dis.*, **22**, 493–510.
30. Ruskaoho, H. (1992) Atrial natriuretic peptide: synthesis, release and metabolism. *Pharmacol. Rev.*, **44**, 479–602.
31. Maack, T. (1992) Receptors of atrial natriuretic factor. *Ann. Rev. Physiol.*, **54**, 11–27.
32. Raine, A.E.G., Firth, J.G. and Ledingham, J.G.G. (1989) Renal actions of atrial natriuretic factor. *Clin. Sci.*, **76**, 1–8.
33. Cogan, M.G. (1990) Renal effects of atrial natriuretic factor. *Ann. Rev. Physiol.*, **52**, 699–708.
34. Cogan, M.G. (1990) Atrial natriuretic peptide. *Kidney Int.*, **37**, 1148–60.
35. Anand-Srivastava, M.B. and Trachte, G.J. (1993) Atrial natriuretic factor receptors and signal transduction mechanisms. *Pharmacol. Rev.*, **45**, 455–97.

36. Davidson, N.C. and Struthers, A.D. (1994) Brain natriuretic peptide. *J. Hypertens.*, **12**, 329–36.
37. Wilkins, M.R., Nunez, D.J. and Wharton, J. (1993) The natriuretic peptide family: turning hormones into drugs. *J. Endrocrinol.*, **137**, 347–59.
38. Moncada, S., Palmer, R.M.J. and Higgs, E.A. (1991) Nitric oxide: physiology, pathophysiology, and pharmacology. *Pharmacol. Rev.*, **43**, 109–42.
39. Ruilope, L.M., Lahera, V., Rodicio, J.L. and Romero, J.C. (1994) Participation of nitric oxide in the regulation of renal function: possible role in the genesis of arterial hypertension. *J. Hypertens.*, **12**, 625–31.
40. Salom, M.G., Lahera, V. and Romero, J.C. (1991) Role of prostaglandins and endothelium-derived relaxing factor on the renal response to acetylcholine. *Am. J. Physiol.*, **260**, F145–F149.
41. Wright, F.S. and Okusa, M.D. (1990) Functional role of tubuloglomerular feedback control of glomerular filtration. *Adv. Nephrol. Necker Hosp.*, **19**, 119–34.
42. Schnermann, J., Häberle, D.A., Davis, J.M. and Thurau, K. (1992) Tubuloglomerular feedback control of renal vascular resistance, in *Handbook of Physiology*, section 8, Renal Physiology (ed. E.E. Windhager) American Physiological Society, New York and Oxford University Press, Oxford, pp. 1675–705.
43. Braam, B., Mitchell, K.D., Koomans, H.A. and Navar, L.G. (1993) Relevance of the tubuloglomerular feedback mechanism in pathophysiology. *J. Am. Soc. Nephrol.*, **4**, 1257–74.
44. Kurokawa, K. (1993) Chloride conductance of mesangial cells. *Renal Physiol. Biochem.*, **16**, 15–20.
45. Kunz, D., Mühl, M., Walker, G. and Pfeilschifter, J. (1994) Two distinct signaling pathways trigger the expression of inducible nitric oxide synthase in rat renal mesangial cells. *Proc. Natl. Acad. Sci. USA*, **91**, 5387–91.
46. Bredt, D.S. and Snyder, S.H. (1994) Nitric oxide: a physiologic messenger molecule. *Ann. Rev. Biochem.*, **63**, 175–95.
47. Raij, L. and Baylis, C. (1995) Glomerular actions of nitric oxide. *Kidney Int.*, **48**, 20–32.
48. Lingrel, J.B., Huysse, J.V., O'Brien, W. *et al.* (1994) Structure–function studies of the Na,K-ATPase. *Kidney Int.*, **45**, suppl. 44, S-32 – S-39.
49. Drenckhahn, D., Jöns, T., Kollert-Jöns, A. *et al.* (1993) Cytoskeleton and epithelial polarity. *Renal Physiol. Biochem.*, **16**, 6–14.
50. Berry, C.A. (1983) Water permeability and pathways in the proximal tubule. *Am. J. Physiol.*, **245**, F279–F294.
51. Beck, J.S., Laprade, R. and Lapointe, J.-Y. (1994) Coupling between transepithelial Na transport and basolateral K conductance in renal proximal tubule. *Am. J. Physiol.*, **266**, F517 – F527.
52. Moe, O.W., Preisig, P.A. and Alpern, R.J. (1990) Cellular model of proximal tubule NaCl and $NaHCO_3$ absorption. *Kidney Int.*, **38**, 605–11.
53. Harris, P.J. (1992) Regulation of proximal tubular function by angiotensin. *Clin. Exp. Pharmacol. Physiol.*, **19**, 213–22.
54. Reeves, W.B. and Andreoli, T.E. (1992) Renal epithelial chloride channels. *Ann. Rev. Physiol.*, **54**, 29–50.
55. Funder, J.W. (1993) Aldosterone action. *Ann. Rev. Physiol.*, **55**, 115–30.
56. Horisberger, J.-D. and Rossier, B.C. (1992) Aldosterone regulation of gene transcription leading to control of ion transport. *Hypertension*, **19**, 221–7.
57. Wehling, M., Christ, M. and Theisen, K. (1992) Membrane receptors for

aldosterone: a novel pathway for mineralocorticoid action. *Am. J. Physiol.*, **263**, E974–E979.
58. Ganguly, A. (1992) Atrial natriuretic peptide-induced inhibition of aldosterone secretion: a quest for mediator(s). *Am. J. Physiol.*, **263**, E181–E194.
59. Zeidel, M.L. (1993) Hormonal regulation of inner medullary collecting duct sodium transport. *Am. J. Physiol.*, **265**, F159–F173.
60. Breyer, M.D. (1991) Regulation of water and salt transport in collecting duct through calcium-dependent signaling mechanisms. *Am. J. Physiol.*, **260**, F1–F11.
61. Smith, P.R. and Benos, D.J. (1991) Epithelial $Na^+$ channels. *Ann. Rev. Physiol.*, **53**, 509–30.
62. Hansell, P. (1992) Evaluation of methods for estimating renal medullary blood flow. *Renal Physiol. Biochem.*, **15**, 217–30.
63. Roman, R.J. and Zou, A.-P. (1993) Influence of the renal medullary circulation on the control of sodium excretion. *Am. J. Physiol.*, **265**, R963–R973.
64. Kriz, W. (1983) Structural organisation of the renal medullary counterflow system. *Fed. Proc.*, **42**, 2379–85.
65. Stephenson, J.L. (1983) The renal concentrating mechanism: fundamental theoretical concepts. *Fed. Proc.*, **42**, 2386–91.
66. Sands, J.M. and Kokko, J.P. (1990) Countercurrent system. *Kidney Int.*, **38**, 695–9.
67. Handler, J.S. (1988) Antidiuretic hormone moves membranes. *Am. J. Physiol.*, **255**, F375–F382.
68. Harris, H.W., Strange, K. and Zeidel, M.L. (1991) Current understanding of the cellular biology and molecular structure of the antidiuretic hormone – stimulated water transport pathway. *J. Clin. Invest.*, **88**, 1–8.
69. Breyer, M.D. and Ando, Y. (1994) Hormonal signaling and regulation of salt and water transport in the collecting duct. *Ann. Rev. Physiol.*, **56**, 711–39.
70. Gellai, M. (1990) Modulation of vasopressin antidiuretic action by renal $\alpha_2$-adrenoceptors. *Am. J. Physiol.*, **259**, F1–F8.
71. Breyer, M.D., Jacobson, H.R. and Hebert, R.L. (1990) Cellular mechanisms of prostaglandin $E_2$ and vasopressin interactions in the collecting duct. *Kidney Int.*, **38**, 618–24.
72. Knepper, M.A. and Star, R.A. (1990) The vasopressin-regulated urea transporter in renal inner medullary collecting duct. *Am. J. Physiol.*, **259**, F393–F401.
73. Bertorello, A.M and Katz, A.I. (1993) Short-term regulation of renal Na-K-ATPase activity: physiological relevance and cellular mechanisms. *Am. J. Physiol.*, **265**, F743–F755.
74. Woolfson, R.G., Poston, L. and De Wardener, H.E. (1994) Digoxin-like inhibitors of active sodium transport and blood pressure: the current status. *Kidney Int.*, **46**, 297–309.
75. Goto, A., Yamada, K., Hagi, N. *et al.* (1992) Physiology and pharmacology of endogenous digitalis-like factors. *Pharmacol. Rev.*, **44**, 377–99.
76. Wang, W. Sackin, H. and Giebisch, G. (1992) Renal potassium channels and their regulation. *Ann. Rev. Physiol.*, **54**, 81–96.
77. Field, M.J., Stanton, B.A. and Giebisch, G.H. (1984) Influence of ADH on renal potassium handling: a micropuncture and microperfusion study. *Kidney Int.*, **25**, 502–11.
78. Dubose, T.D. (1990) Reclamation of filtered bicarbonate. *Kidney Int.*, **38**, 584–9.

79. Schuster, V.L. (1993) Function and regulation of collecting duct intercalated cells. *Ann. Rev. Physiol.*, **55**, 267–88.
80. Capasso, G., Malnic, G., Wang, T. and Giebisch, G. (1994) Acidification in mammalian cortical distal tubule. *Kidney Int.*, **45**, 1543–54.
81. Paillard, M. and Bichara, M. (1989) Peptide hormone effects on urinary acidification and acid base balance: PTH, ADH and glucagon. *Am. J. Physiol.*, **256**, F973–F985.

# 2

# Progression of chronic renal disease

*K.P.G. Harris and J. Walls*

## 2.1 INTRODUCTION

Progressive loss of renal function results in the accumulation of a variety of toxins normally removed by the kidney. This results in the development of the 'uraemic syndrome' and death will result unless renal function is replaced by dialysis. Although it is clear that the degree of renal impairment (and not the underlying renal disease) predicts most accurately the clinical manifestations of patients with the uraemic syndrome, attempts over the decades to identify putative substances that are responsible for the constellation of signs and symptoms which make up this syndrome have met with limited success.

The true incidence of end stage renal failure (ESRF) is not known, but the reported incidence continues to increase by 8–9% a year. The number of people taken on to dialysis each year varies widely from country to country. In Western Europe 60–100 patients per million population start dialysis each year [1], but in the USA the rate is higher. This variation is more likely to reflect underlying attitudes to the provision of dialysis services than true differences in the incidence of the disease, and in any case must represent an underestimate of the problem. One estimate has suggested an expected lifetime incidence of 'end stage' chronic renal failure of 1 in 200 people. Treatment with dialysis is effective but carries a high morbidity and mortality, and results in a high economic cost to providers of health care.

*Renal Disease.* Edited by G. Venkat Raman. Published in 1998 by Chapman & Hall, London. ISBN 0 412 45700 8.

Progressive renal scarring may occur as a result of continuing damage from the underlying renal disease, or as a result of a maladaptive response that occurs in the kidney following renal injury, or both. Clinical observations suggest that once a renal injury has produced a certain degree of renal damage progressive kidney failure is often inexorable [2]. Experimental studies have led support to the hypothesis that once a critical reduction in nephron number has occurred, a maladaptive response occurs in the remaining renal tissue which causes renal failure to progress even when the initial insult is no longer present. Thus therapies for chronic renal failure should be aimed at not only the process which initiates renal injury but also those processes which are responsible for its inexorable progression. Indeed the latter approach is likely to be more effective since most patients present with renal disease long after the initial insult has occurred and once renal scarring and loss of renal function is severe.

In the past two decades much experimental work has been aimed at understanding the pathophysiology of the processes that result in the progressive loss of renal function. Understanding these processes raises the prospect of developing rational and specific therapies to slow (or stop) the inexorable decline in renal function which would otherwise occur. Such strategies would have obvious benefits to patients and health providers alike. More recently attempts have been made to demonstrate the relevance and applicability to humans of strategies which have proved successful in experimental animal models of chronic renal failure.

## 2.2 PATHOPHYSIOLOGY OF CHRONIC RENAL DISEASE

The histology of the kidney in end stage renal disease is characterized by localized areas of cellular proliferation, collapse of the glomerular capillary bed and glomerulosclerosis, together with atrophy of the tubules, which are surrounded by inflammatory cells. There is diffuse fibrosis characterized by increased deposition of collagen and mesenchymal matrix, increased lipid deposition and increased numbers of fibroblasts [3]. The functional unit of the kidney is in essence replaced by scar tissue in response to injury. It is accepted that this histological appearance is not a distinct clinical entity, but the final common outcome of a variety of different clinical renal diseases [3].

Within the glomerulus there are four distinct cell types (endothelial, mesangial, epithelial and macrophages), all of which may participate in the sclerotic process through the excess production and/or decreased degradation of basement membrane and mesangial matrix. An increase in both normal basement membrane and mesangial matrix components (collagens IV and V, laminin and fibronectin, and glycosaminoglycans) and in addition collagens I and III (which are not found in the normal glomerulus) is typically found in the sclerosed glomerulus [3].

Although glomerulosclerosis is considered the histological hallmark of the 'end stage kidney', it should be pointed out that the whole nephron is involved in this process and atrophy of tubules surrounded by inflammatory cells and diffuse fibrosis are also typically seen. Thus a more correct term would be **nephrosclerosis**. Whether glomerulosclerosis leads to tubular atrophy as a consequence of ischaemia 'downstream', or the interstitium is the primary site of the injury with glomerular loss secondary to this, or a combination of both is often impossible to define.

It has been known for many years that tubulo-interstitial disease occurring in chronic renal failure (CRF) is correlated with renal function. In patients with persistent glomerulonephritis the degree of tubular atrophy is a better predictor of renal function, determined by plasma creatinine, than measures of histological changes in the glomeruli [4]. Using a semi-quantitative score of renal biopsy pathology an inverse correlation between the severity of interstitial disease and renal function (measured by inulin clearance) has been demonstrated [5]. The correlation of renal function with glomerular pathology in the same patients was poor. More recently the prognostic importance of interstitial pathology has been reviewed in a number of renal diseases including membranoproliferative glomerulonephritis type I, membranous glomerulonephritis, diabetic nephropathy, focal sclerosing glomerulonephritis and IgA nephropathy [6].

Several mechanisms have been proposed to explain how tubulo-interstitial changes ultimately result in the decreased glomerular filtration rate. It has been suggested that interstitial expansion increases post-glomerular vascular resistance with the effects of decreasing the renal plasma flow and thus decreasing the glomerular filtration rate. During the scarring process both resident cells and infiltrating inflammatory cells may release various cytokines and other substances that have vasoactive effects which may influence post-glomerular vascular tone. It has been proposed that these effects on post-glomerular vasculature contribute to glomerular hypertension which is considered to be a determinant of progressive renal damage (see Section 2.4). It has also been suggested that vasoactive substances released within the interstitium find their way into adjacent glomeruli and thereby exert direct effects on glomerular function.

Whilst it is clear that tubulo-interstitial damage occurs in renal diseases of glomerular origin and that tubulo-interstitial damage may directly contribute to the loss of renal function it is not immediately obvious why the interstitium is damaged at all in most renal diseases and this remains the topic for much current experimental work.

## 2.3 THE MALADAPTIVE RESPONSE – EVIDENCE FROM EXPERIMENTAL ANIMAL MODELS

The observation that nephrosclerosis occurs as a result of a variety of different renal diseases, has led to attempts to define a unifying hypothesis of progressive renal failure. The concept has evolved that once a sufficient reduction in nephron number has occurred as a result of a renal injury, a series of compensatory mechanisms come into play in the remaining nephrons, which are actually maladaptive, and result long term in the development of renal fibrosis and subsequent loss of renal function. This hypothesis has proved attractive to nephrologists as it can explain why the 'end stage kidney' has a similar appearance irrespective of the initial insult and why renal disease can progress even when the initial insult is no longer present.

On the basis of experimental studies many potential 'maladaptive

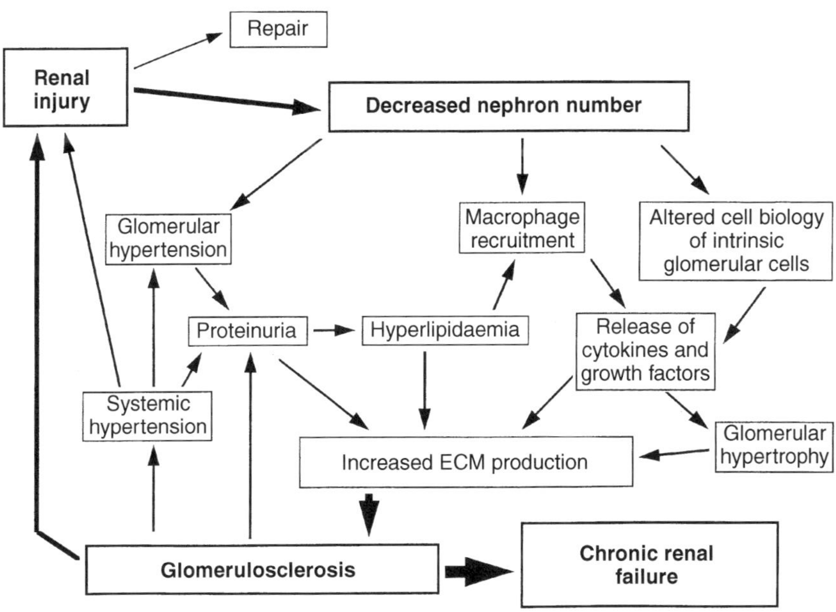


**Figure 2.1** Mechanisms whereby an initial renal injury may lead to glomerulosclerosis. A renal insult may be followed by tissue repair or more commonly a permanent loss of nephrons. As a result of the latter a complex and interacting series of responses is initiated which subsequently results in further nephron destruction and hence progressive chronic renal failure (the maladaptive response).

responses' have been proposed as being key to the development of progressive renal scarring. These include haemodynamic alterations (both systemic and glomerular), alterations in humoral factors such as lipids and parathyroid hormone (PTH), changes in growth factors and cytokines, the role of infiltrating cells and the development of proteinuria. It is likely however that no single factor is responsible for propagating progressive renal injury, but that the aetiology is multifactorial, with several factors acting in concert, all feeding into a final common pathway which results in nephrosclerosis [3] (Figure 2.1).

A large number of experimental models of glomerulosclerosis have been developed to study the pathogenetic factors which may contribute to its development [7]. The most extensively studied model of chronic renal failure is that induced by partial infarction of one kidney combined with contralateral nephrectomy (the so-called remnant kidney model). The model is characterized by the development of systemic hypertension, proteinuria, progressive sclerosis in the remaining nephrons and uraemia [8]. The model of surgical reduction in nephron number has been used most extensively in rats but a variety of species, including cats, rabbits, goats and sheep have also been studied. In addition it is now clear that following a large reduction in renal mass in humans there is an increased incidence in glomerulosclerosis in the remaining tissue [9]. Although surgical reduction in renal mass is unusual in man, by analogy similar pathogenetic mechanisms may play a role however nephron loss has been caused, whether it be by a toxic insult, an immunological insult such as glomerulonephritis, or a metabolic insult such as diabetes.

## 2.4 HAEMODYNAMIC ALTERATIONS

### 2.4.1 Systemic hypertension

Most experimental models of glomerulosclerosis and most human renal diseases are characterized by the presence of systemic hypertension. In the remnant kidney model, control of hypertension has been shown to protect against the development of glomerulosclerosis. This protection has been demonstrated with different classes of antihypertensives, including triple therapy (hydrochlorthiazide, hydralazine and reserpine), calcium channel blockers and angiotensin-converting enzyme (ACE) inhibitors. In experimental models of chronic renal failure it appears that different antihypertensive regimes do not provide equivalent renal protection, with ACE inhibitors consistently conveying greater protection than other classes of antihypertensive agents [10, 11]. This has led to the suggestion that blood pressure-independent mechanisms may be important to the development of glomerulosclerosis. The greater renoprotective properties of ACE inhibitors may be explained by their unique ability to modulate glomerular haemodynamics by reducing the vasoconstrictor tone of angiotensin II on the efferent arteriole of the glomerulus and thus lower glomerular capillary pressure (see below). ACE inhibitors, however, also have the potential to modulate angiotensin II-induced renal growth, modulate local cytokine networks, and reduce leucocyte influx, all of which may contribute to an additional renoprotective action.

In human renal diseases there is a clear association between the level of blood pressure and the rate of decline in renal function with age. In accelerated hypertension it is also apparent that aggressive treatment of the hypertension not only improves survival but also the renal prognosis. Studies have also clearly demonstrated that controlling the blood pressure slows the rate of progression of chronic renal failure in diabetic nephropathy [12] and in a variety of different primary renal diseases [13, 14]. Whether a particular class of antihypertensive agent conveys additional benefit over the control of blood pressure alone in non-diabetic human renal disease remains unclear.

### 2.4.2 Glomerular hypertension

Following a reduction in renal mass, early adaptive changes in the remaining nephrons include an increase in renal plasma flow per nephron and an increase in single nephron glomerular filtration rate (SNGFR) [15]. This is brought about by vasodilation of both the afferent and the efferent arteriole; the afferent arteriole dilates more than the efferent arteriole as the latter is subjected to vasoconstrictor tone by the action of angiotensin II. As a result the glomerular capillary pressure rises and the SNGFR increases. Whilst these changes would be teleologically meaningful in compensating for reduced renal mass, it has been suggested that hyperfiltration in the remaining glomeruli results in the development of progressive glomerulosclerosis.

Elegant studies, particularly by Brenner's group at the Brigham and Women's hospital in Boston, have advanced this theory. Using micropuncture techniques usually in the Munich–Wistar rat (whose superficially placed glomeruli make it ideal for such studies), it has been demonstrated that hyperperfusion, hyperfiltration and intraglomerular hypertension, characterized by an elevated transcapillary hydraulic pressure difference are responsible for the subsequent glomerular damage and increased permeability [15]. The theory is supported by the fact that therapeutic manoeuvres aimed at normalizing glomerular haemodynamics, particularly glomerular capillary pressure such as low-protein diets [15] and ACE inhibitors [10] or angiotensin II receptor antagonists appear to delay or prevent the development of glomerulosclerosis.

However, a variety of other manoeuvres, including heparin (both anticoagulant and non-anticoagulant) and lipid-lowering drugs, which do not appear to have any haemodynamic effects, also appear to provide protection against the development of glomerulosclerosis in the remnant kidney model. In addition, puromycin aminonucleside nephrosis, a model which progresses to glomerulosclerosis, is not characterized by an elevated glomerular pressure at least early in the course of the disease, although it may subsequently develop as the disease progresses.

The important interplay between systemic hypertension and glomerular haemodynamic changes on the development of glomerulosclerosis has been demonstrated in studies in the Wistar–Kyoto rat. In this strain of rat, a reduction in renal mass results in glomerular hyperfiltration without systemic hypertension. As a result there is only a small increase in glomerular capillary pressure and no evidence of morphological damage to the kidney [16]. Furthermore, in a study comparing the effect of ACE inhibition and calcium channel blockade on the development of glomerulosclerosis in the remnant kidney, protection against glomerulosclerosis was directly related to the reduction in glomerular hypertension. ACE inhibition caused efferent arteriolar dilatation, controlled glomerular hypertension and afforded protection against glomerulosclerosis even if blood pressure control was not optimal; calcium channel blockade dilated the afferent arteriole allowing the transmission of systemic blood pressure directly to the glomerular capillary bed and hence provided less glomeruloprotection for a given fall in systemic blood pressure [10].

In the kidney the interstitial blood supply originates from post-glomerular vessels and hence alterations in glomerular haemodynamics are likely to have a profound influence on interstitial blood flow. Oxygen tension in the kidney is known to be less than systemic arterial oxygen tension and hence proximal tubular cells which are highly metabolically active are vulnerable to minor changes in oxygen delivery. In order to explain the interstitial fibrosis that is an inevitable consequence of glomerular disease, Fine *et al.* have proposed that glomerular hypertension results in an increase in blood pressure transmitted to the post-glomerular capillaries, damaging them and causing interstitial ischaemia [17]. Once scarring and increased matrix production have started then the increased distance between tubular cells and peritubular capillaries would further increase the ischaemic injury. Studies of human biopsy specimens have indeed demonstrated a progressive loss of post-glomerular capillaries in progressive renal disease [18].

### 2.4.3 Glomerular hypertrophy

Glomerular hypertrophy is invariably associated with glomerulosclerosis raising the possibility that the two processes may be pathogenetically linked. Glomerular hypertrophy is a characteristic feature of diabetes and precedes the development of nephropathy. In addition glomerular size increases after a reduction in renal mass in both experimental animals and humans. Uninephrectomy which stimulates the hypertrophy of the remaining glomeruli accelerates the development of glomerulosclerosis in a variety of experimental models of renal disease, and glucocorticoids which also promote renal hypertrophy, accelerate glomerulosclerosis.

Glomerular hypertrophy could result from the haemodynamic alterations discussed above. Many renoprotective manoeuvres which alter glomerular haemodynamics such as low-protein diets and ACE inhibitors also modulate the degree of renal hypertrophy that is observed. Yoshida however has been able to dissociate the development of glomerular haemodynamic alterations from glomerular hypertrophy by combining a 2/3 infarction of one kidney with either a contralateral nephrectomy or diversion of the contralateral ureter into the peritoneal cavity. Glomerular hypertension occurred in both models, but glomerular hypertrophy only occurred in the model with the contralateral nephrectomy. In addition the degree of glomerular injury was greatest in the rats with the contralateral nephrectomy suggesting that hypertrophy was an important precursor for any subsequent glomerular scarring [19]. Experiments in which the growth hormone axis has been manipulated so as to either inhibit or enhance the hypertrophic response to renal mass reduction also provide evidence for a pathogenetic link between the development of glomerular hypertrophy and glomerulosclerosis.

Despite these compelling observations the case that glomerular hypertrophy is a unifying hypothesis for the development of glomerulosclerosis remains to be proven, since conflicting results have been obtained depending on the strain of rat studied and the model used. When uninephrectomy was compared to bilateral partial renal infarction, only the latter developed glomerulosclerosis despite the degree of hypertrophy being greater following uninephrectomy. In addition the NAR strain of rat develops rapidly progressive glomerulosclerosis following a reduction in renal mass despite only modest renal hypertrophy and in these rats glomerular hypertension appears to be a better predictor of damage. Further evidence against a critical role for glomerular hypertrophy is provided by the observation that in rats with the remnant kidney, ACE inhibition completely protected against the development of glomerulosclerosis but had no effect on the degree of glomerular hypertrophy; glomerular pressure and not glomerular volume were more consistently associated with glomerulosclerosis [11]. Similar observations have also been made in rats with streptozotocin-induced diabetic glomerulosclerosis.

Support for a pathogenetic role for glomerular hypertrophy in human renal disease has been provided by recent observations by Fogo *et al.* using sequential biopsy material from children with proteinuria in whom a large glomerular tuft area was associated with the subsequent development of focal sclerosis and a more severe clinical course [20]. However, the adverse prognostic significance of glomerular hypertrophy remains to be confirmed in adults with the nephrotic syndrome.

## 2.5 ABNORMALITIES OF HUMORAL FACTORS

Numerous humoral factors have been implicated in the pathogenesis of glomerulosclerosis. Experimental evidence suggests that hyperphosphataemia, elevation of PTH and altered calcium homeostasis, all characteristic features of chronic renal failure, may contribute to progressive renal damage.

Abnormalities of lipid metabolism are common accompaniments of renal damage and could play a role in the progression of renal disease [21]. Hyperlipidaemia aggravates a number of experimental renal diseases and treatment of animals with renal disease with lipid-lowering drugs abrogates the development of glomerulosclerosis. Furthermore glomerulosclerosis has many histological analogies to atherosclerosis leading some workers to suggest a common pathogenesis [22]. The role of lipid and lipoprotein abnormalities in progressive renal injury is discussed in Chapter 9.

Acidosis is a universal finding in chronic renal failure. Acidosis would be expected to lead to enhanced intra-renal ammonia generation which in turn could provoke tubulo-interstitial inflammation by activation of the alternate pathway of complement via the amidation of C3 [23]. Bicarbonate supplementation of animals with a remnant kidney has been shown to result in a decrease in low-molecular-weight proteinuria and tubulo-interstitial disease in the short term but recent observations from our laboratory have been able to demonstrate that long-term acidosis does not cause renal injury, nor does correction of acidosis long term prevent the development of renal injury and chronic renal failure in rats with the remnant kidney [24].

Experimental observations in animals where the growth hormone axis has been manipulated provides evidence for a role of circulating growth factors in the development of glomerular hypertrophy and glomerulosclerosis [25]. Following subtotal nephrectomy, the progression of glomerular sclerosis is markedly attenuated in rats deficient in growth hormone (GH). This attenuation of structural injury correlates with a marked decrease in glomerular hypertrophy suggesting that endogenous GH plays an important determining role in the progression of glomerulosclerosis. Similar observations have also been made in experimental models of diabetic nephropathy. In addition exogenous administration of recombinant GH exacerbates puromycin aminonucleoside nephropathy in rats, increasing urinary protein excretion, decreasing inulin clearance and increasing the extent of segmental glomerulosclerosis and tubulo-interstitial injury. Furthermore, glomerular hypertrophy was enhanced by recombinant GH. In studies using the rat remnant kidney model, the glomerular filtration rate did not appear to be adversely affected by prolonged growth hormone treatment. Survival data, however, in these animals did suggest that the growth stimulating effects of recombinant growth hormone in uraemic animals may be accompanied by a trend toward reduced longevity, and histological evaluation revealed increased glomerular hypertrophy and glomerulosclerosis.

It is less clear whether growth hormone may have a deleterious effect on normal kidneys. Acromegalic patients do not seem to display an increased incidence of glomerulosclerosis and GH administration to normal rats results in an increase in glomerular filtration rate and glomerular planar area without altering blood pressure or inducing proteinuria. However, mice transgenic for bovine growth hormone develop glomerular lesions characterized by a disproportionate increment in glomerular volume and progressive mesangial sclerosis [26]; in contrast mice transgenic for insulin-like growth factor 1 exhibit only slight glomerular hypertrophy and develop little glomerulosclerosis.

It is possible that GH plays a permissive role in the development of renal scarring adversely affecting renal structure and function only in the presence of an underlying nephropathy. If such an adverse effect were found in humans as well as rodents it would have important clinical implications. The growth promoting effects of GH are of potential therapeutic importance to children with chronic renal failure. Fortunately although such renal adverse effects of growth hormone remain of theoretical concern, to date there is no convincing evidence that GH administration accelerates the development of chronic renal failure in either normal children or children with renal disease.

## 2.6 CYTOKINES AND GROWTH FACTORS

A growing body of evidence supports a critical role for cytokines and growth factors in the development of glomerulosclerosis and interstitial fibrosis. It is clear that both intrinsic renal cells and infiltrating cells (see Section 2.7) are capable of producing such factors which may then act in a paracrine or autocrine fashion. Some cytokines including interleukins (Il-1$\beta$, Il-6) and tumour necrosis factor (TNF-$\alpha$) appear to play an important role in the inflammatory response and are unregulated in both experimental and human proliferative glomerulonephritides [27]. Recent evidence would support a pivotal role for other cytokines, such as the platelet-derived growth factor (PDGF) and transforming growth factor (TGF-$\beta$) in the development of renal scarring. These cytokines may induce cell hypertrophy or proliferation and modulate extracellular matrix synthesis and degradation. Expression of both PDGF and its receptor by intrinsic glomerular cells is associated with the early mesangial cell proliferation that follows a critical reduction in renal mass. Furthermore, administration of recombinant PDGF to rats will cause mesangial cell proliferation, and transfection of the PDGF gene into normal rat kidney promotes over-expression of PDGF and the development of glomerular cell proliferation and glomerulosclerosis. PDGF will also upregulate the production of TGF-$\beta$ by mesangial cells.

TGF-$\beta$ is a homodimer of approximately 25 kDa produced by a wide variety of cell types. It is a multifunctional cytokine, but of relevance to the progression of renal disease is its ability to regulate the production and turnover of extracellular matrix. The pathological consequences of increased production of TGF-$\beta$ within the kidney have been termed 'the dark side of wound repair' by Border and his colleagues, since the replacement of the nephron with scar tissue results in the loss of functional units from the kidney and hence chronic renal failure. TGF-$\beta$ enhances the synthesis of many extracellular matrix proteins including collagen, fibronectin and proteoglycans whilst at the same time inhibiting matrix degradation by both decreasing the production of proteases and enhancing the production of their inhibitors.

Constitutive TGF-$\beta$ expression is found in normal glomeruli of mice, rats and humans. Increased expression of TGF-$\beta$ is found in a variety of immunological (anti Thy-1 glomerulonephritis) and toxic (aminonucleoside nephrosis and diabetes) models of renal disease and is associated with the deposition of extracellular matrix proteins. In addition enhanced immunostaining for TGF-$\beta$ has been found in diverse human renal diseases which lead to progressive renal scarring including chronic allograft rejection, diabetic nephropathy, immunoglobulin A (IgA) nephropathy and systemic vasculitis. TGF-$\beta$ production within the kidney may be from a variety of cell types including infiltrating macrophages or platelets as well as intrinsic renal cells such as fibroblasts, tubular cells and mesangial cells.

Compelling evidence for a central role for TGF-$\beta$ in the development of glomerulosclerosis comes from the observation that transfection of the TGF-$\beta$ gene into glomeruli *in vivo* results in the accumulation of extracellular matrix and severe glomerular damage leading to glomerulosclerosis [28]. In addition strategies which block the action of TGF-$\beta$ afford protection against the development of glomerulosclerosis; for example, administration of a neutralizing antibody to TGF-$\beta$ is able to prevent the accumulation of extracellular matrix proteins and proteoglycans seen in experimental glomerulonephritis [29]. Similarly, the administration of the naturally occurring proteoglycan decorin, which acts to bind and neutralize all isoforms of TGF-$\beta$, has the same protective effect.

It is also of note that low-protein diets, whose beneficial effects in experimental renal disease have previously been attributed to haemodynamic alterations, also cause a reduction in TGF-$\beta$ gene expression within the kidney. Furthermore, high glucose stimulates TGF-$\beta$ gene expression by tubular cells in culture, suggesting a possible pathogenetic role for this cytokine in the development of diabetic nephropathy.

## 2.7 INFILTRATING MACROPHAGES

Normal glomeruli contain a small number of resident macrophages. The exact role of these cells remain unclear but they are likely to play a role in maintaining normal glomerular structure and function. Evidence has recently been provided for a critical pathogenetic role of infiltrating macrophages in the development of renal scarring in diverse non-immunologically mediated models of chronic renal failure. In these models their role may be analogous to that in the development of scar tissue elsewhere in the body [30]. In the rat, uninephrectomy (which results in the development of glomerulosclerosis) causes an influx of leucocytes in the remnant glomeruli within one to two weeks. This occurs before light microscopic changes, the development of microalbuminuria or glomerular hypertrophy, suggesting that the leucocyte influx may be a cause, rather than a consequence, of renal damage. An early infiltrate of glomerular macrophages has also been observed in puromycin aminonucleoside nephrosis, an experimental model of non-immune glomerular injury that progresses to glomerulosclerosis. The pathogenetic importance of the infiltrate is demonstrated by the fact that abolition of the infiltrate by X-irradiation or a diet free of essential fatty acids, prevents the development of glomerulosclerosis [31].

The number of macrophages per glomerulus is increased by cholesterol feeding. Such observations may provide the experimental basis for the observation that cholesterol feeding enhances the development of glomerulosclerosis in a variety of animal models of renal disease, and that control of the hypercholesterolaemia is beneficial.

An interstitial accumulation of T cells and macrophages is also a prominent feature of many experimental models of renal disease [30]. It is likely that the presence of these cells within the interstitium provides a potent stimulus to interstitial fibroblasts and promotes fibrosis. Interstitial macrophage accumulation is a characteristic finding in puromycin aminonucleoside nephrosis where it has been shown to modulate glomerular function acutely. Furthermore, in this model the presence of macrophages within the interstitium correlates well with the production of extracellular matrix (ECM) proteins, suggesting that macrophages do induce interstitial fibrosis [32].

The exact mechanisms by which infiltrating cells promote mesangial expansion, tubulo-interstitial damage and increased ECM production remains to be determined. They are known to be a potent source of cytokines and growth factors, some of which are capable of stimulating ECM production by mesangial cells. Macrophages and macrophage-conditioned medium can stimulate the production of the extracellular matrix proteins by mesangial cells in culture [33]. This effect is likely to be the result of a complex network of cytokines acting in both an autocrine and a paracrine fashion. Macrophages are a potent source of TGF-$\beta$ and PDGF, whose role in renal scarring has been discussed previously.

The mechanisms involved in the recruitment of large numbers of these biologically active cells into the kidney have been extensively studied. This process consists of two main parts: (i) the expression of adhesion molecules which facilitate monocyte migration from blood vessels into the kidney and (ii) the release of chemotactic substances. In many rat models of experimental glomerulonephritis there is up-regulation of the intercellular adhesion molecule (ICAM-1) expression both in the glomerulus and the peritubular capillaries, which interacts with its ligand (LFA-1) on leucocytes. The functional importance of this process has been demonstrated in anti-glomerular basement membrane (GBM) glomerulonephritis in the rat with the use of neutralizing antibodies to either ICAM-1 or LFA-1, which inhibit glomerular leucocyte infiltration and renal injury. Expression of adhesion molecules may be induced either by direct immunological insult or indirectly via the production of molecules such as interleukin-1 and tumour necrosis factor.

A diverse array of both immune and non-immune mediated renal insults have been shown to result in the production of chemotactic substances by the glomerulus or its constituent cells. These include a monocyte-specific lipid-like chemoattractant and the chemokines monocyte chemotactic protein 1 (MCP-1) and RANTES. In addition proximal tubular cells can produce both MCP-1 and a lipid-like chemotactic factor. It is likely that no single chemoattractant is responsible for the recruitment of leucocytes into the kidney as demonstrated by the observation that although MCP-1 expression is increased in puromycin aminonucleoside nephrosis, neutralizing antibodies to MCP-1 do not appear to either ameliorate macrophage recruitment in this model or prevent renal injury [32]. A full understanding of the processes involved in the recruitment of cells into the kidney may provide potential therapeutic targets for the prevention of renal scarring.

## 2.8 PROTEINURIA

The development of proteinuria is a universal finding in progressive renal disease. Evidence is now accumulating that proteinuria is of pathogenetic importance to the progression of chronic renal failure, rather than simply a marker of the severity of the renal disease.

Under normal circumstances only low-molecular-weight substances gain access to the urinary space, larger molecules being excluded by an intact glomerular barrier. In glomerular disease the barrier is disrupted and macromolecules, including albumin and larger proteins, gain access to both the mesangium and the tubular fluid. Hence the potential exists for one or more of these abnormally filtered proteins to interact adversely with the mesangium and/or the cells lining the tubular space, promoting further injury. The hypothesis that proteinuria may itself be an independent determinant of the progression of renal disease is strengthened by the observation that the degree of proteinuria can be correlated with the rate of progression of renal failure in both human and experimental renal disease. This is an attractive hypothesis since it not only provides a cause of progression but also a means by which glomerular disease may ultimately result in interstitial scarring.

The pathogenetic significance of proteinuria has recently been further supported by the observation that a reduction in proteinuria by the use of an ACE inhibitor is associated with a slowing of the rate of progression of renal failure [34]. In this study the beneficial effect of ACE inhibition was only observed in those patients in whom the drug brought about a reduction in the level of proteinuria.

The majority of the evidence that proteinuria is a determinant of progression of renal failure remains circumstantial and is predominantly based on correlations. In the past few years several plausible potential mechanisms have been put forward to explain how proteinuria might lead to progressive renal injury. In addition there is now a large body of evidence mostly from *in vitro* studies, suggesting a nephrotoxic potential for proteinuria. Such lines of evidence broadly fall into two main groups: (i) mesangial toxicity as a result of mesangial overload with abnormally filtered macromolecules, and (ii) induction of proximal tubular cell dysfunction as a result of abnormal amounts and/or types of protein being presented to the proximal tubular brush border.

Mesangial accumulation of macromolecules can produce mesangial cell injury, mesangial cell proliferation, increased production of mesangial matrix and hence glomerulosclerosis. In particular lipoproteins have been implicated in this regard (see Chapter 9).

Higher-molecular-weight proteins when filtered by a damaged glomerulus may also interact adversely with tubular cells. They may be reabsorbed and metabolized by the proximal tubule which would then be vulnerable to the effects that these proteins may produce (see Figure 2.2). Adverse effects of proteinuria could result from either the quantity of protein in the tubular fluid or from the effects of a particular biologically active protein, which is not normally found in the urine but may appear following glomerular damage. A variety of proteins have been demonstrated to be directly toxic to tubular epithelial cells, although the mechanism for this is unknown. Tubular injury may result in leakage of lysosomal enzymes into the cytoplasm of the tubular cell and the consequent cell injury could stimulate inflammation and scarring.

Proximal tubular cells have been shown to take part in the process of inflammation and scarring, with the production of matrix proteins, pro-

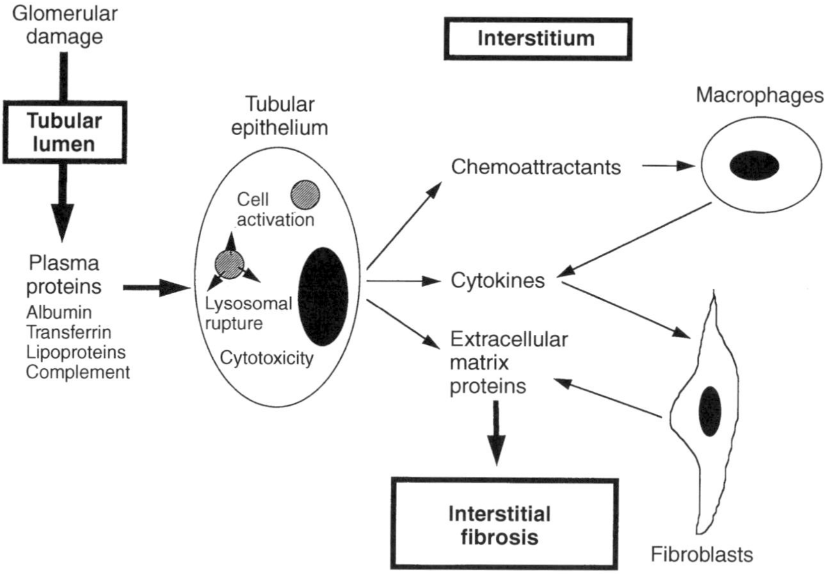


**Figure 2.2** The mechanisms by which proteins filtered as a result of glomerular injury may cause interstitial inflammation and scarring. In glomerular disease filtered proteins in the tubular lumen alter the biology of the tubular epithelium. This results in the release into the interstitium of chemoattractants, cytokines and extracellular matrix proteins. As a result there is accumulation of macrophages which also release cytokines to recruit and stimulate fibroblasts. The resultant increase in extracellular matrix causes scarring.

inflammatory cytokines and chemotactic substances. Proteins may directly modulate tubular cell function, altering both their growth characteristics and their phenotypic expression of cytokines and matrix proteins [35].

As previously discussed ammonia generation within the kidney may play a role in the development of progressive interstitial disease [23]. Increased ammonia production could result from catabolism of the increased amount of reabsorbed proteins, and in patients with glomerulonephritis the level of urinary ammonia correlates well with the level of proteinuria.

Proteinuria may also exert an adverse effect by exacerbating other pathological processes within the tubulo-interstitium. It is for instance possible that in tubular cells that are already stressed by hypoxia, the additional energy required to reabsorb and digest large amounts of proteins could result in damage to those cells, with the subsequent development of fibrosis.

Whether the potential adverse effects of proteinuria are attributable to an individual protein, or the molecules it carries, or due to the combined effects of the many proteins filtered by a damaged glomerulus, remains unknown. Direct toxicity of a number of proteins, including albumin and transferrin, has recently been demonstrated [35]. Since proteinuria is associated with a bad prognosis, therapeutic strategies aimed at non-specific reduction of proteinuria are logical. Further understanding of how subtle differences in the quality of proteinuria may affect the development of renal scarring holds the prospect of developing more specific therapies.

## 2.9 FROM RAT TO MAN – THERAPIES APPLICABLE TO HUMANS

Our understanding of the pathogenesis of the majority of primary renal insults is limited and hence the scope for effective primary prevention is small. Congenital or genetic causes of CRF will not be readily amenable to therapy in the near future. Treatment of glomerulonephritis with immune modulation has met with limited success although some types of glomerulonephritis, such as rapidly progressive glomerulonephritides and those associated with systemic lupus, do appear to benefit from immunosuppression. Many such diseases present late, often after a prolonged asymptomatic phase, when considerable renal damage may already have occurred. Important exceptions to this rule include hypertension, diabetes and chronic pyelonephritis. Effective screening for and treatment of hypertension will protect against end organ damage and renal failure. Diabetic nephropathy typically develops many years after the onset of the disease and is heralded by the development of microalbuminuria, which can be readily detected in the diabetic clinic. It is now clear that effective treatment of diabetes with the establishment of near normoglycaemia has a significant impact on the development of diabetic complications including nephropathy [36].

It remains likely however, that in the majority of cases therapies will have to be aimed at retarding the progression of already established renal injury. Various models of glomerulosclerosis have been extensively studied to examine the mechanisms which may contribute to the development of renal failure, on the assumption that there is a 'final common pathway', and that they can be extrapolated from rat and man. They have also been used to examine potential therapeutic interventions which may interrupt this 'final common pathway' and hence delay or prevent progression. The relevance of the pathogenetic mechanisms worked out in experimental models to human disease remains unclear. Sequential ultrastructural or haemodynamics data are impossible to obtain in humans. However, it seems likely that a similar mechanism may apply. For example following a large reduction in renal mass in humans there is an increased incidence in glomerulosclerosis in the remaining tissue [9]. Thus nephron loss however caused, whether it be by an immunological insult, a toxic insult or a metabolic insult, is likely to initiate further and progressive glomerulosclerosis. It is also interesting to note that the normal human ageing process (as in the rat) leads to glomerulosclerosis, with a slow and progressive decline in GFR, becoming apparent after the age of 70. This process is of no clinical significance in the vast majority of people, but extrapolating the data indicates that, if we were to live to the age of 150 years, many of us would reach ESRF and require dialysis.

Experimental models of renal disease have also been used to examine potential therapeutic manoeuvres, which may be employed in man. Whether such therapies will in time be applicable to man, will depend on the results of proper clinical studies. In the experimental model the exact time of onset of the disease is known and it has a short and predictable time course. These factors do not usually apply in human renal disease, so there needs to be caution in extrapolating the results to humans. The majority of experimental studies have been designed to examine one particular pathogenetic mechanism in isolation. In reality, human disease is likely to be more complicated than this, and this in turn may explain why some of the proposed therapeutic interventions, which appear so dramatically successful in experimental models, have yet to be proven successful in humans.

To date the only therapeutic manoeuvre shown conclusively to be effective in preventing glomerulosclerosis in humans is the control of systemic hypertension. Control of systemic hypertension has been shown to slow the rate of deterioration in the glomerular filtration rate in a variety of primary glomerular diseases [12] and diabetic nephropathy [11]. More recently attention has focused on what should be the target blood pressure and whether the choice of antihypertensive agent is important. Previously most nephrologists would have considered a target blood pressure of 140/90 mm Hg as adequate. Recent evidence from the MDRD study in the USA has demonstrated that a greater degree of renal protection was afforded by achieving a mean blood pressure of 92 mm Hg (i.e. 120/80) compared with 107 mm Hg (i.e. 140/90) [13]. The benefit of improved blood pressure control was only seen in those patients with proteinuria >1 g/24 h (patients with minimal proteinuria already had a very slow rate of progression). Within the first three months of study tight blood pressure control was associated with a more rapid decline in GFR (presumably a result of altered renal haemodynamics), but the rate of deterioration subsequently slowed, such that at 36 months the group with better blood pressure control had a significantly higher GFR than the control group.

Whether a particular class of antihypertensive agent conveys benefit over another remains controversial in many primary renal diseases despite the clear cut advantages of ACE inhibitors in experimental animal studies. Studies in diabetic nephropathy have however demonstrated a benefit for this class of drug, confirming the experimental observations. In one study treatment with captopril resulted in a significant delay in the time to doubling of the serum creatinine and a delay to the onset of the need for dialysis or transplantation [37] compared to placebo treatment, despite comparable blood pressure control (140/90 mm Hg) in the two groups [37]. ACE inhibition also appears to delay the evolution from microalbuminuria to overt proteinuria in diabetic nephropathy in both type I and type II diabetics. The use of ACE inhibitors can be associated with a decline in renal function which may be irreversible in patients with renovascular disease; since vascular disease is common in type II diabetics this group may be prone to such a complication from ACE inhibitors and therefore these agents should be used with caution. These subjects are covered in greater detail in Chapters 3 and 6.

The role of ACE inhibitors in delaying the progression of non-diabetic renal disease is much less clear. Some small studies would support the concept that they are uniquely renoprotective over and above their antihypertensive action. Meta-analyses of such studies would suggest that ACE inhibition is associated with a greater reduction in the level of proteinuria for a given fall in blood pressure than other antihypertensive regimes. It has also been suggested that in IgA nephropathy the protective action of ACE inhibition is seen in association with a particular ACE genotype. However these observations remain to be confirmed in large prospective randomized studies which are currently under way. To date one large study comparing an ACE inhibitor with a calcium channel blocker failed to show any significant difference in the rate of deterioration in renal function after three years [38].

Dietary protein restriction (DPR) has been employed to ameliorate the symptoms of progressive renal failure for many years. More recent observations by Brenner that DPR in the rat affords protection against the development of progressive renal failure have led some nephrologists to advocate the use of low-protein diets in humans with chronic renal failure. There is much anecdotal evidence in the literature in support of such an approach in humans; however much of this was poorly controlled, with small sample size and used crude assessment of renal function (usually reciprocal creatinine plots) to determine the rate of progression. To date there have been three large prospective randomized studies on the effect of low-protein diet on the progression of renal disease, two of which accurately assessed renal function with clearance techniques. One study concluded that dietary protein restriction was effective in slowing the rate of progression [39]. Another concluded that there was little evidence to support the use of low-protein diets [40]. The most recent and largest study – the MDRD study [13] – may have shown a small benefit of dietary intervention in patients with moderate renal impairment but not in those with severe renal impairment. Further secondary analyses of the MDRD study have attempted to define potential groups of patients who may benefit from protein restriction but the power of such secondary analyses is limited. Thus, significant doubts remain as to the value of protein restriction in delaying the progression of CRF.

In addition, there are further unanswered questions, such as what level of protein restriction should be used, when should it be instituted and which renal diseases benefit most? Low-protein diets are frequently poorly tolerated by many patients and compliance is often low. Data from the MDRD study would suggest that a low-protein diet (0.6 g protein per kg body weight per day) instituted and adhered to in patients with moderate renal failure may be beneficial. Although low-protein diets may have a limited effect on the progression of renal failure they may have other benefits which are of potential therapeutic importance. These include:

1. Possible slowing of progression of renal failure.
2. Lessening of 'uraemic' symptoms.
3. Improved carbohydrate metabolism.
4. Improved lipid metabolism.
5. Improved amino acid metabolism.
6. Correction of acidosis.
7. Reduction in proteinuria.
8. Improved hormonal profile including PTH and erythropoietin.

If such diets are to be used, dietetic supervision is mandatory not only to improve compliance, but to ensure that the patient does not become malnourished by adhering inappropriately to the prescribed regime; it is well established that the morbidity and mortality are increased if patients start dialysis in a poor nutritional state.

It is perhaps disappointing that despite extensive research over several decades and our knowledge of the pathophysiology of chronic renal failure, the only proven effective therapeutic tool available to the nephrologist remains the control of blood pressure. Looking to the future it is possible that strategies will be developed to effectively block the fibrogenic response to renal injury within the kidney. Whether these therapies will prove applicable and safe in humans remains a matter of speculation. The demonstration of a beneficial effect of blocking TGF-$\beta$ in experimental models of renal disease shows considerable promise. However, more work is required to define the most efficient way to block harmful unregulated cytokines selectively in renal disease. For the moment the appropriate use of antihypertensive agents must remain our most effective treatment strategy for patients with progressive chronic renal failure.

## REFERENCES


1. Geerlings, W., Tufreson, G., Ehrich, J.H.H. *et al.* (1994) Report on the management of renal failure in Europe. *Nephrol. Dial. Transplant.*, **9**, suppl. 1, 6–25.
2. Holevy, J. and Hayslett, J.P. (1986) Clinical features and course of glomerulosclerosis, in *The Progressive Nature of Renal Disease* (eds W.E. Mitch, B.M. Brenner and J.H. Stein), Churchill Livingstone, New York, pp. 189–201.
3. Klahr, S., Schreiner, G. and Ichikawa, I. (1988) The progression of renal disease. *N. Engl. J. Med.*, **318**, 1657–66.
4. Risdon, R.A., Sloper, J.C., de Wardener, H.E. (1966) Relationship between renal function and histological changes found in renal-biopsy specimens from patients with persistent glomerular nephritis. *Lancet*, **2**, 363–6.
5. Schainuck, L.I., Striker, G.E., Cutler, R.E. and Benditt, E.P. (1970) Structural–functional correlations in renal disease. Part II: the correlations. *Hum. Pathol.* **1**, 631–41.
6. Burton, C.J. and Walls, J. (1994) Proximal tubular cell, proteinuria and tubulointerstitial scarring. *Nephron*, **68**, 287–93.
7. Furness, P.N., Harris, K.P.G. (1994) An evaluation of experimental models of glomerulonephritis. *J. Exp. Pathol.*, **75**, 9–22.
8. Chanutin, A. and Ferris, E. (1932) Experimental renal insufficiency produced by partial nephrectomy. *Arch. Intern. Med.*, **49**, 767–87.
9. Novick, A.C., Gephardt, G., Guz, B. *et al.* (1991) Long term follow-up after partial removal of a solitary kidney. *N. Eng. J. Med.*, **325**, 1058–62.
10. Anderson, S., Rennke, H.G. and Brenner, B.M. (1986) Therapeutic advantage of converting enzyme inhibitors in arresting progressive renal injury associated with systemic hypertension in the rat. *J. Clin. Invest.*, **77**, 1993–2000.

11. Griffin, K.A., Picken, M.M. and Bidani, A.K. (1995) Deleterious effects of calcium channel blockade on pressure transmission and glomerular injury in rat remnant kidneys. *J. Clin. Invest.*, **96**, 793–800.
12. Bakris, G.L. (1993) Hypertension in diabetic patients. An overview of interventional studies to preserve renal function. *Am. J. Hypertens.*, **6**, 140S–147S.
13. Alverstand, A., Gutierrez, A., Bucht, H. and Bergstrom, J. (1988) Reduction of blood pressure retards the progression of chronic renal failure in man. *Nephrol. Dial. Transplant*, **3**, 624–31.
14. Klahr, S., Levey, A.S., Beck, G.J. *et al.* (1994) The effects of dietary protein and blood pressure control on the progression of chronic renal disease. *N. Engl. J. Med.*, **330**, 877–84.
15. Hostetter, T.H., Olson, J.L., Rennke, H.G. *et al.* (1981) Hyperfiltration in remnant nephrons: a potentially adverse response to renal ablation. *Am. J. Physiol.*, **241**, F85–F93.
16. Bidani, A.K., Mitchell, K., Schwartz, M.M. *et al.* (1990) Absence of glomerular injury or nephron loss in a normotensive rat remnant kidney model. *Kidney Int.*, **38**, 28–38.
17. Fine, L.G., Ong, A.C.M. and Norman, J.T. (1993) Mechanisms of tubulo-interstitial injury in progressive renal diseases. *Eur. J. Clin. Invest.*, **23**, 259–65.
18. Bohle, A., Gise, H.V., Mackensen-Haen, S. and Stark-Jacob, B. (1981) The obliteration of the postglomerular capillaries and its influence upon the function of both glomeruli and tubuli. *Klin. Wochenschr.*, **59**, 1043–51.
19. Yoshida, Y., Fogo, A. and Ichikawa, I. (1989) Glomerular hemodynamic changes vs. hypertrophy in experimental glomerular sclerosis. *Kidney Int.*, **35**, 654–60.
20. Fogo, A., Hawkins, E.P., Berry, P.L., *et al.* (1990) Glomerular hypertrophy in minimal change disease predicts subsequent progression to focal glomerular sclerosis. *Kidney Int.*, **38**, 115–23.
21. Moorhead, J.F., Chan, M.K. and Varghese, Z. (1986) The role of abnormalities of lipid metabolism in the progression of renal disease, in *Contemporary Issues in Nephrology. The Progressive Nature of Renal Disease*, Vol. 14, (eds W.E. Mitch, B.M. Brenner and J.H. Stein), Churchill Livingstone, New York, pp. 133–48.
22. Diamond, J.R. and Karnovsky, M.J. (1988) Focal and segmental glomerulosclerosis: Analogies to atherosclerosis. *Kidney Int.*, **33**, 917–24.
23. Clark, E.C., Nath, K.A., Hostetter, M.K. and Hostetter, M.D. (1991) Role of ammonia in progressive interstitial nephritis. *Am. J. Kidney Dis.*, **17**, suppl. 1, 15–19.
24. Throssell, D., Brown, J., Harris, K.P.G. and Walls, J. (1995) Renal acidosis does not contribute to chronic renal injury in the rat. *Clin. Sci.*, **89**, 643–50.
25. El Nahas, Am, Bassett, A.H., Cope, G.H. and Le Carpentier, J.E. (1991) Role of growth hormone in the development of experimental renal scarring. *Kidney Int.*, **40**, 29–34.
26. Yang, C.W., Striker, L.J., Kopchick, J.J. *et al.* (1993) Glomerulosclerosis in mice transgenic for native or mutated bovine growth hormone gene. *Kidney Int.*, **39**, suppl. S90–S94.
27. Noronha, I.L., Niemir, Z., Stein, H. and Waldherr, R. (1995) Cytokines and growth factors in renal disease. *Nephrol. Dial. Transplant.*, **10**, 775–86.
28. Isaka, Y., Fujiwara, Y., Ueda, N. *et al.* (1993) Glomerulosclerosis induced by *in vivo* transfection of transforming growth factor-$\beta$ or platelet-derived growth factor gene into rat kidney. *J. Clin. Invest.*, **92**, 2952–3062.

29. Border, W.A., Okuda, S., Languino, L.R. *et al.* (1990) Suppression of experimental glomerulonephritis by antiserum against transforming growth factor $\beta$1. *Nature*, **346**, 371–4.
30. Nikolic-Paterson, D.J., Lan, H.Y., Hill, P.A. and Atkins, R.C. (1994) Macrophages in renal injury. *Kidney Int.*, **45**, suppl. S79–S82.
31. Diamond, J.R., Pesek, I., Ruggieri, S. and Karnovsky, M.J. (1989) Essential fatty acid deficiency during acute puromycin nephrosis ameliorates late renal injury. *Am. J. Physiol.*, **257**, F798–F807.
32. Eddy, A.A. (1995) Interstitial macrophages as mediators of renal fibrosis. *Exp. Nephrol.*, **3**, 76–9.
33. Harris, K., Pawlucyzk, I.Z.A., Throssell, D. and Furness, P. (1995) Role of the macrophage in the development of glomerulosclerosis. *Exp. Nephrol.*, **3**, 87.
34. Praga, M., Hernandez, E., Montoyo, C. *et al.* (1994) Long-term beneficial effects of angiotensin-converting enzyme inhibition in patients with nephrotic proteinuria. *Am. J. Kidney Dis.*, **20**, 240–8.
35. Burton, C.J., Walls, J. and Harris, K.P.G. (1996) Fibronectin production by human tubular cells: the effect of apical protein. *Kidney Int.*, **50**, 760–7.
36. Feldt-Rasmussen, B., Mathiesen, E.R., Jensen, T. *et al.* (1991) Effect of improved metabolic control on loss of kidney function in type 1 (insulin dependent) diabetic patients: an update of the Steno studies. *Diabetologia*, **34**, 164–70.
37. Lewis, E.J., Hunsicker, L.G., Bain, R.P. and Rhode, R.D. (1993) The effect of angiotensin converting-enzyme inhibition on diabetic nephropathy. *N. Engl. J. Med.*, **329**, 1456–62.
38. Zucchelli, P., Zuccala, A., Borghi, M. *et al.* (1992) Long-term comparison between captopril and nifedipine in the progression of renal insufficiency. *Kidney Int.*, **42**, 452–8.
39. Ihle, B.E., Becker, G.J., Whitworth, J.A. *et al.* (1989) The effect of protein restriction on the progression of renal insufficiency. *N. Engl. J. Med.*, **321**, 1773–7.
40. Locatelli, F., Alberti, D., Graziani, G. *et al.* (1991) Prospective, randomised, multicentre, trial of the effect of protein restriction on progression of chronic renal insufficiency. *Lancet*, **337**, 1299–304.

# 3

# Hypertensive/ischaemic nephropathy

*G.Venkat Raman*

## 3.1 INTRODUCTION

Hypertension is almost invariably encountered at some stage in the natural history of chronic renal disease. It is probably the single most important factor in determining the progression of renal failure. However, there is an important interaction with ethnicity. In white Caucasians, essential hypertension rarely leads to end stage renal failure (ESRF), particularly owing to the wide availability of efficient antihypertensive drugs – though hypertension frequently appears as a secondary phenomenon, and certainly contributes to the development of ESRF. It is primary accelerated hypertension which is commonly associated with renal failure. On the other hand, it is now well recognized that 'benign' essential hypertension is a particularly common and severe cause of renal failure in Afro-Caribbeans. In people from the Indian sub-continent, hypertension associated with obesity and diabetes is a prominent cause of ESRF. Hypertension is frequently associated with ischaemic nephropathy, and together, they account for some 20% of ESRF in Western populations.

There is a fundamentally close relationship between blood pressure and the kidney, with strong arguments in support of the hypothesis that essential hypertension is, indeed, the end result of a subtle renal abnormality. The leading causal hypotheses include the following.

1. Failure in the renal autoregulatory function in terms of salt and water excretion [1].

*Renal Disease.* Edited by G. Venkat Raman. Published in 1998 by Chapman & Hall, London. ISBN 0 412 45700 8.

2. Excessive production of a circulating inhibitor of the Na/K ATPase, possibly ouabain released from the hypothalamus [2, 3].
3. Accumulation of cytosolic calcium in the vascular smooth muscle cell [4].
4. Sympathetic hyperactivity related to intracranial/cerebral ischaemia [5].
5. Hyperinsulinaemia leading to both central sympathetic overactivity and sodium retention by the kidneys [6].
6. Genetic factors such as enhanced activity of $Na^+/H^+$ exchanger-1, and related G-proteins [7].

A wide variety of endocrine and paracrine/autocrine agents have been implicated in the genesis of hypertension (Table 3.1) in various experimental models, but none of them has been consistently shown to be causal in essential hypertension. A detailed discussion of these mechanisms is beyond the scope of this chapter. Whatever the mechanisms, there is a striking relationship between blood pressure control and the kidney as shown by the ability of a kidney transplant to 'cure' long-standing hypertension, as well as by its ability to produce hypertension. Thus hypertension has been shown to 'travel' with the kidney, both experimentally and clinically [8].

There are clearly identified forms of hypertension secondary to parenchymal diseases of the kidney, and in chronic renal failure, of different origins. In these situations, renal abnormalities may be responsible for hypertension by two well-established mechanisms, and several other possible mechanisms.

**Table 3.1** Hormonal factors implicated in the pathogenesis of hypertension

| |
|---|
| Catrecholamines |
| Adrenaline |
| Noradrenaline |
| Renin system |
| Angiotensin II |
| Aldosterone |
| Endothelins |
| Nitric oxide (endothelium-derived relaxing factor) |
| Atrial natriuretic peptide |
| Kallikrein–kinin system |
| Prostaglandins |
| Growth hormone |
| Corticosteroids |
| Parathyroid hormone |

1. Increased production of a systemic vasopressor, e.g. activation of the renin–angiotensin–aldosterone system.
2. Salt and water retention leading to volume overload.

Other potential mechanisms include the following.

3. Tonic sympathetic afferent stimulation by scarred or damaged kidneys.
4. Impaired production of an endogenous vasodilator hormone, e.g. prostaglandins, kinins, medullipin.
5. Uraemic accumulation of asymmetric dimethyl arginine, which competes with L-arginine, impairing generation of endothelium-derived nitric oxide.
6. Endothelial dysfunction, with over-generation of endothelins.
7. Reduction of intracellular magnesium in uraemia (shown by nuclear magnetic resonance spectroscopy).
8. Uraemic impairment of baroceptor/chemoreceptor function.

**Table 3.2** Causes of chronic renal ischaemia

(a) Macrovascular disease
   1. Hypertension
   2. Atherosclerotic renal arterial/aortic disease
   3. Fibromuscular dysplasia of renal arteries
   4. Large vessels vasculitis
      Classical polyarteris nodosa
      Kawasaki disease
   5. Renal artery stenosis in transplanted kidney
   6. Mechanical arterial obstruction
      e.g. aortic dissection, renal artery aneurysm, embolism, trauma

(b) Microvascular disease
   1. Hypertension
   2. Vasculitis group
      Renal micropolyarteritis, Wegener's granulomatosis
   3. Microangiopathic haemolytic anaemia
   4. Systemic sclerosis
   5. End stage of severe parenchymal disease

(c) Circulatory failure – low cardiac output states

(d) Drug-induced
   1. Cyclosporin
   2. ACE inhibitors

It is very likely that a number of these factors operate simultaneously in any individual. Whatever the underlying mechanism, hypertension itself can directly lead to chronic renal failure (CRF) over a period of time, if undetected or inadequately treated. Furthermore, it can significantly accelerate the progression of CRF caused by other primary diseases, notably diabetic nephropathy. Thus, there is the potential for a vicious cycle, hypertension and renal impairment mutually aggravating each other. The classic example of this is seen in malignant or accelerated hypertension.

Parenchymal renal ischaemia, or ischaemic nephropathy, is steadily increasing in incidence as a cause of CRF. This is largely due to the increase in longevity, and more effective treatment of potentially lethal conditions. Though ischaemia may be caused by a number of mechanisms (Table 3.2), the major contributors in this disease process are hypertension and atherosclerosis. Less commonly, fibromuscular dysplasia (FMD) may cause unilateral disease in younger individuals.

## 3.2 PATHOGENESIS

The role of the kidney in causing essential hypertension will not be discussed in any further detail. Discussion will be confined to the renal aspects of hypertension and ischaemia. While hypertension may be the most important adjunct to the genesis of renal ischaemia, ischaemic nephropathy can manifest itself even in the absence of hypertension. There is a clear analogy with ischaemic heart disease, where atherosclerotic disease is the major underlying pathology, without the necessity for coexistent hypertension. Though the list of causes of renal ischaemia is long, in practice the vast majority of cases of ischaemic nephropathy are due to hypertension and atherosclerosis.

The pathological components of the hypertensive process include:

1. increased vascular smooth tone/contractility;
2. vascular smooth muscle hypertrophy;
3. smooth muscle and endothelial cell hyperplasia/proliferation;
4. fibrinoid necrosis;
5. vascular/capillary luminal occlusion.

The outcome for renal survival is determined by a complex interaction between hypertensive damage to the glomeruli and ischaemia due to impaired flow. On the one extreme there is the severe hypertensive damage with an acute diminution of flow as seen in accelerated hypertension, leading to ESRF within a matter of months. At the other extreme there is the slow and gradual onset of renal ischaemia seen as part of the normal ageing process, which may not quite reach the stage of ESRF. In between there is a wide range of degrees of progression, depending on the nature and severity of the renal disease and the degree of hypertension.

It may be helpful to consider the renal damage as occurring in three stages. A number of diseases may pass through these stages, which may be a final common pathway.

- Stage 1: glomerular hypertension. This is the stage of mechanical glomerular damage caused as a direct consequence of sustained hypertension, often associated with glomerular hyperperfusion. This has been shown to be an important pathogenetic process in a variety of renal diseases, including glomerulonephritis and diabetic nephropathy, and may be present even without systemic hypertension. It represents a critical loss of nephrons, leaving the rest to undergo compensatory changes. Glomerular filtration rate (GFR) may be supranormal or normal.
- Stage 2: glomerular ischaemia. This second stage is due to a net diminution of blood flow and filtration across the glomerular filter, such that renal impairment becomes manifest biochemically. In ischaemic nephropathy, without previous hypertension, stage 1 may be bypassed. GFR is reduced, and may diminish progressively, the rate being accelerated by hypertension or other forms of renal insult.
- Stage 3: progressive glomerular sclerosis. The end result of both forms of injury is progressive glomerulosclerosis, and it will be evident that when the two processes are combined the rate of sclerosis will be considerably accelerated. The rate of progression is determined by the severity of the disease process, and efficacy of the treatment given. The various aspects of the progression of renal disease are considered elsewhere (Chapter 2) and will not be taken up in any further detail here.

Chronic systemic arterial hypertension leads to benign nephroarteriosclerosis, leading to glomerular ischaemia and progressive sclerosis. However, prior to the stage of ischaemia, chronic elevation of systemic blood pressure leads to glomerular hypertension, leading to hyperperfusion and this in itself can accelerate glomerulosclerosis. This initial stage of glomerular hypertension is thought to be a final common pathway for progressive renal failure occurring as a consequence of many forms of parenchymal renal disease including glomerulonephritis and diabetes [9, 10], all of which have a high incidence of associated hypertension.

A more serious illness is represented by the development of malignant or accelerated hypertension, which may arise *de novo*, or secondary to some underlying renal parenchymal disease. The condition is usually mediated by an excessive activation of the renin–angiotensin–aldosterone system (RAAS). Pathologically it leads to severe nephroarteriosclerosis, leading to the rapid development of renal failure. The histological appearances are characterized by marked medial hypertrophy, fibrinoid necrosis in the walls of the vessels and glomerular ischaemia. The glomeruli present an onion skin appearance. Similar appearances are seen in progressive systemic sclerosis with renal involvement, haemolytic uraemic syndrome and thrombotic microangiopathy, and acute cyclosporin toxicity.

A more well-defined entity is that of renovascular hypertension, caused by unilateral or bilateral renal artery stenosis. Typically this used to be seen in young adults, due to congenital fibromuscular hyperplasia involving the renal arteries. However there is an increasing incidence of bilateral atherosclerotic renal arterial disease causing a similar syndrome in older patients. The condition is characterized by renal ischaemia, leading to excessive activation of the RAAS and resultant hypertension. The degree of hypertension is highly variable and it may present as anything ranging from mild benign hypertension to life-threatening accelerated hypertension.

With increasing longevity in the last two decades, there has been a striking increase in the incidence of 'ischaemic nephropathy'. The pathogenesis of this entity is basically no different from that of the bilateral atherosclerotic renovascular disease, but hypertension may be absent. Indeed, ischaemic nephropathy is nothing more than the expression of the normal ageing process, whereby the kidneys become gradually ischaemic and there is a slowly progressive decline in renal function in patients in their eighth and ninth decades. While some patients may be normotensive and some hypertensive, there is quite often isolated systolic hypertension, which is also a manifestation of the atherosclerotic process. Histological examination in these cases reveals glomerular ischaemia, tubular atrophy and narrowing of the arterioles. The situation may be complicated by the coexistence of glomerular hypertension and ischaemia in different areas, thus making it difficult to tailor therapy to the pathophysiological change.

## 3.3 PATHOPHYSIOLOGY

Most forms of renal parenchymal disease tend to produce hypertension at some point in their natural history. This is usually renin mediated, as a response by the juxtaglomerular apparatus to a perceived fall in renal arterial perfusion pressure. Hypertension tends to appear early in glomerulonephritis and diabetic nephropathy, and somewhat later in polycystic renal disease and chronic pyelonephritis. The best example of renin-mediated hypertension occurs in the rare renin-producing tumours. Long-standing essential hypertension can develop a secondary renin-mediated element to it, if atherosclerotic renal artery stenosis develops as a complication. This is a situation where after many years the hypertension can switch from being benign to malignant.

When renal disease progresses to the point of oliguria (relative to fluid intake), circulatory volume and salt retention become the major mediators of hypertension. At this stage renin secretion may be suppressed by the volume expansion. In end stage renal failure treated by dialysis, typically renin secretion may decline and blood pressure is simply determined by the circulatory volume. More importantly, by this stage there is often the development of secondary vascular smooth muscle hypertrophy (VSMH), which maintains a hypertensive state irrespective of the volume status or other hormonal factors. Thus, many patients require maintenance antihypertensive treatment in spite of adequate volume contraction on dialysis, a fact that is particularly applicable to black subjects.

In ischaemic nephropathy associated with ageing, reduced arterial compliance predisposes to systolic hypertension, irrespective of renin secretion or the volume status. Typically, plasma renin activity diminishes with advancing age.

In a minority of patients with tubulo-interstitial renal disease (including a small proportion with chronic pyelonephritis) there exists a salt-losing state, which tends to keep the patient normotensive with recurrent episodes of salt and water depletion, hypotension and the potential for transient acute tubular necrosis. If the renal disease progresses to the point of relative oliguria, then these patients may become hypertensive late in the natural history of their disease.

Lastly, there may be a significant contribution to the development of hypertension by iatrogenic factors. For example, corticosteroids may be used in high dose and for prolonged periods for different forms of vasculitis, glomerulonephritis and after transplantation. Cyclosporin, which is a standard immunosuppressive agent for transplant recipients, is increasingly used for treatment of autoimmune diseases, both renal and non-renal. Both these drugs, cyclosporin in particular, have a significant potential for producing sustained hypertension. Non-steroidal anti-inflammatory drugs (NSAIDs) are also well known to precipitate or aggravate hypertension, in established renal disease.

Post-transplant hypertension is very common and has several potential pathogenetic mechanisms, including the immunosuppressive drugs mentioned above. The presence of the host kidneys is often an important factor, probably through hypersecretion of renin. In addition, hypersecretion of renin from the graft itself is an important mechanism, particularly in the presence of rejection or transplant renal artery stenosis. An additional volume-mediated component may supervene when graft function fails. The topic is reviewed in detail elsewhere [11].

### 3.3.1 Role of the renin–angiotensin system

Angiotensin II (Ang II) has been known to be one of the most potent endogenous vasoconstrictors and was considered for some time to be involved in the genesis of essential hypertension, but a definitive link has not been established. Most studies have concentrated on circulating RAAS and Ang II, and it has only recently been recognized that vascular or tissue RAAS may play a fundamental role in hypertensive pathology and progressive renal failure. In this context, Ang II is now recognized as a potent stimulus for hypertrophy and cellular proliferation. Thus Ang II plays a significant role within various tissues and treatment with angiotensin-converting enzyme (ACE) inhibitors is thought to have the effect of ameliorating Ang II toxicity at the tissue level, notably cardiac and renal tissue.

It is now recognized that in addition to the ACE, there are other chymases which can carry out the same process in their ability to convert the relatively inert Ang I to the highly active Ang II. This non-ACE pathway explains one reason for failure of ACE inhibitors in certain individuals, and the possible superiority of the new Ang II receptor antagonists, such as losartan.

## 3.4 MECHANISMS OF PROGRESSION

The wide variety of mechanisms that have been shown to be of importance in the progression of renal failure are comprehensively covered in Chapter 2. However there are specific issues related to hypertension and ischaemic renal disease which need to be addressed. It is important to distinguish the difference between lowering blood pressure and ameliorating the target organ damage caused by high blood pressure. The former is relatively easy to monitor and is the gold standard by which treatments are assessed. We are all familiar with the somewhat disappointing results obtained from the many large-scale clinical trials of hypertension, in terms of the less than expected benefit in reducing cardiac events. Therefore, with the increasing incidence of hypertensive/ischaemic nephropathy as a cause of ESRF, one has to address the question of whether antihypertensive treatment is merely successful in reducing blood pressure, and perhaps not so effective in terms of reducing the target organ damage – in this case the kidney. The next point to consider is whether a particular drug or class of drugs has a beneficial effect on renal survival mediated by mechanisms other than mere reduction of blood pressure.

Haemodynamic injury is thought to be the most important pathophysiological factor in determining the progression of renal failure [10]. Thus glomerular hypertension and hyperperfusion are thought to be a prerequisite for the development of progressive glomerulosclerosis, resulting in ESRF. It is a false assumption that systemic hypertension equals glomerular hypertension. Therefore reduction of systemic blood pressure may not necessarily lead to a corresponding decrease in glomerular pressure. Furthermore, different classes of antihypertensive drugs exert differential effects in various vascular regions. Thus it is important to make the distinction between systemic and glomerular hypertension, which may each exist independent of the other.

Glomerular damage and progressive sclerosis are due to an interplay between two critical factors – the hydraulic pressure of the blood acting on the glomerular wall, and the different pathological processes directly affecting the glomerular filtration barrier (diseases such as glomerulonephritis). This interaction manifests as proteinuria, beginning initially with a phase of microalbuminuria (defined arbitrarily as a urinary albumin excretion rate of greater than 20 $\mu$g/min). The filtered albumin is reabsorbed from the tubular lumen and this in turn stimulates mesangial cells and macrophages to release cytokines such as tumour necrosis factor and interleukin-2, which produce further inflammation, local damage, and lead to a decrease in the filtration rate, surface area and coefficient of filtration. Thus proteinuria can set up a vicious cycle and it will be apparent that a drug that lowers systemic blood pressure, without concomitantly reducing proteinuria, is less likely to be effective in retarding progression of renal disease.

Risk factors for the progression of renal failure include, in addition to hypertension, obesity, glucose intolerance, smoking and hyperlipidaemia. Indeed, there is a strong interaction between hypertension and obesity, with the combination leading to an increase in the degree of proteinuria and the progression of renal failure. Both complications are significantly accelerated by the coexistence of diabetes mellitus.

Ischaemic nephropathy, also termed atherosclerotic renovascular disease or atheroembolic renal disease, has two components to it:

1. stenosis of one or both renal arteries, or major aortic atherosclerosis and
2. atheromatous embolism or cholesterol embolization.

## 3.5 PHARMACOLOGICAL MANIPULATION

Antihypertensive drugs may exert their beneficial renal protective effects in one or more of the following ways.

1. Reduction of glomerular pressure secondary to a reduction of systemic arterial pressure.
2. Reduction of glomerular pressure by direct modulation of the balance between the afferent and efferent arterial pressures.

3. Repair of ongoing glomerular damage by the modulation of other adverse local factors (cytokines) which promote inflammation and tissue damage.
4. Reversing atherosclerosis – the single most important associated factor in producing ischaemic nephropathy.

The antihypertensive effect of a drug is likely to lower the intraglomerular pressure, but this effect may be negated if the drug preferentially dilates the afferent and not the efferent arteriole. A drug which is able to produce dilatation on both arterioles is likely to achieve the expected reduction in intraglomerular pressure (IGP). A drug that selectively dilates or relaxes the efferent arteriole is likely to have a powerful effect in terms of reducing IGP, and consequently proteinuria. Indeed these concepts have been borne out by a number of studies which show striking differences in the effects of different drugs.

Calcium channel blockers (CCB) have differing effects on glomerular vessels. Nifedipine, whilst lowering blood pressure, increases IGP and the urinary albumin excretion rate (AER). Verapamil and diltiazem, which have an effect in dilating both sets of arterioles, have a beneficial effect in lowering IGP and AER. ACE inhibitors, because of their selective action on the efferent arteriole, produce a more striking beneficial effect in reducing IGP and AER.

## 3.6 CLINICAL SYNDROMES

### 3.6.1 Hypertensive nephropathy

This is typically characterized by a long-standing history of hypertension, with some evidence of target organ damage. Poor blood pressure control is frequently associated, and poor compliance is often a feature. There may be significant proteinuria, which rarely reaches nephrotic proportions. Renal function may be normal or impaired. Hypokalaemia should trigger suspicions of an underlying primary cause, such as mineralocorticoid excess (unless the patient is on diuretics). Obesity, hyperlipidaemia and glucose intolerance (insulin resistance) frequently coexist. Other vascular problems – cardiac, cerebral, peripheral – may be evident.

### 3.6.2 Renal hypertension

This is due to an underlying primary renal disease, and is characterized by other signs, such as haematuria, proteinuria, abnormal biochemistry, imaging abnormalities, etc. Glomerulonephritis may present with an active urinary sediment and heavy proteinuria, and is diagnosed by kidney biopsy. Polycystic disease often presents with just hypertension and the diagnosis depends on family history, palpation of the enlarged organs and ultrasound examination. Chronic pyelonephritis is diagnosed by history, combined with evidence of renal scarring on imaging. Renovascular disease may be suspected by the finding of upper abdominal bruits and smooth shrunken kidneys on ultrasonography. A detailed discussion of the individual diseases is beyond the scope of this book.

Autoimmune diseases may declare themselves by their systemic signs such as the butterfly rash of lupus or the peripheral features of scleroderma. Supporting tests include appropriate immunological screening for antibodies, e.g. antibodies to double-stranded DNA and antibodies to neutrophil cytoplasmic antigen. Often tell-tale clues may be lacking and the only abnormality may be non-specific findings on ultrasound examination, namely a bright hyperechoic appearance, poor corticomedullary demarcation and reduced renal size.

### 3.6.3 Malignant (accelerated) hypertension (MHT)

This is a medical emergency, which typically presents with severe headaches and serious target organ involvement:

- retinopathy – visual impairment, grade III/IV changes (essential criterion for the diagnosis);
- cardiac – congestive failure or crescendo angina;
- vascular – dissecting aneurysms;
- cerebral – fits or focal neurological signs due to hypertensive encephalopathy, cerebral or subarachnoid haemorrhage;
- renal – proteinuria (mild to heavy), renal impairment (which may range from near normal to oliguric acute renal failure);
- hypokalaemia is often seen due to secondary hyperaldosteronism.

A striking feature of MHT is the potential for reversing the acute renal damage by aggressive antihypertensive therapy. This is one condition where 'end stage renal failure' can be rescued, and the patient can recover sufficient renal function to become independent of dialysis, even after months of dialysis support.

### 3.6.4 Ischaemic nephropathy

This typically presents in the elderly, with a combination of systolic hypertension, minimal proteinuria, impaired renal function, epigastric bruits and a strong association with peripheral vascular disease or claudication. This is an exaggeration of the so-called 'normal ageing kidney', with slow progression of renal failure.

### 3.6.5 Hypertension in diabetes

This condition deserves special mention, because of the frequency of the association and the overriding importance of blood pressure in the pathogenesis of diabetic nephropathy. Hypertension usually correlates with the degree of microalbuminuria, and is a forerunner of renal failure. Blood pressure control is of vital importance in preventing progression.

## 3.7 AIMS AND TARGETS OF ANTIHYPERTENSIVE THERAPY

Lowering blood pressure is not an end in itself. When hypertension exists as a disease in its own right because of its severity and target organ damage, as in accelerated hypertension, lowering of the blood pressure levels becomes the imperative. Fortunately this occurrence is relatively rare, and more commonly seen are patients with mild to moderate asymptomatic hypertension, which exists as a risk factor rather than a disease. The purpose of treatment therefore is to achieve protection for vital organs against chronic hypertensive damage.

From a renal standpoint the most important aim is to prolong renal survival. In order to achieve that we need to be able to monitor certain parameters. The degree of proteinuria, as microalbuminuria, is a useful marker of early disease. Overt proteinuria may not occur until relatively late in the disease. An important goal is to reduce proteinuria, as this has been associated with retarding the progression of renal failure. Furthermore, successful treatment must ensure that the reduction in proteinuria achieved is maintained.

Short-term changes in GFR are not as important as the long-term preservation. Thus, in hypertensive patients with glomerular hyperperfusion and hypertension, successful treatment of blood pressure reduces proteinuria, as well as the hyperfiltration, into the normal range. Similarly in subjects with loss of functioning renal mass, the baseline GFR may be low (though the single nephron GFR may be high) and successful treatment may reduce proteinuria, and reduce the GFR further, with the promise of long-term preservation. Therefore short-term reduction of GFR, typically seen with ACE inhibitor treatment, does not imply an adverse effect on renal survival.

On the contrary, a drug that reduces blood pressure but increases the single nephron GFR and IGP may be expected to produce an increase in proteinuria and a negligible (or even adverse) effect on the progression of renal failure. A clear distinction between the total GFR and single nephron GFR is critical to a proper understanding of the pathophysiology and successful medical treatment.

This concept applies to ischaemic nephropathy as well, where the ischaemia has produced a low IGP. Any treatment that reduces the single nephron GFR further can accelerate the progression of renal failure. It is in this group that ACE inhibitors should be avoided, and CCB are potentially more beneficial.

As will be evident from the foregoing discussion on the conflicting effects of ACE inhibition on renal circulation and that of calcium antagonists on proteinuria, the aim of treatment should be to maintain (or lower) the IGP to an optimal level, with minimal effect on glomerular filtration. Effective treatment thus requires the achievement of this balance, which often has a narrow margin within which to operate.

What is the target blood pressure to achieve? The current recommendation would be lower than 140/90 mmHg, and preferably 130/80 mmHg. Refractory hypertension requires multiple drug therapy and even maximal treatment may not be adequate to control blood pressure. In this case minoxidil, a potent vasodilator, is often invaluable. In making the choice of drug, all the other relevant factors should be taken into consideration. In particular, current thinking dictates that the cardiovascular risk factor profile should be assessed and the treatment threshold should be lowered as the risk factors add up. Thus, it is very important to measure the lipid profile, in particular it is well known that the nephrotic syndrome produces a very significant rise in cholesterol and this could be of clinical importance in precipitating coronary events. For years physicians have neglected the lipid abnormalities in patients with renal disease, but there is no longer any justification for this. The question of lipid abnormalities being potentially important in the progression of renal disease is considered in detail in Chapter 9.

## 3.8 MONITORING RENAL FUNCTION

Control of blood pressure should be accompanied by critical assessment of the progress of the disease. The serum creatinine remains the single most practical measurement in nephrology. The GFR may be measured crudely by means of creatinine clearance, and more accurately by chemical (inulin, iohexol) or isotope (EDTA/DTPA) clearance techniques, which tend to be laborious and expensive. Serial documentation of the reciprocal of serum creatinine concentration has been used as one way to monitor the progress, and may be useful as a predictor of the duration before reaching ESRF. However, the slope of reciprocal creatinine is by no means infallible and can be misleading. Proteinuria should also be measured routinely and the conventional method is to estimate the protein content of a 24 hour collection of urine. This method is again laborious and often inaccurate. A simpler alternative method consists of measuring the albumin-to-creatinine concentration ratio in a random sample of urine or, in the presence of concomitant renal failure, the measurement of fractional albumin excretion (albumin:creatinine clearance ratio). Adequate treatment of blood pressure should be associated with a reduction in urinary protein excretion in most cases.

Much interest has been focused in the recent years on microalbuminuria, defined as abnormally high excretion of albumin, in the face of a negative dipstix or other test for protein in the urine. In quantitative terms, this is defined as an albumin excretion rate of greater than 20 $\mu$g/min (30 mg/day), which is approximately equivalent to 2 mg of albumin/mmol of creatinine in the urine. Proteinuria has two components to it – that due to the primary renal disease and that due to the high blood pressure. Therefore, good blood pressure control might reduce the proteinuria, but may not abolish it if there is active underlying disease.

Electrolytes should be monitored regularly, and in particular while using ACE inhibitor treatment (for reasons to be discussed). The renal function (serum creatinine or GFR) should be measured immediately prior to starting treatment, and repeated within three to four weeks and then followed up once every six to 12 months, depending on the pre-existing renal function. For reasons mentioned above, the lipid profile must be measured, including the high-density lipoprotein (HDL) cholesterol. Hyperlipidaemia should be actively treated.

## 3.9 PREVENTION AND TREATMENT

Adequate management of hypertension is probably the single most important measure in slowing the progression of renal disease. Quite apart from this, adequate treatment of hypertension is also of crucial importance in the prevention of coronary and cerebrovascular disease. Considerable evidence suggests that different antihypertensive agents can reduce proteinuria and slow the rate of progression of renal disease in a number of situations, particularly diabetes mellitus [12–17], non-diabetic conditions [18–21] and even when blood pressure was 'normal' to start with [22, 23]. Thus there are very compelling reasons for attempting to achieve meticulous blood pressure control.

> The level at which to intervene is arbitrary. The threshold recommended in **essential** hypertension varies between 140/90 mm Hg (USA), 150/95 mm Hg (WHO) and 160/100 mm Hg (UK) [24–26]. In the presence of coexistent vascular risk factors such as diabetes and hyperlipidaemia, one would be advised to err on the lower side of the recommended levels for intervention. Arguably, concomitant renal disease should therefore encourage clinicians to adopt lower thresholds.

It is important to follow the guidelines with respect to the diagnosis of hypertension by means of three separate readings on three occasions at least a week apart [26], except when there is obvious clinical evidence of hypertensive target organ damage, or accelerated hypertension. In borderline cases ambulatory blood pressure monitoring may be invaluable in excluding 'white coat hypertension'.

### 3.9.1 Non-pharmacological treatment

It is now widely accepted that in mild to moderate essential hypertension (without target organ damage) the first step should be to apply non-pharmacological methods and lifestyle modification. These include:

1. weight reduction for obesity;
2. moderate alcohol consumption (<14 units per week);
3. increase in dynamic physical exercise;
4. reduction of salt intake;
5. fat-modified low-cholesterol diet;
6. cessation of smoking.

The last two measures may not directly lower blood pressure, but are crucial adjuncts for the prevention of cardiovascular disease, and probably renal progression. There is preliminary evidence that increasing the intake of potassium and magnesium may be of benefit in lowering blood pressure. These methods may be applied in hypertension associated with renal disease, though they are likely to be less successful.

### 3.9.2 Pharmacological methods

All the currently used antihypertensive drugs can be used effectively in renal hypertension. From the point of view of cardiovascular prevention in **essential** hypertension, current recommendations [24–26] favour first-line use of thiazides (particularly in the elderly) and beta-blockers, based on large-scale trial evidence [27–30]. Though the newer classes, namely ACE inhibitors, CCB and alpha-blockers, have a number of theoretical advantages over the older drugs, their superiority in essential hypertension has not yet been validated in clinical trials. A number of intervention studies using these agents are currently in progress.

From the **renal** standpoint different criteria are applicable, in contrast to essential hypertension. Proteinuria has been shown to be effectively reduced by most antihypertensives, though most attention has focused on ACE inhibitors and CCB. Diuretics, beta-blockers and alpha-blockers have been inadequately evaluated so far. ACE inhibitors have been the most extensively studied and have shown unequivocal benefits, particularly in diabetic nephropathy.

### 3.9.3 Diuretics

Thiazides, which are quite effective in essential hypertension, are likely to be effective in renal hypertension only in the early stages of the disease, before renal impairment sets in. However, there may be special situations where thiazides could have a special role, such as in hypertension coexisting with hypercalciuria (in calcium oxalate stone formers), where thiazides may also reduce calcium excretion. Thiazides tend to produce glucose intolerance and may aggravate insulin resistance. They may also produce or aggravate hyperlipidaemia and hyperuricaemia. As renal failure is commonly associated with these abnormalities, thiazides are generally avoided.

Frusemide and bumetanide (loop diuretics) may contribute to the control of hypertension by increased urine output and consequent reduction of volume-mediated hypertension. In order to achieve the latter effect, in the later stages of renal failure, frusemide may have to be employed in large doses, up to 500 mg a day. In the generalized oedema associated with renal failure, there is often a considerable amount of gut oedema, which may impair the absorption of many drugs. Therefore, if the oedema is resistant to oral treatment, intravenous frusemide should be employed in doses of up to 250 mg daily. It is also worth noting that in general, intravenous dosage should not exceed this ceiling, because of the potential for direct nephrotoxicity and deafness. In combination with ACE inhibitors, loop diuretics have a synergistic antihypertensive effect.

### 3.9.4 Beta-blockers

These drugs are generally safe and effective in the treatment of most forms of hypertension, including renal disease. They have obvious additional advantages in terms of treatment of ischaemic heart disease, both in a symptomatic sense and in terms of secondary prevention. Beta-blockers have relatively little direct effect on renal function, though they generally reduce renin secretion and some of them have been shown to reduce renal blood flow. However, these are minor variations on a theme and there is no definite agent of choice in renal disease. Cardioselectivity may be of advantage because of the reduced side-effect profile. There is some evidence that beta-blockade can reduce proteinuria and retard progression of renal failure [12, 13, 31] but appears less striking in comparison with ACE inhibitors and CCB.

### 3.9.5 Alpha-blockers

These drugs, which are potentially very effective, have been generally undervalued and poorly studied. Apart from being effective in lowering blood pressure in most forms of hypertension, they have been shown to improve the lipid profile, with an increase in the HDL:total cholesterol ratio. The newer longer acting agents are generally safe and well tolerated. There is very little trial-based data on their long-term efficacy in reducing renal or cardiovascular morbidity and mortality. Much work remains to be done. There may be a particular advantage with these drugs when hypertension coexists with prostatism, which may be relieved concomitantly.

### 3.9.6 Calcium channel blockers (CCB)

This group of drugs has become exceedingly popular in the management of all forms of hypertension. In addition to lowering blood pressure they have additional beneficial effects in angina, though with the disadvantage that they are generally contraindicated in heart failure. They are safe in most situations and the main limitation to their use remains intolerance. They are also particularly effective in lowering systolic blood pressure, and therefore may be superior to other drugs in isolated systolic hypertension, which is frequently associated with ischaemic nephropathy. In these situations they are clearly superior to ACE inhibitors.

The renal effects of CCB are generally neutral, in the presence of normal kidneys. GFR is usually not affected. IGP may be affected variably. A fall in systemic blood pressure leads to a fall in IGP, but this effect may be annulled by opposite effects on the balance between the afferent and efferent arteriolar tone. Nifedipine, for example, dilates only the afferent vessel, and may thus lead to a transmission of systemic pressure and actually raise IGP. On the other hand, verapamil and diltiazem dilate both arterioles, and therefore tend to lower IGP, irrespective of systemic pressure. These differences may have important clinical implications.

However, in parenchymal renal disease, particularly with significant proteinuria, CCB should be used with caution. Studies with nifedipine have given conflicting results, with one showing benefit [32] and others a significant deleterious effect on proteinuria, as well as rate of progression, particularly in diabetics [33, 34]. There is some evidence that verapamil and diltiazem [35, 36] may be able to reduce proteinuria and retard progression of renal failure, but more definite evidence is required before these benefits can be attributed to them (see below).

There is some interesting evidence to suggest that CCB may

produce regression of atherosclerosis, and if this is borne out, these agents may have a special significance in the treatment of ischaemic nephropathy.

### 3.9.7 ACE inhibitors

These are an effective group of drugs with multiple sites of pharmacological action. They are useful in most categories of hypertension and in all ages. In particular, they lack the systemic side effects of many of the other antihypertensives and generally produce a better quality of life, compared to their rivals. In addition, they may be able to restore insulin sensitivity and this may be important in slowing down atherogenesis. However, they are drugs which require particular caution, as in the presence of bilateral renal artery stenosis (or unilateral stenosis in a single kidney) they can precipitate a dramatic fall in glomerular perfusion, resulting in renal failure. Hence they have to be used with caution, particularly in the elderly and those with obvious arteriopathy.

In terms of renal effects, ACE inhibitors produce efferent arteriolar dilatation, a fall in IGP and trans-capillary glomerular pressure, a rise in renal plasma flow and no net change in GFR in normal kidneys. In chronic parenchymal disease there may be a small fall in GFR, which is either transient, or otherwise stable and insignificant. It is in subjects with significant renovascular disease (with resultant angiotensin II-induced efferent vasocostriction) that ACE inhibitors produce a serious fall in GFR.

It is this ability of ACE inhibitors to lower IGP that is thought to contribute to their ability to reduce proteinuria, slow down the rate of glomerulosclerosis, and prolong renal survival [37, 38]. ACE inhibitors may also have beneficial effects on reducing basement membrane pore size, without a change in blood pressure [39]. Thus they have a protective effect over and above the effect attributable to blood pressure lowering.

Pre-existing renal failure is not a contraindication to their use, although it increases their predilection for producing hyperkalaemia. They have been shown to have beneficial effects on the progression of kidney disease, particularly diabetic nephropathy, where they can reduce proteinuria and prolong renal survival. Similar benefits may be obtained in a variety of progressive renal diseases, but the evidence is still awaited. ACE inhibitors should be used with caution in some diabetics, and others with renal tubular acidosis and pre-existing hyperkalaemia.

In addition to hypertension, the other major area where ACE inhibitors have been shown to significantly improve survival is in heart failure (with systolic dysfunction). Thus in the coexistence of hypertension and heart failure, ACE inhibitors must be considered the drugs of choice, unless there are specific contraindications.

The prototype captopril has to be used at least twice a day and, because of its rapid absorption and short duration of action, it has a tendency to produce a powerful first-dose effect in susceptible individuals – those with severe or accelerated hypertension, high-dose diuretics and heart failure. Enalapril is usually effective given once daily. A number of long-acting once-daily preparations are now available. As a general rule patients being started on ACE inhibitors should have renal function and electrolytes measured before and within three to four weeks of starting treatment, particularly in individuals at risk. Sometimes ACE inhibition can induce a gradual decline in renal function over several weeks. While they can be prescribed routinely on an outpatient basis for mild to moderate hypertension, treatment must always be given under careful supervision if the hypertension is either severe or there is associated heart failure.

Recent studies [40, 41] using losartan, an angiotensin II receptor blocker (selective for the AT-1 receptor), have demonstrated an almost identical protective effect, both in lowering blood pressure and proteinuria, establishing the fundamental importance of angiotensin II in progression of renal failure. There are three potential mechanisms by which this drug (and its successors) may be superior to ACE inhibitors.

1. Greater efficacy because of their ability to block non-ACE pathways.
2. Greater efficacy because of the unopposed stimulation of the AT-2 receptor, which has the effect of producing vasorelaxation.
3. Absence of cough as a side effect (present in roughly 15% of patients given ACE inhibitors.

### 3.9.8 Choice of drug therapy

There is now strong evidence showing that treating hypertension adequately in diabetes can significantly reduce proteinuria and prolong renal survival. Also, there is evidence that in essential hypertension, adequate treatment can produce renal survival that matches that of normotensive controls. Thus, there is strong evidence that hypertension should be treated actively.

What of the choice of drug? From the cardiovascular point of view, large-scale studies over the last 20 years have shown unequivocal benefit obtained using thiazides and beta-blockers. The recent studies and recommendations support the use of thiazides as standard first-line treatment for essential hypertension. Alpha-blockers, CCB and ACE inhibitors appear to have theoretical advantages, but trial evidence of their superiority remains to be demonstrated.

**Table 3.3** Results from a meta-analysis of trials in diabetic nephropathy

| Treatment | Percentage change | | |
|---|---|---|---|
| | Blood pressure | Proteinuria | GFR |
| Placebo | −2 | +39 | −0.7 |
| Diuretics/beta-blockers | −10 | −20 | −0.8 |
| Nifedipine | −12 | −2 | −4.0 |
| CCB (except nifedipine) | −16 | −42 | +0.2 |
| ACE inhibitors | −16 | −53 | −0.1 |

From the point of view of renal protection, however, a large number of studies in the last five to 10 years have shown some of the newer classes to be superior. Two major meta-analyses [42, 43] in diabetes have shown a significantly greater anti-proteinuric effect with ACE inhibitors compared to CCB, with diuretics and beta-blockers in third place. In several experimental studies again it has been established beyond doubt that ACE inhibitors are able to protect the kidneys from different models of progressive glomerulosclerosis (see Chapter 2).

The effects shown in a meta-analysis of trials in diabetic nephropathy are given in Table 3.3 [43].

Successful prolongation of renal survival is predicted by the degree of fall in proteinuria caused by the intervention. Thus, proteinuria is a useful surrogate endpoint to monitor in the treatment of hypertension. More interestingly, clinical and experimental studies have demonstrated the ability of ACE inhibitors to reduce proteinuria and prolong renal survival, even in the absence of a blood pressure-lowering effect. Thus ACE inhibitors clearly have additional protective effects, probably mediated by their ability to suppress angiotensin II formation.

A detailed meta-analysis of comparative trials of antihypertensives in proteinuria has recently been published [44]. A very recent landmark study [45] showed that benazepril (an ACE inhibitor), compared to placebo, regardless of blood pressure status, conferred a significant protective effect on renal survival over a three-year period, in a variety of renal diseases – blood pressure control being achieved to an equivalent extent in both groups by other classes of drugs. The risk reduction was greatest in males and those with glomerular diseases and diabetes; there was no benefit in polycystic disease. There are suggestions that ACE inhibitors and CCB (verapamil or diltiazem) may be more effective in combination than the individual components [46].

### 3.9.10 Treatment of ischaemic nephropathy

Analogous to ischaemic heart disease it is interesting to postulate that aspirin might be of benefit in retarding ischaemic renal disease. However, more evidence is required before making a general recommendation. Nevertheless there would appear to be no contraindication to using low-dose aspirin in patients with ischaemic nephropathy. Novel treatments, such as antibodies directed against platelet-derived growth factor and platelet glycoprotein IIb/IIIa receptor (which promote platelet aggregation), are currently being evaluated [47, 48].

The role of lipid-lowering therapy in retarding the progression of renal failure remains a subject of debate and is discussed more fully in Chapter 9. In addition to their potential for reversing atherosclerotic lesions, lipid-lowering drugs may have anti-proliferative and anti-oxidant properties [47, 48]. In any case lipid-lowering treatment should be actively considered, if only for general cardiovascular protection.

*Renal angioplasty*

Earlier unsatisfactory attempts at open surgical revascularization for renal artery stenosis (RAS) have now given way to the well-established method of percutaneous transluminal renal angioplasty (PTRA). This procedure in experienced hands, can certainly restore function to a poorly functioning kidney. The major problem is patient selection, and identifying those most likely to benefit.

There is little evidence to support PTRA in unilateral disease, particularly when hypertension is not a major problem. Even in refractory hypertension, PTRA may only provide short-term benefit, and in the most severe cases, uninephrectomy may be the best solution.

In bilateral RAS there is good reason to attempt PTRA, with a view to preserving renal function for as long as possible, and avoiding or postponing end stage renal failure. This would seem a common sense approach, particularly in light of publications [49, 50] which have shown that angioplasty may allow patients with 'ESRF' to become dialysis-independent. At least in the transplant situation, PTRA is well accepted as treatment of significant RAS.

The gold standard for diagnosis remains renal angiography, though duplex Doppler scanning may provide useful information in a non-invasive way. Captopril-enhanced renography may also help, though this latter method lacks sensitivity. It may still be valuable in terms of predicting outcome of intervention; thus it has been suggested that a positive result should indicate intervention by PTRA, and a negative result should exclude intervention [51]. Magnetic resonance angiography is non-invasive, sensitive, and may yet become the investigation of choice.

## 3.10 SUMMARY AND CONCLUSIONS

1. Adequate control of blood pressure is of crucial importance in retarding the progression of renal failure, whatever the cause.
2. In the presence of renal impairment or other cardiovascular risk factors, the treatment threshold should be lowered to 140/90 mm Hg, (particularly in younger individuals), the target being 130/80 mm Hg.
3. The initial choice of drug may not be of importance in essential hypertension, but special considerations apply in the presence of proteinuria or renal failure.
4. ACE inhibitors appear to be the most useful agents in general, particularly in the presence of significant proteinuria and in hypertension associated with diabetic nephropathy. However, they have a dangerous potential for precipitating acute renal failure in the presence of renal artery stenosis, and should be used with caution, particularly in the elderly.
5. Calcium channel blockers are probably the safest drugs to use in ischaemic nephropathy, in the elderly, when proteinuria is not significant and when the cause of renal failure is obscure. Nifedipine is best avoided in the presence of significant proteinuria and in diabetics.
6. Combination therapy with an ACE inhibitor and a CCB (verapamil or diltiazem) may be very effective, and should be used when the response to monotherapy appears inadequate.
7. Associated cardiovascular risk factors, in particular the lipid profile, should be monitored and treated.
8. Ischaemic nephropathy should be actively treated by attempts to correct systolic hypertension and hyperlipidaemia. The role of aspirin is uncertain, but it may be used as a non-specific measure.

## REFERENCES


1. Guyton, A.C., Hall, J.E., Lohmeier, T.E. *et al.* (1981) The concept of whole body autoregulation and the dominant role of the kidneys for long-term blood pressure regulation, in *Frontiers in Hypertension Research* (eds J.H. Laragh, F.R. Buhler and D.W. Seldin), Springer-Verlag, New York, pp. 125–34.
2. MacGregor, G.A. and de Wardener, H.E. (1981) Is a circulating sodium transport inhibitor involved in the pathogenesis of essential hypertension? *Clin. Exp. Hypertens.*, **3**, 815–30.
3. Woolfson, R.G., Poston, L. and de Wardener, H.E. (1994) Digoxin-like inhibitors of active sodium transport and blood pressure: the current status. *Kidney Int.*, **46**, 297–309.

4. Blaustein, M.P. and Hamlyn, J.M. (1983) Sodium transport inhibition, cell calcium, and hypertension. The natriuretic hormone/$Na^{+}-Ca^{2+}$ exchange/hypertension hypothesis. *Am. J. Med.*, **77**, 45–59.
5. Dickinson, C.J. (1995) Cerebral oxidative metabolism in essential hypertension: a meta-analysis. *J. Hypertens.*, **13**, 653–8.
6. Reaven, G.M., Lithell, H. and Landsberg, L. (1996) Hypertension and associated metabolic abnormalities – the role of insulin resistance and the sympathoadrenal system. *N. Engl. J. Med.*, **334**, 374–81.
7. Siffert, W. (1996) Essential hypertension – are we on the way to identify primary defects? *Nephrol. Dial. Transplant.*, **10**, 1975–6.
8. Rettig, R. and Uber, A. (1995) Hypertension and the kidney: new insights from results of renal transplantation studies. *Nephrol. Dial. Transplant.*, **10**, suppl. 9, 9–16.
9. Brenner, B.M., Meyer, T.W. and Hostetter, T.H. (1982) Dietary protein intake and the nature of progressive nature of kidney disease: the role of haemodynamically mediated glomerular injury in the pathogenesis of progressive glomerular sclerosis in aging, renal ablation and intrinsic renal disease. *N. Engl. J. Med.*, **307**, 652–9.
10. Anderson, S. and Brenner, B.M. (1986) The role of intraglomerular pressure in the initiation and progression of renal disease. *J. Hypertens.*, suppl. 4, S236–8.
11. Venkat Raman, G. (1991) Post-transplant hypertension. *J. Human Hypertens.*, **5**, 1–6.
12. Mogensen, C.E. (1981) Long-term antihypertensive therapy inhibits progression of diabetic nephropathy. *Acta Endocrinol.*, **S242** 31–5.
13. Parving, H.H., Anderson, A.R., Schmidt, U.M. and Svendsen, P.A. (1983) Early aggressive antihypertensive treatment reduces rate of decline in kidney function in diabetic nephropathy. *Lancet*, **i**, 1175–9.
14. Bjork, S., Nyberg, G., Mulec, H. *et al.* (1986) Beneficial effects of angiotensin converting enzyme inhibition on renal function in patients with diabetic nephropathy. *Br. Med. J.*, **293**, 471–4.
15. Marre, M., Chatellier, G., Leblanc, H. *et al.* (1988) Prevention of diabetic nephropathy with enalapril in normotensive diabetics with microalbuminuria. *Br. Med. J.*, **297**, 1092–5.
16. Lewis, E.J., Hunsicker, L.G., Bain, R.P. and Rohde, R.D. (1993) The effect of angiotensin-converting-enzyme inhibition on diabetic nephropathy. *N. Engl. J. Med.*, **329**, 1456–62.
17. Velussi, M., Brocco, E., Frigato, F. *et al.* (1996) Effects of cilazapril and amlodipine on kidney function in hypertensive NIDDM patients. *Diabetes*, **45**, 216–22.
18. Bianchi, S., Bigazzi, R., Baldari, G. and Campese, V.M. (1991) Long term effects of enalapril and nicardipine on urinary albumin excretion in patients with chronic renal insufficiency: a 1 year follow up. *Am. J. Nephrol.*, **11**, 131–7.
19. Maschio, G., Alberti, D., Janin, G. *et al.* (1996) Effect of the angiotensin-converting-enzyme inhibitor benazepril on the progression of chronic renal insufficiency. *N. Engl. J. Med.*, **334**, 939–45.
20. Kamper, A.L., Strandgaard, S. and Leyssac, P.P. (1995) Late outcome of a controlled trial of enalapril treatment in progressive chronic renal failure. Hard end-points and influence of proteinuria. *Nephrol. Dial. Transplant.*, **10**, 1182–8.
21. Kamper, A.L., Strandgaard, S. and Leyssac, P.P. (1992) Effect of enalapril on

the progression of chronic renal failure. A randomised controlled trial. *Am. J. Hypertens.*, **5**, 423–30.

22. Maschio, G., Cagnoli, L., Claroni, F. *et al.* (1994) ACE inhibition reduces proteinuria in normotensive patients with IgA nephropathy: a multicentre, randomised, placebo-controlled study. *Nephrol. Dial. Transplant.*, **9**, 265–9.
23. Hannedouche, T., Landais, P., Goldfarb, B. *et al.* (1994) Randomized controlled trial of enalapril and beta blockers in non-diabetic chronic renal failure. *Br. Med. J.*, **309**, 833–7.
24. The fifth report of the Joint National Committee on Detection, Evaluation, and Treatment of High Blood Pressure (JNCV) (1993) *Arch. Intern. Med.*, **153**, 154–83.
25. WHO/ISH Guidelines Subcommittee (1993) Guidelines for the management of mild hypertension. *Bull. Int. Soc. Hypertens.*, 3–16.
26. Sever, P., Beevers, G., Bulpitt, C. (1993) Management guidelines in essential hypertension: report of the second working party of the British Hypertension Society. *Br. Med. J.*, **306**, 983–7.
27. Medical Research Council Working Party (1985) MRC trial of treatment of mild hypertension. *Br. Med. J.*, **291**, 97–104.
28. SHEP Cooperative Research Group (1991) Prevention of stroke by antihypertensive drug treatment in older persons with isolated systolic hypertension. *J. Am. Med. Assoc.*, **265**, 3255–64.
29. Dahlof, B., Lindholm, L.H., Hansson, L. *et al.* (1991) Morbidity and mortality in the Swedish Trial in old patients with hypertension (STOP-Hypertension). *Lancet*, **338**, 1281–5.
30. Wijkstrand, J., Warnold, I., Olsson, G. *et al.* (1988) Primary prevention with metoprolol in patients with hypertension. Mortality results from the MAPHY study. *J. Am. Med. Assoc.*, **259**, 1976–82.
31. Christensen, C.K. and Mogensen, C.E. (1985) Effect of antihypertensive treatment on progression of incipient diabetic nephropathy. *Hypertension*, **7**, II 109–13.
32. Zucchelli, P., Zuccala, A., Borghi, M. *et al.* (1992) Long term comparison between captopril and nifedipine in the progression of renal insufficiency. *Kidney Int.*, **42**, 452–8.
33. Mimran, A., Insua, A., Ribstein, J. *et al.* (1988) Contrasting effects of captopril and nifedipine in normotensive patients with incipient diabetic nephropathy. *J. Hypertens.*, **6**, 919–23.
34. Demarie, B.K. and Bakris, G.L. (1990) Effects of different calcium antagonists on proteinuria associated with diabetes mellitus. *Ann. Intern. Med.*, **113**, 987–8.
35. Bakris, G.L., Barnhill, B.W. and Sadler, R. (1992) Treatment of arterial hypertension in diabetic humans: Importance of therapeutic selection. *Kidney Int.*, **41**, 912–9.
36. Slataper, R., Vicknair, N., Sadler, R. and Bakris, G.L. (1993) Comparative effects of different antihypertensive treatments on progression of diabetic renal disease. *Arch. Intern. Med.*, **153**, 973–80.
37. Zatz, R., Dunn, B.R., Meyer, T.W. *et al.* (1986) Prevention of diabetic glomerulopathy by pharmacological amelioration of glomerular capillary hypertension. *J. Clin. Invest.*, **77**, 1925–30.
38. Anderson, S. and Brenner, B.M. (1988) Therapeutic benefit of converting-enzyme inhibition in progressive renal disease. *Am. J. Hypertens.*, **1**, 380S–383S.
39. Remuzzi, A., Perticucci, E., Ruggenenti, P. *et al.* (1991) Angiotensin

converting enzyme inhibition improves glomerular size-selectivity in IgA nephropathy. *Kidney Int.*, **39**, 1267–73.

40. Gansevoort, R.T., de Zeeuw, D. and de Jong, P.E. (1994) Is the antiproteinuric effect of ACE inhibition mediated by interference in the renin–angiotensin system? *Kidney Int.*, **45**, 861–7.
41. Gansevoort, R.T., de Zeeuw, D., Shahinfar, S. *et al.* (1994) Effects of the angiotension II antagonist losartan in hypertensive patients with renal disease. *J. Hypertens.*, suppl., **12**, S37–42.
42. Kasiske, B.L., Kalil, R.S., Ma, J.Z. *et al.* (1993) Effect of antihypertensive therapy on the kidney in patients with diabetes: a meta-regression analysis. *Ann. Intern. Med.*, **118**, 129–39.
43. Weidman, P., Schneider, M. and Bohlen, L. (1995) Therapeutic efficacy of different antihypertensive drugs in human diabetic nephropathy: an updated meta-analysis. *Nephrol. Dial. Transplant.*, **10**, suppl 9, 39–45.
44. Gansevoort, R.T., Sluiter, W.J., Hemmelder, M.H. *et al.* (1995) Antiproteinuric effect of blood pressure lowering agents: a meta-analysis of comparative trials. *Nephrol. Dial. Transplant.*, **10**, 1963–74.
45. Maschio, G., Alberti, D., Janin, G. *et al.* (1996) Effect of the angiotensin-converting-enzyme inhibitor benazepril on the progression of chronic renal insufficiency. *N. Engl. J. Med.*, **334**, 939–45.
46. Bakris, G. and Williams, B. (1995) Angiotensin converting enzyme inhibitors and calcium antagonists alone or combined: does the progression of diabetic renal disease differ? *J. Hypertens.*, suppl., **13**, S95–101.
47. Gotto, A.M. Jr (1993) Dyslipidaemia and atherosclerosis. A forecast of pharmaceutical approach, *Circulation*, **87**, suppl III, III54–III59.
48. Dzau, J.V., Gibbons, G.H., Cooke, J.P. and Omoigui, N. (1993) Vascular biology and medicine in the 1990s: scope, concepts, potential, and prospectives. *Circulation*, **90**, 2070–84.
49. Kaylor, W.M., Novick, A.C., Ziegelbaum, M. and Vidt, D.G. (1989) Reversal of end stage renal failure with surgical revascularisation in patients with atherosclerotic renal artery occlusion. *J. Urol.*, **141**, 486–8.
50. Scoble, J.E. and Hamilton, G. (1990) Atherosclerotic renovascular disease: remediable cause of renal failure in the elderly. *Br. Med. J.*, **300**, 1670–1.
51. Zuccala, A. and Zucchelli, P. (1995) Atherosclerotic renal artery stenosisi – when is intervention by PTA or surgery justified? *Nephrol. Dial. Transplant.*, **10**, 585–7.

# 4

# Glomerulonephritis

*P.D. Mason and C.D. Pusey*

## 4.1 INTRODUCTION

The term 'glomerulonephritis' is often used loosely to cover all types of glomerular disease although not all are associated with inflammation of the glomerulus. It is more accurate to refer to non-proliferative glomerular disease as glomerulopathy or nephropathy. Furthermore, the term glomerulonephritis (GN) does not convey the fact that there is often associated interstitial inflammation or that the vessels may also be involved, particularly in the secondary glomerulonephritides. Immunological processes are implicated in the pathogenesis of most forms of glomerular disease, although the precise mechanisms are understood in only a few. Early referral for evaluation and diagnosis is important since timely treatment, when indicated, may slow or prevent progression to end stage renal failure (ESRF).

## 4.2 PRESENTATION AND DIAGNOSIS OF GLOMERULONEPHRITIS

Glomerular disease may present in a variety of ways:

- asymptomatic proteinuria;
- asymptomatic haematuria;
- nephrotic syndrome;
- nephritic syndrome;
- acute/rapidly progressive renal failure;
- end stage chronic renal failure;
- hypertension.

*Renal Disease.* Edited by G. Venkat Raman. Published in 1998 by Chapman & Hall, London. ISBN 0 412 45700 8.

Although specific histological types of glomerulonephritis often present with characteristic clinical features, it is not generally possible to predict the histological diagnosis accurately – hence the need for renal biopsy. Many patients come to medical attention following the incidental detection of haematuria or proteinuria. Referral is indicated for patients with proteinuria, once infection has been excluded, and for those with impaired renal function or hypertension. The assessment of haematuria is more difficult, but patients under 50 years with isolated asymptomatic haematuria should generally be referred to a nephrologist, while those over 50 years are more likely to have a urological cause and should initially be referred to a urologist.

Patients present with a wide spectrum of disease from asymptomatic

**Table 4.1** Useful blood tests in the investigation of glomerular disease

| Test | Interpretation |
|---|---|
| *Non-specific* | |
| Full blood count | High white blood count in vasculitis, infection |
| Electrolytes, urea and creatinine | Severity of renal impairment |
| Albumin | ↓ in nephrotics, chronic infection |
| Immunoglobulins | ↑ in vasculitis, SLE, post-infectious GN<br>IgA raised in ~50% of IgA nephropathy and HSP<br>IgM paraprotein in MEC |
| Complement | Low C4 $\pm$ C3: MEC, SLE, post-infectious GN, MCGN-I<br>Low C3, normal C4: MCGN-II and sometimes SLE<br>High C3, C4: systemic vasculitis |
| *Specific* | |
| Anti-GBM antibody | Goodpasture's disease |
| ANCA | Systemic vasculitis |
| Anti-dsDNA antibody | SLE |
| Cryoglobulins | MEC (low levels in SLE and post-infectious GN) |
| C3 nephritic factors | MCGN-II (and occasionally SLE) |

SLE = systemic lupus erythematosus.
HSP = Henoch–Schönlein purpura.
MEC = mixed essential cryoglobulinaemia.
MCGN = mesangiocapillary glomerulonephritis.
GBM = glomerular basement membrane.
ANCA = antineutrophil cytoplasmic antibodies.

urinary abnormalities to full blown nephritic or/and nephrotic syndromes, while other patients have features of both. The nephritic syndrome is characterized by abrupt onset of haematuria (often with red blood cell casts), proteinuria (usually moderate), and reduced renal function with salt and water retention causing oedema and hypertension. The nephrotic syndrome is characterized by heavy proteinuria ($>3\,g/24\,h$) associated with hypoalbuminaemia, oedema and usually hypercholesterolaemia. Occasionally, patients may present with acute renal failure, secondary to a rapidly progressive GN. Although the history, examination, urinalysis and blood investigations (Table 4.1) may suggest a likely cause, definitive diagnosis requires a renal biopsy. Glomerulonephritis is considered to be the cause of end stage renal failure in about 25–35% of patients accepted on to dialysis programmes in the West. Since the progression of glomerulonephritis may be insidious, some patients present in chronic renal failure with small kidneys. By this stage renal biopsy is more hazardous and often reveals only sclerosed glomeruli and tubular atrophy with interstitial fibrosis, making the precise diagnosis difficult or impossible to confirm. Whenever a renal biopsy is contemplated the risks must be weighed against the benefits, despite the attraction of making a tissue diagnosis. Although the incidence of significant complications is low, the findings, especially in patients with mild disease, may be non-specific and of little prognostic value. Many nephrologists therefore only biopsy patients in whom specific treatment is likely to be indicated or when assessment of prognosis is important [1]. Mild haematuria and/or low-level proteinuria (less than 2 g/day) in the absence of renal impairment or hypertension are associated with a good long-term prognosis. Such patients can be safely managed with regular monitoring. An increase in proteinuria, the development of hypertension, or deterioration of renal function would then be the indications for renal biopsy.

## 4.3 CLASSIFICATION OF GLOMERULONEPHRITIS

Ideally glomerular disease should be classified according to the underlying immunopathological process, but this is possible in only a few conditions [2]. Currently the most satisfactory classification depends upon the histological appearances, which divide the glomerulonephritides into proliferative and non-proliferative types. The former may then be subdivided depending on the proliferating cell types, and qualified by the pattern of involvement. The terms 'diffuse' or 'focal' refer to the proportion of glomeruli involved, while 'segmental' (rather than 'global') implies the involvement of only a segment of each affected glomerulus. Extraglomerular proliferation is the accumulation of cells within Bowman's capsule. If this is extensive, occupying more than one

**Table 4.2** Classification of glomerular disease

| *Non proliferative* | *Proliferative* |
|---|---|
| Minimal change nephropathy | Mesangial proliferative GN (IgA nephropathy) |
| Focal segmental glomerulosclerosis | Mesangiocapillary GN |
| Membranous nephropathy | Diffuse proliferative GN |
| | Focal segmental GN |
| | Crescentic GN |

half of Bowman's space, it is referred to as a 'crescent' – hence the term crescentic nephritis. In addition the pattern, distribution and nature of immune deposits as determined by immunostaining and electron microscopy (EM) may aid diagnosis. Table 4.2 gives a brief classification of the primary glomerulonephritides. Secondary glomerular disease may be associated with multisystem disorders, including mixed essential cryoglobulinaemia, systemic vasculitis and systemic lupus erythematosus, and with infection, malignancy and drugs.

## 4.4 GENERAL ASPECTS OF MANAGEMENT

Several aspects of treatment are common to patients with different forms of glomerular disease. These include the control of hypertension, the management of salt and water retention and the nephrotic syndrome, and strategies to slow or prevent the progressive renal deterioration that commonly accompanies chronic renal disease irrespective of the aetiology.

Glomerular diseases, particularly the proliferative types, are often associated with hypertension. Vigorous blood pressure control is important at every stage of management and there is a strong impression that effective control slows the rate of progression of renal failure irrespective of the underlying cause [3] as well as reducing the risk of cardiovascular disease and cerebrovascular events. The blood pressure to aim for is controversial and should probably depend upon the age of the patient. It has recently been demonstrated that patients with chronic renal failure and an average blood pressure equivalent to 125/75 mm Hg (145/75 in those >60 years) had a slower rate of decline in renal function than patients with an average blood pressure of 140/90 (160/90 in those >60 years) [4]. These data suggest that the target blood pressure should be less than 130/80 at least in younger patients, which is lower than many nephrologists have hitherto recommended.

The pathogenesis of hypertension (see also Chapter 3) in renal disease is complex, multifactorial and likely to vary between patients, but sodium and water retention and renin-dependent mechanisms are probably the predominant factors. There are clearly a large number of available treatments. Sometimes there is a clear indication for a particular group of drugs, such as diuretics if fluid retention is evident, although these agents may also be effective when fluid retention is not overt. Beta-blockers are effective and commonly used, but are associated with a moderately high incidence of side effects. Alpha-blocking and directly acting vasodilators are also useful in the treatment of hypertension, but usually in combination with other drugs. The calcium antagonists are also generally well tolerated alternatives.

Angiotensin-converting enzyme inhibitors (ACEI) are generally well tolerated and are clearly a logical choice in patients in whom renin is an important factor in causing hypertension, though they may also be effective in patients with low circulating renin levels. They have also been suggested to have an additional beneficial effect by lowering intraglomerular capillary pressure as well as systemic hypertension. Treatment with ACEI has been proven to reduce the rate of progression of renal failure in animals with chronic renal failure, especially when diabetic nephropathy is responsible. There are now controlled clinical trial data suggesting that ACEI have an advantage over other antihypertensive drugs in terms of reducing proteinuria and delaying the progression of diabetic nephropathy [5]. Superiority of ACEI over other agents has not however been proven in patients with chronic glomerulonephritis, and the effectiveness of blood pressure control is probably more important than the type of drugs used. ACEI should be avoided in patients with proven or suspected renal artery stenosis since reduction of the angiotensin II-induced efferent artery vasoconstriction results in a fall in glomerular filtration and renal failure. The topic is dealt with in greater detail in Chapter 3.

Nephrotic patients should be prescribed a low-salt, but normal-protein diet. Control of oedema may be accomplished with diuretics, and loop diuretics are usually necessary, especially when renal function is reduced. Refractory oedema may be treated by the addition of metolazone, which has a synergistic effect with the loop diuretics, although patients treated with both agents should be carefully monitored for hypovolaemia, hyponatraemia and hypokalaemia. ACE inhibitors may significantly reduce proteinuria and are useful when an antihypertensive effect is also necessary. Non-steroidal anti-inflammatory drugs (NSAID) reduce proteinuria and act synergistically with ACEI. Although useful in selected patients, care must be taken since NSAID may cause a marked fall in glomerular filtration rate (GFR) and diminish the effectiveness of diuretics and antihypertensives. Severely nephrotic patients may need prophylactic anticoagulants and antibiotics [6], and if the underlying cause of the nephrotic syndrome cannot be cured, then treatment of the hypercholesterolaemia should also be considered.

The role of low-protein diets in patients with chronic renal failure has been highly controversial. Such diets have been suggested to slow the progression of chronic renal failure [7] but a recent large controlled study did not find that protein restriction was beneficial in the majority of patients [4] (Chapter 2).

## 4.5 SPECIFIC TREATMENT OF GLOMERULONEPHRITIS

Although a similar range of immunosuppressive agents has been used in most types of glomerulonephritis, the treatment regimens and results of treatment vary considerably. We shall therefore discuss the diagnosis, aetiology, presentation and management of the common histological types separately.

### 4.5.1 Minimal change nephropathy

Minimal change nephropathy (MCN) is responsible for 90% of nephrotic syndrome in children and about 20% in adults. In children, MCN occurs most often under the age of six years and boys are affected twice as commonly as girls. In older children and adults the sex ratio is 1:1. Clinically it is usually characterized by the abrupt onset of oedema, which can be gross, with ascites, and pleural and pericardial effusions. In about half of the patients the initial attack and subsequent relapses follow an upper respiratory tract infection. Whether these are pathogenetically relevant or coincidental is not clear.

Children presenting with the nephrotic syndrome are generally treated with steroids, and renal biopsy is reserved for non-responders. The glomeruli are normal on light microscopy (LM) with widespread fusion of epithelial foot processes on EM. Occasionally mild mesangial proliferation on LM and small amounts of immunoglobin M (IgM) on immunostaining may be seen in patients who respond like those with minimal change disease (see below). The topic is discussed in greater detail in Chapter 15.

An immunological pathogenesis has been proposed on the basis of the response to cyclophosphamide, steroids and cyclosporin A, the induction of remission following measles (since the virus infects lymphocytes and impairs cell-mediated immunity), and the association with T cell lymphomas. In the vast majority of patients the condition is idiopathic, but before treatment is commenced underlying causes of MCN should be considered (Table 4.3). The association with atopy and

**Table 4.3** Secondary causes and associations of glomerulonephritis

---

*Minimal change*
- Drugs: Non-steroidal anti-inflammatory drugs
  - Lithium
  - Gold
  - Rifampicin
  - Recombinant interleukin-2 and interferon
- Hodgkin's disease
- Atopy

*Focal segmental glomerulosclerosis*
- Intravenous drug abuse
- HIV infection
- Malignancy
- Following focal necrotizing glomerulonephritis
- Lithium

*IgA nephropathy*
- Hepatic cirrhosis
- Coeliac disease/dermatitis herpetiformis
- Seronegative arthritis (especially ankylosing spondylitis)
- Tuberculosis
- Oat cell carcinoma
- Mycosis fungoides
- HIV infection

*Membranous nephropathy*
- Tumours – 15% of cases, proportion increasing with age
- Drugs – especially gold and penicillamine
- Infectious – hepatitis B, syphilis, quartan malaria
- Systemic lupus erythematosus
- Sickle cell disease

*Mesangiocapillary glomerulonephritis*
- Tumours, especially malignant melanoma
- Chronic lymphatic leukaemia
- Infections, e.g. endocarditis, hepatitis B, schistosomiasis
- Mixed essential cryglobulinaemia
- Systemic lupus erythematosus
- $\alpha_1$-antitrypsin disease
- Inherited complement deficiencies
- Chronic transplant rejection

---

raised IgE levels is interesting. Occasionally allergens are identified which trigger MCN and their avoidance results in remission, although the mechanisms involved are not understood. T cell lymphomas (including Hodgkin's disease) and mesotheliomas are also occasionally associated with MCN. Familial cases have been reported and there is an association with HLA-DR7 and DR3 (DR8 in Japan).

*Children*

Children are treated with prednisolone 1 mg/kg/day (or 2 mg/kg alternate days) for eight to 12 weeks or for one week after induction of remission. Half the induction dose is then given for up to one month with subsequent tapering over several months. More than 90% of children respond within eight weeks (80% within four weeks). The risk of relapse is higher if therapy is stopped after four weeks (81% at 12 months) rather than 12 weeks (36% at 12 months) [8], without a greater incidence of side effects. Failure to respond after one month is managed by some nephrologists with three pulses of methyl prednisolone (1 g/ 1.73 $m^2$) on alternate days.

About 30% of responders never have a relapse, another 10–20% are cured after one to four steroid-responsive episodes, while the remainder are frequent relapsers or become steroid-dependent. Several studies have suggested that the duration of steroid therapy required to induce remission from a relapse is similar to that required for the first attack. However, prolonged, high steroid doses are not associated with a subsequent lower risk of further relapse. Some authors prefer a short sharp course of prednisolone (60 mg/$m^2$/day) until three days after clinical remission has been established, followed by alternate day 40 mg/$m^2$ for four weeks. Others prefer a gradual tapering after remission to the 'threshold' level at which previous relapses occurred, with continuation of this dose for 12–18 months. The former approach appears to be associated with more relapses, although the total amount of steroids administered may be less, depending on the threshold dose. If the threshold dose is high or relapses frequent, alkylating agents are indicated to avoid chronic steroid toxicity.

The question of using alkylating agents in children with steroid-responsive disease is controversial and the risks have to be weighed against those of steroid toxicity or uncontrolled nephrotic syndrome. Children that require a dose of steroids likely to interfere with growth ($>$0.5 mg/kg on alternate days) probably demand alternative treatment [9]. An eight-week course of cyclophosphamide (2–2.5 mg/kg/day) is effective at inducing longer-lasting remissions, and there is some evidence that 12 weeks' treatment results in fewer relapses [10]. Children who relapse frequently are more likely to respond with a permanent remission than those who are steroid dependent. Chlorambucil (0.2 mg/kg/day) for two months appears to have a similar effect to cyclophosphamide and is widely used in some countries as an alternative. Nitrogen mustard (mechlorethamine) given intravenously 0.8 mg/kg daily for four days and repeated after one month generally induces rapid remissions – typically in seven days even without steroids. It is rarely used nowadays but may be worth considering for patients in whom high-dose steroids carry extra risks (e.g. diabetes mellitus), and for those with serious complications in whom a rapid response is particularly desirable. It does not produce a high rate of long-lasting remission in patients with steroid-dependent disease.

Cyclosporin A (up to 150 mg/m$^2$/day and aiming for trough levels of 100–200 ng/ml) is usually effective in children with both steroid-dependent and frequently relapsing nephrotic syndrome [11]. The response correlates with the initial steroid responsiveness, but relapse is almost inevitable within three months of stopping treatment, and there is a risk of nephrotoxicity. Cyclosporin A is therefore usually reserved for patients who have failed to respond to other treatments, and whose steroid dose is likely to result in long-term toxicity. Levamisole has also been used successfully in steroid-dependent children, as demonstrated by a multicentred double-blind trial of 2.5 mg/kg on alternate days for four to 12 months. The mechanism of action is obscure and most patients relapse within three months following the course of treatment. Since it appears to be a safe drug it is sometimes used as an alternative to steroids in children with milder disease.

Children with steroid-resistant nephrotic syndrome should have a renal biopsy to exclude other causes of nephrotic syndrome. A variety of other treatments including high-dose pulse methylprednisolone and aggressive cytotoxic regimes have been tried with variable success in uncontrolled series. It is probably prudent to avoid prolonged steroid therapy, although a recent French study reported complete remission in nearly half of a group of 61 children treated with cyclosporin A and steroids over a six-month period. Such a relatively benign regime may be indicated in view of the potential long-term complications of uncontrolled nephrotic syndrome. Children are also discussed in Chapter 15.

### *Adults*

Initially adults are treated with steroids (1 mg/kg/day), but respond more slowly than children and only 75% finally respond even after four months. However, those that do respond relapse less often than children (30–50%). Bowel oedema, which is sometimes severe enough to cause diarrhoea, may limit the absorption of steroids, especially the enteric coated preparations which should therefore be avoided. Frequently relapsing and steroid-dependent patients should be treated with cyclophosphamide (2–2.5 mg/kg/day) for eight to 12 weeks, which induces a permanent remission more often than in children (75% at two years). There is some evidence that a permanent remission is more likely with a 12-week rather than eight-week course. Adults may develop transient non-nephrotic relapses, and therefore re-treatment should generally await the development of the nephrotic syndrome.

As in children, cyclosporin A (4–6 mg/kg/day) is effective, but relapse generally follows dose reduction or withdrawal. It may be worth considering as a short to medium-term management strategy, since there is evidence that remission eventually occurs in 50–75% of patients even without treatment [12]. However, careful monitoring is required since nephrotoxicity is common after more than one year's treatment [13].

### 4.5.2 Focal segmental glomerulosclerosis (FSGS)

This relatively common type of glomerular disease causes up to 15% of cases of the nephrotic syndrome. It is more commonly associated with hypertension than MCN. The characteristic pathological features are of focal and segmental glomerular scars/sclerosis and hyalinosis, containing IgM and C3 on immunostaining. The EM changes of extensive foot-process fusion are the same as in minimal change nephropathy. Juxtamedullary glomeruli are affected first, and sometimes focal areas of interstitial fibrosis with tubular fall-out are clues to early disease in the absence of affected glomeruli. The LM changes are not specific and a similar appearance may be the end result of focal segmental or even diffuse proliferative GN, and may also be seen in hypertension and other causes of chronic renal impairment. However, widespread foot-process fusion and nephrotic range proteinuria are not characteristic in these other conditions.

The aetiology of FSGS is unknown although primary epithelial cell damage has been proposed. Most cases are idiopathic but there are several reported associations (Table 4.3), although the pathogenesis of the disease in these circumstances may be different. Genetic and racial factors may also be important, since FSGS in HIV-infected patients and in intravenous drug abusers occurs almost exclusively in Afro-Caribbeans. In HIV-associated FSGS the sclerosis is often global rather than segmental and the glomerular tufts are shrunken ('collapsing FSGS'). Tubuloreticular inclusions within endothelial cells are also characteristic. This pattern carries a grave prognosis and rapid progression to renal failure within four months is common with no response to treatment. When FSGS is associated with pathological obesity, an elevated GFR has sometimes been reported and a haemodynamic explanation has been proposed.

Until relatively recently, FSGS, especially in nephrotic patients, was considered to have a grim prognosis with a poor response to treatment and a high rate of progression to end stage renal failure (50% in 10 years). However, it is now recognized that up to 40% of both adults and children remit in response to steroids, and the five-year actuarial renal survival in responders exceeds 95%. Even in non-responders the renal survival is 55% at five years [14]. Banfi *et al.* reported that only 30% of patients treated with steroids and/or immunosuppressive drugs developed chronic renal failure after a mean follow-up of 75 months [15]. In this series some patients received prednisolone alone (either 1 mg/kg/day for eight weeks followed by a tapered dose or three i.v. pulses of methylprednisolone followed by 0.5 mg/kg/day). Others were treated with steroids plus an immunosuppressive drug (chlorambucil, cyclophosphamide or azathioprine) given concurrently or during alternate months. Patients who responded to treatment were less likely to develop progressive renal impairment. Others have reported similar experiences [16].

We therefore recommend that patients with FSGS should initially be treated with steroids, as for minimal change nephropathy. It is worth giving cyclophosphamide (dose and duration as for MCN) to those who respond but subsequently relapse, since a proportion can expect a sustained remission [17]. Steroid-unresponsive patients are unlikely to respond to cyclophosphamide and the decision to treat must be carefully considered for individual patients. Cyclosporin A is sometimes effective, as demonstrated in two controlled trials when administered for six months (150–200 mg/m$^2$/day or 5–6 mg/day). As in MCN, relapse is common following drug withdrawal. However, cyclosporin A may have a role in patients with refractory nephrotic syndrome and normal renal function.

### 4.5.3 IgA nephropathy (Berger's disease)

IgA nephropathy was first described just 26 years ago, but is now recognized as the most common form of glomerulonephritis, at least in developed countries. The typical presentation is with recurrent episodes of macroscopic haematuria in young men. Episodes occur at the same time (synpharyngitic) or several days after an upper respiratory tract infection, much earlier than in post-streptococcal nephritis. Presentation may be with persistent microscopic haematuria or proteinuria, and occasionally with nephrotic syndrome or rapidly progressive renal failure.

It is characterized histologically by mesangial hypercellularity and matrix expansion, with diffuse mesangial deposits of IgA, and often small amounts of IgG and complement C3. There are a number of diseases associated with this histological picture (Table 4.3). The pathogenesis is unknown, although up to 50% of patients have elevated IgA levels, and IgA deposition in normal skin may be seen. It has been suggested that infection at a mucosal site might trigger IgA disease although the IgA response is from bone marrow-derived cells. The deposits are mostly $IgA_1$ subclass, often associated with the J chain, and polymeric, and it is possible that they contain antigen(s), although this has not been convincingly demonstrated. Glomerular damage is believed to be complement-mediated [18], either following alternative pathway activation by IgA containing complexes or classical pathway activation by the smaller amounts of IgG that are usually also present. The pathogenic role of IgA is by no means established; for example in patients with advanced liver disease heavy IgA (but not IgG) deposits in the mesangium (and at other sites) are frequently seen although clinical evidence of renal disease is uncommon. Genetic factors have been implicated with a reported association with DR4 and DQw7, but not all studies have found this. There is also an intriguing association with certain polymorphisms at the IgA heavy chain switch region.

Although originally thought to follow a benign course, it is now clear that the development of end stage renal failure is a significant risk, occurring in about 15% of patients at 10 years and 20–30% or more at 20 years, with rapid deterioration in some patients. The presence of hypertension, nephrotic syndrome and persistent heavy haematuria or proteinuria is indicative of a poorer prognosis. Few controlled trials of therapy have been performed, and those that have are generally insufficiently 'powerful' to answer the question of whether treatment is effective. Steroids, cyclophosphamide, dipyridamole and warfarin have all been tried in patients with mild to moderate proteinuria. The published trials provide little convincing evidence of efficacy, except perhaps for long-term cyclophosphamide although this carries significant risks. Until patients who are likely to have an aggressive course can be predicted reliably, no specific treatment is recommended for the majority with low levels of proteinuria [19]. It is probably worth treating patients with severe nephrotic syndrome (affecting about 5%) with a limited course of prednisolone since they sometimes (especially those with mild histological lesions) respond like those with MCN [19, 20]. Patients with rapidly progressive disease and crescentic nephritis are another subgroup potentially worth treating with steroids and cytotoxic drugs. There are anecdotal reports and uncontrolled trials suggesting benefit from pulse steroids, cyclophosphamide and plasma exchange, alone or in combination. Finally, there have been recent reports of beneficial effects of low-antigen diets [21] and intravenous immunoglobulin [22] in patients with poor prognostic indicators, but further and longer-term studies are required. As in other glomerular diseases, cyclosporin A may reduce proteinuria, but there is no evidence that it has an effect on the natural history of the disease.

### 4.5.4 Mesangial proliferative GN (other types)

Mesangial proliferation is a relatively non-specific finding seen in many forms of glomerular disease. It has been observed as an isolated feature, without immune deposits in patients with proteinuria (which may be of nephrotic range) or haematuria. Some such patients present with haematuria (like those with IgA disease, but without deposits) and they are said to have a good prognosis. It has been proposed that patients presenting with nephrotic syndrome have a severe form of MCN. It seems more likely that this group is heterogeneous. More than half respond as if they had MCN, but up to one third subsequently develop features of FSGS and renal impairment.

Mesangial proliferation with IgM deposition is a relatively uncommon entity, sometimes called IgM nephropathy. Whether this should be considered a separate entity is not clear, particularly since small amounts of IgM are commonly found on immunostaining in various types of glomerular disease including MCN. Patients with this entity may be steroid responsive, steroid dependent or steroid resistant in fairly equal proportions [23] and some respond to cyclophosphamide. The actuarial renal survival has been estimated in one study as 80% and 64% at five and 10 years respectively. Nephrotic patients should be given a trial of steroids.

### 4.5.5 Membranous nephropathy

Membranous nephropathy (MN) is the commonest cause of nephrotic syndrome in adults. Pathologically it is characterized by relatively normal glomerular cellularity, but a thickened basement membrane. Fine granular peripheral deposits of immunoglobulin and complement are seen on immunostaining, with subepithelial deposits on EM. The aetiology is unknown although it is believed to have an immunological basis in view of the immune deposits found in the kidney and by analogy with the Heymann model of nephritis. The pathological appearances of this model are strikingly similar to human MN and are due to autoantibodies against a glycoprotein (gp330) found on tubular and glomerular epithelial cells. However, as yet, there is no convincing evidence implicating any particular antigen in man. Susceptibility to the disease is linked to the major histocompatibility complex (MHC) genes and the human disease is associated with HLA-DR3 in Europeans. A variety of target antigens have been proposed but, even in hepatitis B or tumour-associated disease, activation of the complement system with the generation of the membrane attack complex (C5b-9) is necessary for the development of experimental nephritis and it seems likely that it is also involved in human disease. There is some evidence that the measurement of C5b-9 in the urine may give an indication of ongoing damage, and it may help to identify patients who should be treated more aggressively (see below).

In the majority of patients, membranous nephropathy is idiopathic but a number of underlying causes and associations are known (Table 4.3). The incidence of occult malignancy in patients with MN is <2% overall, although this percentage increases with age. Lung cancer is the commonest associated tumour followed by carcinoma of the colon, rectum, kidney, breast and stomach. Opinion varies as to the extent to which patients should be investigated for malignancy. Investigations beyond a careful examination, biochemical screen and chest X-ray should probably be reserved for patients with additional symptoms or signs such as weight loss or anaemia. Removal of the tumour often results in remission of nephrotic syndrome and relapse has been associated with tumour recurrence.

Hepatitis B virus is the most commonly reported infective association of membranous nephropathy and is a particularly frequent association in children and in Americans. Most patients do not have overt liver disease but they often have detectable surface antigen, e-antigen and anticore antibodies. Although the e-antigen and cationic anti-e antibodies have been demonstrated in the glomeruli of affected patients, this is not proof of a primary aetiological role. Patients with hepatitis B virus-associated MN may have hypocomplementaemia which is unusual in idiopathic cases. Children generally do well, with spontaneous remission within 12 months of diagnosis in two thirds, and less than 5% develop renal failure. Adults fare less well with persistence of the disease being the rule, and up to one third develop progressive renal impairment or failure. Treatment with alpha-interferon and antiviral agents has been tried but with disappointing results. Steroids should not be used since they may allow enhanced viral replication and chronic active hepatitis. The outcome of membranous nephropathy associated with other infections is often favourable but depends on the infection. For instance, although antimalarial treatment usually results in remission of *Plasmodium*-associated nephrotic syndrome, renal impairment is often progressive. Drug-associated disease usually resolves following drug withdrawal.

A substantial proportion (20–30%) of patients with idiopathic membranous nephropathy (IMN) remit spontaneously, up to 40% have a partial remission or remain stable, and up to 30% develop progressive renal failure. A poor prognosis is more likely to be associated with male sex, age >50 years and heavy proteinuria, although impaired or deteriorating renal function is the best predictor of progressive disease [24, 25]. This natural history has made assessment of treatment regimens difficult.

Steroids alone may diminish proteinuria (by up to 30%) during treatment and a reduced rate of progression of renal failure was reported in one controlled trial, although this was not confirmed in two subsequent trials. However, treatment with steroids and cytotoxic drugs has been demonstrated to increase the likelihood of remission and preservation of renal function in controlled trials [26, 27]. Patients were given alternating months of steroids (0.5 mg/kg/day prednisolone following methylprednisolone 1 g i.v. for the first three days) and chlorambucil (0.2 mg/kg/day), while the control groups received placebo or steroids alone. This approach has become known as the 'Ponticelli' regimen after the principal author. In the first trial, at five years 22/30 treated versus 10/25 control patients were in remission and the renal function of those treated was better preserved. The second trial suggested that patients given chlorambucil and steroids were more likely to remit, but the difference was not statistically significant at four years. Furthermore, although there was a trend suggesting that the chlorambucil group had less decline of renal function, this also failed to reach statistical significance. Cyclophosphamide has been used in various regimens with reported success, but has not been subjected to adequate controlled trials.

Because of the natural history of the disorder and the potential toxicity of the Ponticelli regimen, most nephrologists are unwilling to treat aggressively all patients with membranous nephropathy. Ponticelli's trials specifically excluded patients with a creatinine level of >150 μmol/l. There have been a number of uncontrolled trials and anecdotal reports of steroid and cytotoxic drug regimens in patients with deteriorating renal function. Most have suggested that treatment reduces the rate of deterioration of renal function or even improves it, as well as reducing proteinuria. There has been one prospective randomized trial, in 26 patients, which failed to find a benefit. However, this may have been because the patients included had advanced disease, and they received only six pulses of cyclophosphamide. Our current recommendation is not to treat non-nephrotic patients with normal renal function. Those with impaired renal function in whom other causes have been excluded (especially renal vein thrombosis, interstitial nephritis and acute tubular necrosis) are offered the Ponticelli regimen. We believe patients should be treated as soon as the renal function begins to deteriorate. We are currently studying the effect of three months of cyclophosphamide followed by a change to azathioprine together with tapering steroids, in an open trial. Such treatments are probably also indicated for severely nephrotic patients, even if their renal function is preserved, because of the inherent risks of the nephrotic syndrome. In these cases, the clinician has to make a value judgement, balancing the risks versus the benefits of treatment.

Methods of assessing disease activity and identifying patients who are likely to respond to treatment would be undoubtedly valuable. Some groups recommend monitoring the disease by the measurement of urinary C5b-9 complement complex, which is believed play a role in the glomerular damage (see above) [28]. It is certainly elevated in some patients with IMN, especially those with progressive renal impairment. However, urinary C5b-9 may be present in other conditions (particularly FSGS and diabetic nephropathy) and its prognostic value remains to be established. Others have suggested that in the absence of evidence of complement activation and deposition (by immunostaining for complement components, especially C3c), the disease is immunologically inactive and unlikely to respond. As in other conditions causing nephrotic syndrome, cyclosporin A reduces proteinuria and it may be worth using cautiously in patients with severe proteinuria. There is little evidence to support a role of cyclosporin A modifying the natural history of IMN, although controlled trials to address this question and to establish safety are in progress. Intravenous immunoglobulin has also been used and some but not all reports have claimed a high degree of success; however, controlled trials are needed.

### 4.5.6 Mesangiocapillary glomerulonephritis (MCGN)

Idiopathic mesangiocapillary (or membranoproliferative) glomerulonephritis is relatively uncommon and occurs mainly in young adults or children. It may present with asymptomatic proteinuria and/or haematuria, nephrotic syndrome, acute or chronic renal failure, with hypertension being a common feature. Thirty per cent of patients present with rapidly deteriorating renal function.

The findings on LM are of global proliferation of mesangial cells with an increase in mesangial matrix and thickening of the glomerular basement membrane. In addition there is often infiltration with mononuclear cells, and the hypercellularity characteristically results in a lobular glomerular appearance. The two main types of MCGN are distinguished on the basis of the EM findings. Type I is characterized by subendothelial and mesangial immune deposits, while in Type II ('dense deposit disease') linear electron-dense deposits are found within the basement membrane. In addition the basement membrane characteristically has a double contour caused by immune deposits and interposition of mesangial cells. Crescents are seen, especially in patients presenting with rapidly progressive disease. There is a less well-defined Type III MCGN, characterized by some authors as having subepithelial deposits, but this entity is not widely recognized and will not therefore be addressed further.

This form of nephritis is associated with many conditions (Table 4.3). Type I MCGN is the commonest variety and is usually accompanied by depletion of complement via the classical pathway (with a low C4 and C3), possibly initiated by immune complexes. Worldwide, the majority of cases are associated with infectious and other diseases, though most cases in the West are labelled idiopathic. There is often a preceding respiratory illness, not proven to be streptococcal. Type II MCGN is often associated with C3 nephritic factor (C3NeF) which is an autoantibody to the C3-convertase, C3bBb. C3NeF stabilizes C3bBb, preventing dissociation by the inhibitory factor H, and alternative pathway complement activation (with a low C3 with normal C4) proceeds unrestrained. A proportion of these patients also have partial lipodystrophy, but the mechanisms resulting in glomerulonephritis or partial lipodystrophy are unknown.

Clearly, if an underlying cause, such as infection or chronic lymphatic leukaemia is identified, this should be treated appropriately and the outcome is then usually favourable. In patients with no apparent underlying cause, the probability of developing end stage renal failure is about 50% and 90% at 10 and 20 years respectively. However, spontaneous remission rates of up to 20% have been reported, making interpretation of uncontrolled trials difficult. Furthermore, most data relate to type I MCGN since type II is rare. A wide variety of treatments have been tried, mostly in uncontrolled settings, including steroids, cytotoxic drugs, anticoagulants, antiplatelet drugs and cyclosporin A [29].

The rationale for giving steroids is their anti-inflammatory effects. Most of the early reports were in children who were given quite large doses of steroids (starting at 2 mg/kg on alternate days) for prolonged periods of several years. These and other uncontrolled studies concluded that steroids were beneficial in terms of patient and renal survival, and severity of nephrotic syndrome. Repeat renal biopsies often revealed less proliferation compared with the initial biopsy. The only controlled trial included 80 children followed for a mean of 41 months. Although there was a modest reduction in incidence of renal failure there was a high morbidity from steroid side effects [30]. There have been no controlled trials of steroids in adults with MCGN but retrospective studies have failed to provide convincing support for a role for steroids [31].

Cytotoxic drugs have mostly been used in combination with steroids and often with other drugs. Although early uncontrolled studies reported that cyclophosphamide, prednisolone and dipyridamole were of benefit, these have not been confirmed by subsequent (but small) controlled trials. Antiplatelet and anticoagulant drugs were tried because abnormalities of platelets and platelet consumption are detectable in patients with MCGN as well as in experimental models of the disease. A reduced rate of decline of renal function was observed in a controlled trial of dipyridamole and aspirin in 40 patients at three and five years, although the effect had disappeared by 10 years [31]. There have been two controlled trials of warfarin therapy in addition to dipyridamole, with conflicting results, and there was a high incidence of bleeding complications.

A recent review of the published controlled trial data of treatment for MCGN failed to support claims for any form of specific treatment [31]. Therefore we do not generally recommend specific treatment of patients with MCGN. However, patients with a rapidly progressive course and crescentic nephritis (a subgroup in which controlled trials are unlikely to be organized) are often given a trial of prednisolone and cyclophosphamide, with variable results.

### 4.5.7 Diffuse proliferative glomerulonephritis

Acute glomerulonephritis following infection with certain strains of Group A streptococci is the archetypal example of this form of nephritis, but it is also seen following a variety of other bacterial, viral and parasitic infections. Although globally post-streptococcal nephritis remains a common entity (particularly in childhood), it is now relatively rare in the West. It is more likely to occur following skin rather than upper respiratory tract infection. Subclinical nephritis is much commoner than clinical disease which typically presents with the nephritic syndrome one to three weeks after an infection. The creatinine level is usually elevated, hypocomplementaemia with a low C3 and normal C4 (suggesting alternative pathway activation) is present in 90% of patients, and rheumatoid factor and cryoglobulins are commonly found. When associated with streptococcal infection, the anti-streptolysin O (ASO) titre is elevated in 75% of patients with upper respiratory tract infection but in only 40% of those with skin infection.

Pathologically it is characterized by enlarged hypercellular glomeruli with proliferation of endothelial and mesangial cells which often occlude the capillary lumina. There is infiltration with neutrophils and monocytes which may be intense, particularly early in the course of the disease, and red cells are frequently seen in Bowman's space. Extraglomerular proliferation and crescent formation may occur, but they are not common. The histology is sometimes described as 'acute diffuse endocapillary proliferative glomerulonephritis'. There is usually an accompanying interstitial nephritis and the intensity of this correlates better with reduced function than the glomerular disease. The findings on immunostaining are variable, but usually consist of fine granular deposits along the basement membrane and in the mesangium, of complement C3, properdin and terminal complement pathway components, together with immunoglobulins G and M. Ultrastructurally, subepithelial deposits or 'humps' are typical, although these may also occur in systemic lupus erythematosus (SLE) and endocarditis. Less prominent subendothelial and intramembranous deposits may also be seen.

The renal injury has traditionally been thought to be immune complex mediated, whether or not these are deposited or formed *in situ*. However, why the pathology should be confined to the kidney is unknown. Potential target streptococcal antigens have been the subject of intensive investigation. Probably the best candidate has been called 'endostreptosin', which is present in nephritogenic (and some other) strains and has been detected within affected glomeruli [32]. Significantly, however, this antigen has not been demonstrated to be present within the basement membrane-associated immune deposits. A second putative protein is antigenically related to streptokinase and has chemical characteristics similar to endostreptosin. A cationic proteinase with epitopes similar to those present in the glomerular basement membrane has also been proposed, especially since cationic proteins readily penetrate the anionic glomerular basement membrane. The immunopathology may be due to cross-reactivity between streptococcal and autoantigens. The role of complement components in mediating glomerular damage is unclear. Alternative pathway activation generates the terminal complement C5-9 complex which may be directly toxic. Furthermore anaphylatoxins and chemotaxins such as C3a and C5a may also contribute to initiation of the inflammatory response.

Although the nephritis almost certainly becomes apparent after eradication of the infecting organism, penicillin is usually recommended. Specific treatment directed against the immunological underlying process is not indicated, although clearly control of hypertension and fluid retention is important. The prognosis remains somewhat controversial with a reported long-term incidence of renal abnormalities ranging from $<5\%$ to 60%, although the latter figure is probably biased by more severely affected patients, and possibly by the inclusion of some patients with MCGN [33]. The prognosis appears to be worse in adults and in those presenting with the nephrotic syndrome, but overall less than 2% of patients develop end stage renal failure after 20 years. Nonetheless, long-term follow-up of these patients is recommended.

**Table 4.4** The main forms of crescentic glomerulonephritis

| |
|---|
| Antiglomerular basement membrane disease |
| Primary systemic vasculitis |
| Microscopic polyangiitis |
| Wegener's granulomatosis |
| Churg–Strauss syndrome |
| Systemic disorders |
| Systemic lupus erythematosus |
| Essential mixed cryoglobulinaemia |
| Henoch-Schönlein purpura |
| Behçet's syndrome |
| Rheumatoid disease |
| Primary glomerulonephritis |
| Mesangiocapillary glomerulonephritis |
| Mesangial IgA nephropathy |
| Membranous nephropathy |
| Infection-associated |
| Post-infectious glomerulonephritis |
| Endocarditis |
| Malignancy |
| Carcinoma |
| Lymphoma |
| Drugs |
| Hydralazine |
| Penicillamine |

### 4.5.8 Crescentic glomerulonephritis

This is a histopathological description of a disease in which the clinical features and diagnostic criteria depend upon the underlying cause of the condition [34] (Table 4.4). The rate of deterioration is variable but loss of renal function may occur over days or weeks, and progress to ESRF. Idiopathic rapidly progressive glomerulonephritis is an example of this condition, where no other primary disease is identified. There are however, grounds for considering this a forme fruste of vasculitis (Section 4.7). Treatment consists of aggressive immunosuppression, with or without plasma exchange. The details are discussed under the respective sections.

## 4.6 ANTIGLOMERULAR BASEMENT MEMBRANE (OR GOODPASTURE'S) DISEASE

This condition presents with rapidly progressive glomerulonephritis, often accompanied by lung haemorrhage, and is due to autoantibodies against the glomerular basement membrane (GBM). The target antigen has been demonstrated to be within the C-terminal end of the $\alpha$-3 chain of type IV collagen. The antibodies cross-react with lung basement membrane leading to pulmonary haemorrhage, especially in patients who smoke. The histological picture is of a crescentic nephritis, affecting a large proportion of glomeruli, usually at a similar stage of evolution. Immunofluorescence reveals linear staining of the GBM with immunoglobulins and sometimes complement, and circulating antibodies to the GBM can be detected.

Ultrastructurally, the GBM may be irregularly widened with occasional deposits and frequent breaks in the GBM. The damage is complement dependent although serum complement levels are generally normal. There is a striking association with HLA-DR2(w15) (present in 90% of patients), and a weaker association with HLA-DR4.

Untreated, all patients died rapidly from pulmonary haemorrhage or renal failure. The prognosis has improved following the introduction of plasma exchange and immunosuppression. Plasma exchange is used to remove anti-GBM antibodies, and is combined with steroids (prednisolone 1 mg/kg/day) and cyclophosphamide (2.5–3 mg/kg/day) to treat the glomerular inflammation and prevent resynthesis of antibody [35]. We recommend daily 4 l exchanges for 4.5% human albumin for 14 days or until anti-GBM antibody levels are suppressed (to background levels). Fresh frozen plasma should be given within three days of an invasive procedure (e.g. renal biopsy) to replace clotting factors. Although similar regimens are widely used and there is strong clinical impression of efficacy, they have not been subjected to controlled trials. One controlled study found only equivocal benefit from plasma exchange, but the numbers in this study were small (17 patients) and a non-intensive plasma exchange regimen ($1 \times 4$ l exchange every three days) was used. However, their data revealed that only 1/9 control patients compared with 4/8 plasma-exchanged patients showed improved renal function after treatment.

The majority of patients treated early (creatinine $<600\,\mu$mol/l) are likely to recover renal function, but early series suggested that oligo-anuric patients and those on dialysis before treatment rarely improved, even with plasma exchange. Treatment of such patients was therefore proposed only if they also had pulmonary haemorrhage. Subsequently, several groups have reported that occasional patients with advanced disease do respond – particularly if they are not anuric or if the biopsy reveals a low crescent score and/or low proportion of sclerosed glomeruli. For this reason, the risks of treatment in advanced cases should be assessed for each individual. An additional indication is to reduce anti-GBM antibody levels prior to renal transplantation if they do not spontaneously disappear. The long-term prognosis of successfully treated patients is good and recurrence of the disease, although described, is exceptional.

## 4.7 PRIMARY SYSTEMIC VASCULITIS

The primary vasculitides are a group of disorders associated with necrotizing inflammation of vessels in any organ of the body. One classification is based on the size of the affected vessels and the presence or absence of granulomata (Table 4.5). The clinical manifestations of the vasculitides are described elsewhere [36]. The small vessel vasculitides, including Wegener's granulomatosis (WG) and microscopic polyangiitis (MP), frequently cause a focal necrotizing glomerulonephritis (FNGN) with crescent formation and a similar picture is sometimes seen in Churg–Strauss syndrome. This is usually associated with the rapid development of renal failure, and the clinical description of rapidly progressive glomerulonephritis (RPGN) is sometimes used. Antineutrophil cytoplasmic antibodies (ANCA) are present in around 90% of cases of active small vessel vasculitis. A similar syndrome, occurring in the absence of extrarenal involvement and ANCA, is the so-called 'idiopathic' RPGN, although this probably represents renal-limited small vessel vasculitis. Assays for ANCA are now accepted as of diagnostic importance in vasculitis, but a positive ANCA may also occur in several other disorders. There are two principal patterns of ANCA on indirect immunofluorescence – cytoplasmic (c-ANCA) and perinuclear (p-ANCA). Most patients with Wegener's have c-ANCA, whereas p-ANCA predominate in microscopic polyangiitis and idiopathic RPGN.

**Table 4.5** Classification of primary vasculitis

| *Vessel size* | *No granulomata* | *With granulomata* |
|---|---|---|
| Small | Microscopic polyangiitis | Wegener's granulomatosis |
| Medium | Polyarteritis nodosa | Churg–Strauss syndrome |
| Large | Giant cell arteritis*<br>Takayasu's arteritis* | |

*Giant cell and Takayasu's arteritis are sometimes associated with granulomata.

The characteristic renal pathology is a focal segmental and necrotizing glomerulonephritis. Crescent formation is frequently seen, but overt vasculitis is less common and granulomata in WG occur only occasionally. There is usually evidence of lesions of differing ages in contrast to the findings in Goodpasture's disease. Early changes with focal segmental and mild extraglomerular proliferation coexist with cellular crescents compressing the glomerular tufts and sclerosed glomeruli. Neutrophils are often present and there is usually an extensive interstitial infiltrate. The presence of a large number of eosinophils may suggest the diagnosis of the Churg–Strauss syndrome. Immunostaining is mostly negative for immunoglobulins although fibrin is prominent, and electron-dense deposits are usually absent on EM.

The aetiology of the vasculitides is poorly understood and there are no good animal models. There is accumulating evidence, from clinical and *in vitro* studies, that ANCA are directly involved in pathogenesis. Clinically, levels of ANCA correlate with disease extent and activity and rising levels predict relapse. The major target antigens of c-ANCA and p-ANCA are proteinase 3 and myeloperoxidase respectively, although other targets of p-ANCA sera include elastase and lactoferrin. These enzymes are predominantly located within neutrophil granules but have been detected on the surface of cells. There are reports that ANCA may activate neutrophils to release destructive lysosomal contents, may induce neutrophil cytotoxicity to endothelial cells, and may directly react with target antigens on endothelial cells.

The standard therapy for vasculitis is a combination of steroids and an alkylating agent. Our regimen consists of prednisolone 60 mg/day, tapering rapidly to 20 mg/day and more slowly thereafter, and oral cyclophosphamide (2.5 mg/kg/day, or 2 mg/kg/day if >55 years) for three months. After three months the cyclophosphamide is substituted by azathioprine (2 mg/kg/day) which is continued for at least a year after remission because of the tendency to relapse. A large number of successfully treated patients using a similar regimen, but maintaining therapy with cyclophosphamide until they have been in remission for more than one year, have recently been described from the National Institutes of Health [37]. The regimen that we recommend is associated with a similar incidence of relapse, but with a lower incidence of the long-term morbidity associated with cyclophosphamide, including urothelial toxicity and cancer, gonadal failure, myelodysplasia and haematological malignancies. Relapses generally respond rapidly to re-induction with cyclophosphamide, and some patients need to be maintained on this long-term.

Immunosuppressive drugs can be discontinued in a proportion of patients, but relapses can occur several years later. There has been a suggestion that long-term full-dose co-trimoxazole might reduce the risk of recurrence. However, adequate controlled trial data are not available, and the benefit seems to be restricted to patients with localized upper respiratory disease with few systemic features.

The role for plasma exchange is more controversial. It was introduced because of the then current belief that immune complexes played a pathogenic role in RPGN, and in view of the successful treatment of anti-GBM disease. Initial, uncontrolled reports from several centres suggested benefit from plasma exchange. We have reviewed our own data together with ten uncontrolled series of patients with RPGN (excluding, where possible, anti-GBM disease, SLE, Henoch–Schönlein purpura, infection related and underlying primary glomerulonephritis) treated with plasma exchange [38]. Improvement in renal function was reported to have occurred in 79% overall (range 60–100%) even in those patients on dialysis or with very advanced renal failure. The initial improvement was often maintained medium or long-term. These results compare favourably with 78 'historical control' patients with RPGN who received various combinations of cytotoxic drugs and steroids, but not plasma exchange or pulse methylprednisolone [39]. Three quarters of our 78 patients presenting on dialysis recovered independent renal function by two months, and most maintained function or improved further between two months and one year, comparing favourably with published data on patients treated with cytotoxic drugs alone [39].

Several randomized trials of plasma exchange have been reported. The smaller of these was a multicentre study, which included various types of RPGN treated with a variety of drugs and a non-intensive plasma exchange regimen. A larger proportion of patients receiving plasma exchange improved by four weeks, but no statistically significant benefit could be demonstrated [40]. Another trial involved 48 patients with vasculitis-associated or idiopathic RPGN but excluded other known causes. Patients were stratified for renal function on entry and were randomized to receive a standard drug regimen with or without plasma exchange. Patients who were not on dialysis did well in both treatment groups, but those on dialysis were significantly more likely to recover renal function if they received plasma exchange [41]. However, the number of patients was too small for adequate comparison of long-term outcome. A third trial involved 32 similar patients, but the treatment protocol differed in that pulse methylprednisolone was the initial steroid therapy in both arms of the trial. The results confirmed that plasma exchange provided no additional benefit over drug therapy in non-dialysis-dependent patients [42]. A larger proportion of those on dialysis recovered renal function after plasma exchange, but numbers were too small for adequate analysis. Pooling the results of dialysis-dependent patients from all three trials, 78% improved following plasma exchange with immunosuppression, compared with 42% receiving immunosuppressive drugs alone.

Thus, the evidence supporting a role for plasma exchange in ANCA-associated RPGN or focal necrotizing GN is still not clear-cut, but it seems likely that dialysis-dependent patients are the only group who may benefit. Our practice is to plasma exchange 60 ml/kg (4 l for the average patient) seven to 10 times over two weeks. Cytotoxic chemotherapy should generally be given in these situations whether or not plasma exchange is available. A trial comparing plasma exchange with pulse methylprednisolone is in progress. Our indications for plasma exchange can be summarized as follows:

1. dialysis-dependent renal failure;
2. severe systemic disease unresponsive to drugs;
3. when cytotoxic treatment has to be temporarily withdrawn because of myelotoxicity in patients with uncontrolled disease.

## 4.8 SYSTEMIC LUPUS ERYTHEMATOSUS

Lupus nephritis takes many forms. The World Health Organization (WHO) classification describes five types: I – minimal change; II – mesangial GN; III – focal proliferative GN; IV – diffuse proliferative GN (of varying severity from mild proliferation to marked proliferation with inflammation, fibrinoid necrosis, haematoxylin bodies, wire loops and crescents); V – membranous nephropathy. The problems with this classification are firstly that it is purely descriptive of the predominant type of glomerular involvement, without reference to the other changes, and secondly that many patients have renal lesions combining different WHO types. Activity/chronicity scores take into account tubular, interstitial, vascular and chronic (presumably irreversible) changes, and may correlate better with clinical outcome. There is controversy regarding the value of renal biopsy, but we believe that it is essential in patients who have significant renal involvement to define the pathology and plan treatment.

Renal involvement may be the primary indication for therapy and much circumstantial and some trial data suggest that steroids and cytotoxic drugs are effective. However, because of the heterogeneity of lupus nephritis, trials are difficult to design and interpret, and controlled data are lacking, although few dispute that treatment of diffuse proliferative disease with cytotoxic drugs and steroids greatly reduces the incidence of renal failure [43]. Management needs to be considered in the different clinical settings of acute, severe disease and more chronic indolent nephritis.

Acute severe disease with impaired or deteriorating renal function, and a diffuse proliferative nephritis with or without crescents, may be treated with oral prednisolone (1 mg/kg/day) and cyclophosphamide (2 mg/kg/day) for about 12 weeks, followed by a change to azathioprine, while the prednisolone dose is tapered. The use of monthly pulses of cyclophosphamide (10–15 mg/kg) together with oral steroids is an alternative approach [44]. The role of other therapies, including pulse methylprednisolone and plasma exchange, is controversial. Several studies have suggested that plasma exchange is not beneficial, but these have specifically excluded the most ill patients with high creatinine levels who, anecdotally at least, are those most likely to respond. There is a controlled trial in progress which should answer the question of efficacy in this group. Until the results are available we feel that it is reasonable to manage fulminant disease, and patients unable to receive cyclophosphamide, with plasma exchange and/or pulse methylprednisolone, although the latter may be associated with severe hypertension.

The choice of longer-term maintenance treatment is controversial with little helpful data in the literature. Some nephrologists would never stop azathioprine and low-dose steroids, but we believe that it is reasonable to withdraw these drugs, particularly in young patients, unless several severe relapses of disease have been suffered. Patients with indolent disease or recurrent relapse are currently managed with monthly pulses of cyclophosphamide for six months, followed by three two-monthly pulses. After one year most such patients are converted to azathioprine and managed as above.

All patients are carefully followed up in the clinic, and encouraged to seek an immediate appointment if they have concerns about lupus activity (and many patients are sensitive to early symptoms). Clinic assessment involves symptomatic enquiry and measurement of laboratory parameters including complements, DNA binding, antinuclear antibody titre, ESR, C-reactive protein immunoglobulins, full blood count, renal function and urinary sediment. However, treatment should only be escalated with evidence of clinical disease, and the use of substantially increased steroids and immunosuppression reserved for major organ involvement (not generally skin or joint exacerbation).

There is little guidance in the literature regarding treatment of mild focal proliferative glomerulonephritis. Depending on its severity, we use prednisolone alone or in combination with azathioprine. Membranous lupus nephropathy generally responds poorly to steroids, azathioprine and cyclophosphamide, although some patients respond to a four to eight week course of prednisolone 45–60 mg/day. Cyclosporin A may also be effective, but dose reduction usually results in relapse and long-term usage requires careful consideration because of the potential risks.

## 4.9 HENOCH–SCHÖNLEIN PURPURA

Henoch–Schönlein purpura (HSP) is a small vessel vasculitis associated with immune complexes containing IgA. It typically affects children under 10 years, and is characterized by a purpuric rash around the ankles, buttocks and elbows, arthritis, abdominal pain and glomerulonephritis. Occasionally, the nervous system, heart or lungs may be affected. The renal disease usually presents with haematuria and proteinuria with hypertension, fluid retention and an elevated creatinine, but the nephrotic syndrome may occasionally occur. The renal pathology is similar or identical to that in mesangial IgA disease, although biopsy is usually unnecessary in children presenting with the typical clinical features. Mesangial proliferation may be both segmental and focal when mild, and when florid may have a 'pseudo-MCGN' pattern. Crescent formation in a proportion of glomeruli is not uncommon, especially in patients with macroscopic haematuria. Immunofluorescence and EM in HSP are similar to those found in IgA nephropathy. Interstitial disease and hypertensive changes are common although renal vasculitis is rare.

The pattern, subclass and nature of the deposited IgA are similar to those seen in IgA nephropathy, and similar aetiological hypotheses have been suggested. It is unknown why some patients develop renal disease alone while others have an associated vasculitis. A genetic basis for a difference has been suggested but is unlikely, since there is a case report of both occurring in one child two years apart. Furthermore the simultaneous development of HSP in one monozygotic twin and IgA nephropathy in the other, following a proven adenovirus infection, has also been described.

Most patients (both children and adults) recover completely with normal renal function, although up to 15% may have persisting urinary abnormalities. Occasional patients develop rapidly progressive renal failure and this is usually associated with florid crescents on biopsy and macroscopic haematuria. Patients with haematuria but no proteinuria usually follow a benign course, but in others presenting features are not reliable indicators of long-term outcome. Several studies suggest that long-term outcome is best predicted by the renal function more than one year after onset. For example, in the series reported by Bunchman *et al.*, progression to chronic renal failure was inevitable in patients with a creatinine clearance (CrCl) of $<80\,ml/min/1.73m^2$ three years after presentation, while none with a CrCl of $>110\,ml/min/1.73m^2$ progressed [45].

No treatment has been demonstrated to affect the natural history of HSP. Steroids, cytotoxic therapy, plasma exchange and high-dose pulse methylprednisolone have been tried in patients with rapidly progressive disease with crescents on biopsy but with equivocal results, and no controlled trial has been performed. However, the rarity of these patients makes a trial difficult to organize. Moderately strong circumstantial evidence supporting a role for pulse methylprednisolone has been presented by the Guy's group in children with progressive renal impairment or >75% crescents, although plasma exchange may be equally effective [46].

## 4.10 CRYOGLOBULINAEMIA

Cryoglobulins are immunoglobulins which precipitate from serum in the cold, and may be classified on the basis of their content. Type I cryoglobulinaemia consists of a monoclonal immunoglobulin of unknown specificity, and is often associated with myeloma or leukaemia. In type II cryoglobulinaemia, a monoclonal antibody (usually IgM$\kappa$) with rheumatoid factor activity appears in the circulation and forms complexes with autologous normal immunoglobulin. The clinical manifestations of a purpuric vasculitic skin rash, arthralgia, peripheral neuropathy (often mononeuritis multiplex) and glomerulonephritis, are associated with deposition of immune complexes in the vessels and glomeruli. Whether these are formed *in situ* or deposited from the circulation is unclear. The aetiology in most cases is obscure, though a proportion of patients have, or develop, lymphoma.

The renal disease is most commonly a type I mesangiocapillary glomerulonephritis, but differs from the 'idiopathic' variety in a number of ways. A monocytic infiltrate is commonly prominent and large amorphous intraluminal deposits which are PAS-positive, sometimes referred to as 'intraluminal thrombi', are present. These consist of IgG and IgM and are believed to be deposited cryoglobulin. EM may reveal characteristic 'fingerprint' subendothelial deposits. Mesangio-proliferative, diffuse and focal segmental glomerulunephritis have also been described in association with mixed essential cryoglobulinaemia (MEC).

MEC is the classic example of an immune complex-mediated disease in which the antigen (IgG) is known. Deposition of cryoglobulin complexes occurs in the vessels and in the glomeruli, where they are presumed to activate the classical complement pathway explaining the characteristic low C4 with low/normal C3. Complement activation induces an inflammatory response. There have been two recent reports suggesting a strong association with hepatitis C virus (HCV) exposure with the presence of anti-HCV antibodies. These antibodies, perhaps not surprisingly, have been found in the polyclonal component of the cryoprecipitate together with HCV-DNA. These data, although of great interest, do not prove that HCV is a causative agent and it is possible that, since many MEC patients are treated with plasma exchange, they may have been exposed to HCV in unscreened plasma used as replacement fluid.

Irrespective of the mechanism, because of their predominantly intravascular distribution, circulating complexes and the IgM monoclonal rheumatoid factor are efficiently removed by plasma exchange. However, the rate of recurrence of cryoglobulins (with or without other therapy) following plasma exchange is highly variable, and cryoglobulin levels do not always correlate with symptoms [47].

Type III cryoglobulinaemia consists of polyclonal mixed immunoglobulin, often associated with hyperglobulinaemia and present in a wide variety of infective, inflammatory and neoplastic conditions. It is often an epiphenomenon and usually does not cause symptoms separate from the underlying condition, but may do so. In these circumstances plasma exchange would seem a logical adjunct to therapy.

There have been many reports of the benefit of plasma exchange in MEC, using a variety of treatment regimens [47], but there are no published controlled series. Plasma exchange has been used alone, or in combination with immunosuppressive drugs, for the maintenance of chronic 'stable' disease and for acute therapy in cases with rapidly progressive renal failure. Many clinical features, particularly Raynaud's phenomenon, skin lesions and arthralgia, are rapidly relieved following a small number of plasma exchanges. Patients vary considerably in the rate of re-synthesis of cryoglobulins and recurrence of symptoms; in some, intermittent plasma exchange (for example one or two treatments every month) may give symptomatic improvement, while in others symptoms recur rapidly. Improvement in renal function, an important marker of prognosis, has been reported in some patients treated with plasma exchange and immunosuppressive drugs, although long-term benefit has not been convincingly demonstrated. In view of the lack of controlled data and variability of the disease, clear-cut guidelines for the use of plasma exchange are not possible. Our practice is to assess each patient individually, and tailor treatment accordingly. Patients are given an initial trial of five 4 l plasma exchanges with steroids and cytotoxic drugs (in patients with severe disease). Maintenance management, including frequency of plasma exchange, then depends on the clinical response and rate of cryoglobulin resynthesis.

## REFERENCES


1. Madio, M.P. (1990) Renal biopsy. *Kidney Int.*, **38**, 529–43.
2. Williams, D.G. and Peters, D.K. (1987) Glomerulonephritis and renal manifestations of systemic disease, in *Oxford Textbook of Medicine* (eds D.J. Weatherall, J.G.G. Ledingham, and D.A. Warrell), Oxford University Press, Oxford, pp. 18.36–51.

3. Klahr, S. (1991) Chronic renal failure: management. *Lancet*, **338**, 423–7.
4. Klahr, S., Levey, A.S., Beck, G.J. *et al.* (1994) The effects of dietary protein restriction and blood pressure control on the progression of chronic renal disease. *N. Engl. J. Med.*, **330**, 877–84.
5. Lewis, E.J., Hunsicker, L.G., Bain, R.P. and Rohde, R.D. (1993) The effect of angiotensin-converting enzyme inhibition on diabetic nephropathy. *N. Engl. J. Med.*, **329**, 1456.
6. Bernard, D.B. (1988) Extrarenal complications of the nephrotic syndrome. *Kidney Int.*, **33**, 1184.
7. Fouque, D., Laville, M., Boissel, J.P. *et al.* (1992) Controlled low protein diets in chronic renal insufficiency: Meta-analysis. *Br. Med. J.*, **304**, 216.
8. Arbeitsgemeinschaft für Pädiatrische Nephrologie (1988) Short versus standard prednisolone therapy for initial treatment of idiopathic nephrotic syndrome in children. *Lancet*, **1**, 380.
9. Trompeter, R.S. (1986) Minimal change nephrotic syndrome and cyclophosphamide. *Arch. Dis. Child.*, **61**, 727–9.
10. Arbeitsgemeinschaft für Pädiatrische Nephrologie (1987) Cyclophosphamide treatment of steroid-dependent nephrotic syndrome: comparison of eight weeks with 12 weeks course. *Arch. Dis. Child.*, **62**, 1102–6.
11. Niaudet, D., Broyer, M. and Habib, R. (1991) Treatment of idiopathic nephrotic syndrome with cyclosporin A in children. *Clin. Nephrol.*, **35**, 831–6.
12. Nolasco, F., Cameron, J.S., Heywood, E.F. *et al.* (1986) Adult-onset minimal change nephrotic syndrome: a long term follow-up. *Kidney Int.*, **29**, 1215–23.
13. Melocoton, T.L., Vanni, E.S., Cohen, A.S. and Fine, R.N. (1991) Long-term cyclosporin A treatment of steroid-resistant nephrotic and steroid-dependent nephrotic syndrome. *Am. J. Kidney Dis.*, **18**, 583.
14. Pei, Y., Cattran, D., Delmore, T. *et al.* (1987) Evidence suggesting undertreatment in adults with idiopathic focal segmental glomerulosclerosis. Regional glomerulonephritis registry study. *Am. J. Med.*, **82**, 938–44.
15. Banfi, G., Moriggi, M., Sabadini, E. *et al.* (1991) The impact of prolonged immunosuppression on the outcome of idiopathic focal-segmental glomerulosclerosis with nephrotic syndrome in adults. A collaborative retrospective study. *Clin. Nephrol.*, **36**, 53.
16. Korbet, S.M., Schwartz, M.M. and Lewis, E.J. (1986) The prognosis of focal segmental glomerular sclerosis of adulthood. *Medicine*, Baltimore, **65**, 304.
17. Siegal, N.J., Gaudio, K.M., Krassner, L.S. *et al.* (1981) Steroid-dependent nephrotic syndrome in children: histopathology and relapses after cyclophosphamide treatment. *Kidney Int.*, **19**, 454–9.
18. Emancipator, S.N. (1990) Immunoregulatory factors in the pathogenesis of IgA nephropathy. *Kidney Int.*, **38**, 1216.
19. Schena, F.P., Montenegro, M. and Scivittaro, V. (1990) Meta-analysis of randomised controlled trials in patients with primary IgA nephropathy (Berger's disease). *Nephrol. Dial. Transplant.*, suppl. 1, 47–52.
20. Mustonen, J., Pasternack, A. and Rantala, A. (1983) The nephrotic syndrome in IgA glomerulo-nephritis: response to corticosteroid therapy. *Clin. Nephrol.*, **20**, 172–6.
21. Ferri, C., Puccini, R., Langombardo, G. *et al.* (1993) Low-antigen-content diet in the treatment of patients with IgA nephropathy. *Nephrol. Dial. Transplant.*, **8**, 1193.
22. Rostoker, G., Desvaux-Belghiti, D., Pilatte, Y. *et al.* (1994) High-dose immunoglobulin therapy for several IgA nephropathy and Henoch–Schönlein purpura. *Ann. Intern. Med.*, **120**, 476.

23. Border, W.A. (1988) Distinguishing minimal change disease from mesangial disorders. *Kidney Int.*, **34**, 419.
24. Donadio, J.V. Jr, Torres, V.E., Velosa, J.A. *et al.* (1988) Idiopathic membranous nephropathy: The natural history of untreated patients. *Kidney Int.*, **33**, 708.
25. Schieppati, A., Mosconi, L., Perna, A. *et al.* (1993) Prognosis of untreated patients with idiopathic membranous nephropathy. *N. Engl. J. Med.*, **329**, 85.
26. Ponticelli, C., Zucchelli, P., Imbasciati, E. *et al.* (1984) A controlled trial of methylprednisolone and chlorambucil in idiopathic membranous nephropathy. *N. Engl. J. Med.*, **310**, 946–50.
27. Ponticelli, C., Zucchelli, P., Passerini, P. *et al.* (1989) A randomized trial of methylprednisolone and chlorambucil in idiopathic membranous nephropathy. *N. Engl. J. Med.*, **320**, 8.
28. Brenchley, P.E., Coupes, B., Short, C.D. *et al.* (1992) Urinary C3dg and C5b-9 indicate active immune disease in human membranous nephropathy. *Kidney Int.*, **41**, 933.
29. D'Amico, G. (1992) Influence of clinical and histological features on actuarial renal survival in adult patients with idiopathic IgA nephropathy, membranous nephropathy and membranoproliferative glomerulonephritis: survey of the recent literature. *Am. J. Kidney Dis.*, **20**, 315–23.
30. Tarshish, P., Berstein, J., Tobin, J. and Edelmann, C. (1992) Treatment of mesangiocapillary glomerulonephritis with alternate-day prednisone: a report of the international study of kidney disease in children. *Pediatr. Nephrol.*, **6**, 123.
31. Donadio, J.V. Jr and Offord, K.P. (1989) Reassessment of treatment results in membranoproliferative glomerulonephritis, with emphasis on life-table analysis. *Am. J. Kidney Dis.*, **14**, 445.
32. Cronin, W., Deal, H., Azadegan, A. and Lange, K. (1989) Endostreptosin: isolation of the probable immunogen of acute post-streptococcal glomerulonephritis. *Clin. Exp. Immunol.*, 198.
33. Tejani, A. and Ingulli, E. (1990) Poststreptococcal glomerulonephritis. Current clinical and pathologic concepts. *Nephron*, **55**, 1.
34. Rees, A.J. and Cameron, J.S. (1992) Crescentic glomerulonephritis, in *Oxford Textbook of Clinical Nephrology*, Vol. 1 (eds J.S. Cameron, A.M. Davison, J.-P. Grünfeld *et al.*), Oxford University Press, Oxford, pp. 318–38.
35. Turner, A.N. and Rees, A.J. (1992) Antiglomerular basement membrane disease, in *Oxford Textbook of Clinical Nephrology*, Vol. 1 (eds J.S. Cameron, A.M. Davison, J.-P. Grünfeld *et al.*), Oxford University Press, Oxford, pp. 438–56.
36. Gaskin, G. and Pusey, C.D. (1992) Systemic vasculitis, in *Oxford Textbook of Clinical Nephrology*, Vol. 1 (eds J.S. Cameron, A.M. Davison, J.-P. Grünfeld *et al.*), Oxford University Press, Oxford, pp. 612–36.
37. Hoffman, G.S., Kerr, G.S., Leavitt, R.Y. *et al.* (1992) Wegener's granulomatosis: An analysis of 158 patients. *Ann. Intern. Med.*, **116**, 488.
38. Mason, P.D. and Pusey, C.D. (1993) Plasma exchange in immunological diseases, in *Clinical Aspects of Immunology*, 5th edn (eds P. Lachmann, D.K. Peters, F.S. Rosen and M.W. Walport), Blackwell Scientific, Oxford.
39. Couser, W.G. (1988) Rapidly progressive glomerulonephritis. Classification, pathogenic mechanisms and therapy. *Am. J. Kidney Dis.*, **11**, 449.
40. Glockner, W.M., Sieberth, H.G., Wichmann, H.E. *et al.* (1988) Plasma exchange and immunosuppression in rapidly progressive nephritis: a controlled, multi-center study. *Clin. Nephrol.*, **29**, 1.

41. Pusey, C.D., Rees, A.J., Evans, D.J. *et al.* (1991) Plasma exchange in focal necrotizing glomerulonephritis without anti-GBM antibodies. *Kidney Int.*, **40**, 757.
42. Cole, E., Cattran, D., Magil, A. *et al.* (1992) A prospective randomized trial of plasma exchange as additive therapy in idiopathic crescentic glomerulonephritis. *Am. J. Kidney Dis.*, **20**, 261.
43. Glassock, R.J., Cohen, A.H., Adler, S.G. and Ward, H.J. (1991) Secondary glomerular disease: systemic lupus erythematosus, in *The kidney*, 4th edn (eds B.M. Brenner and F.C. Rector), W.B. Saunders, Philadelphia, pp. 1280–98.
44. Austin, H.A. III, Klippel, J.H., Balow, J.B. *et al.* (1986) Therapy of lupus nephritis: controlled trial of prednisolone and cytotoxic drugs. *N. Engl. J. Med.*, **314**, 614–24.
45. Bunchman, T.E., Mauer, S.M., Sibley, R.K. and Vernier, R.L. (1988) Anaphylactoid purpura; characteristics of 16 patients who progressed to renal failure. *Pediatr. Nephrol.*, **2**, 393–7.
46. Haycock, G.B. (1992) The nephritis of Henoch–Schönlein purpura, in *Oxford Textbook of Clinical Nephrology* Vol. 1 (eds J.S. Cameron, A.M. Davison, J.-P. Grünfeld *et al.*), Oxford University Press, Oxford, pp. 595–612.
47. Frankel, A.H., Singer, D.R.J., Winearls, C.G. *et al.* (1992) Type II essential mixed cryoglobulinaemia: presentation, treatment and outcome in 13 patients. *Q. J. Med.*, **82**, 101–24.

# 5

# Urinary tract infection and pyelonephritis

*R. Maskell*

Urinary tract infection (UTI) affects people of both sexes and all ages throughout the world. Despite the advantages in diagnosis and therapy made over the past fifty years it still presents a continuing problem to patients, doctors and laboratories. With better understanding of the pathogenesis of the condition have come opportunities for prevention, both of the troublesome, but relatively benign, symptoms that affect so many people, and also of the serious renal damage that can occur in a minority of patients. At present, infection and infection-related disease are among the few preventable causes of end stage renal failure. Estimates of the proportion of patients coming onto renal replacement therapy (RRT) programmes in whom the primary renal disease was infection-related vary. From a figure of about 20% when such figures were first collected [1] it has now fallen in some countries, in particular those such as Sweden who have highly developed programmes for identification and management of children with vesicoureteric reflux (VUR) [2].

UTI accounts for the use of very large quantities of antibacterial agents. It is only slowly being recognized, however, that their therapeutic advantages must be balanced against the disadvantages. Induction of bacterial resistance and disruption of the balance of commensal flora are of considerable relevance to the pathogenesis and management of UTI. In a condition usually caused by commensal organisms and which, by its nature, tends to be recurrent, these properties are particularly important.

*Renal Disease.* Edited by G. Venkat Raman. Published in 1998 by Chapman & Hall, London. ISBN 0 412 45700 8.

Nephrologists have not always concerned themselves with UTI. At the time when it was believed to be a common cause of renal failure, some undertook combined studies with laboratories with the purpose of improving diagnosis and identifying patients at risk. With the passage of time came the realization that the prevention of renal failure from UTI rested mainly with paediatricians, working closely with general practitioners. Furthermore, the increasing financial pressures on microbiology laboratories and the emergence of newer infections resulted in a diminution of laboratory interest in UTI and the introduction of cheaper and less reliable diagnostic techniques. The adult patient with UTI is now likely to be referred to a urologist if the general practitioner needs further advice, and surgical methods of investigation and management are often employed. An attempt will be made in this chapter to assess the role of the medical management of UTI, and to make the case that this is an important function of the clinical nephrologist.

## 5.1 CLASSIFICATION OF URINARY TRACT INFECTION

So far as is known at present no microorganisms are present in the normal urinary tract, or its communicating structures, above the level of the distal urethra. The lower one third of the urethra is colonized by commensal flora made up of several bacterial species which are known, in the female, to vary at different stages of life. The flora of the male urethra has not been extensively studied but what evidence there is suggests that it is made up of several species of Gram positive bacteria. The function of this commensal flora is to protect against invasion by potentially pathogenic organisms from the bowel, perineum or, in males, the preputial sac. The mechanisms of this protective function include production of inhibitors, coaggregation of commensal species with each other or with potential pathogens and colonization of epithelial surfaces and competition with potential pathogens for sites of adhesion. In the rare event of infection via the bloodstream, or when, for whatever reason, the protective mechanisms against ascending infection break down, microorganisms gain access to the urinary tract and sometimes thence to its communicating structures.

It is convenient to divide UTI into upper tract infection, involving the kidneys, and lower tract infection, involving the bladder, urethra, prostate or paraurethral glands of the female. It will become apparent, however, that this distinction is sometimes difficult to make clinically, that non-invasive definitive tests are lacking and that, in view of the dynamic nature of its pathogenesis, infection may be present at different levels at different times in the natural history of the condition.

## 5.2 UPPER TRACT INFECTION

Microorganisms may reach the kidney via the bloodstream or by direct inoculation during an invasive procedure. More commonly, however, they gain access by the ascending route from the bladder.

### 5.2.1 Haematogenous infection

The types of haematogenous urinary tract infection are listed in Table 5.1. Neonatal haematogenous urinary infection, in which clinical evidence of infection and a positive blood culture precede a positive urine culture, occurs more commonly in boys than in girls.

Although *Salmonella* is usually excreted without damage to the urinary tract the presence of this organism in renal tissue can rarely precipitate a severe acute glomerulonephritis.

Tuberculous infection of the urinary tract is invariably blood-borne. Some patients who present with urinary tuberculosis have a history of previous infection elsewhere in the body, but in others the primary focus has healed and remains undetected. Trends, both upward and downward, in the incidence of tuberculous infection affect the incidence of urinary tuberculosis after a lag period. In 1980 it was reported to account for 1% of patients reaching renal replacement programmes. Even with the increasing incidence of tuberculous infection in recent years effective chemotherapy should ensure that serious urinary tract damage is prevented. The infecting organism is usually *Mycobacterium tuberculosis*, but there have been occasional isolations of *M. bovis* and *M. fortuitum*. Renal changes in the untreated case include the formation of

**Table 5.1** Haematogenous renal infections

| | | |
|---|---|---|
| **Secondary to bacteraemia** | Neonatal | *Escherichia coli*<br>Group B streptococci |
| | Other | *Staphylococcus aureus*<br>*Mycobacterium* spp<br>*Salmonella* spp<br>*Brucella* spp |
| **Secondary to viraemia** | | Probably many viruses<br>e.g. hanta virus, cytomegalovirus<br>Polyoma virus |
| **Secondary to fungal infection** | | *Candida* spp |

caseating abscesses in the cortex and medulla and, rarely, an interstitial nephritis. When infection spreads to the renal pelvis, ureters and bladder, obstruction due to granulation tissue or fibrosis develops and renal function is gradually lost.

In 20–50% of cases of brucellosis urine cultures may be positive for the organism [3], but pathological changes have only rarely been reported. Renal infection occurring in the course of *Staphylococcus aureus* or *Candida* septicaemia can result in the formation of multiple renal abscesses which, if not successfully treated, may progress to perinephric abscess. This, however, is more likely to occur as a result of infection by the ascending route [4]. Rarer now than in the pre-antibiotic era, renal abscess usually occurs in adults, but there have been reports of the condition in the neonatal period and in young children.

Viruses enter the bloodstream in the course of many viral illnesses, including measles, mumps, cytomegalovirus and Coxsackie infections. Indeed, viraemia is such a prominent feature of viral infection that urinary excretion of viruses probably occurs far more often than is generally realized. Urinary symptoms are rare; the condition is self-limiting, and few studies have been undertaken. Rarely renal function may be acutely and temporarily deranged by exotic viruses, such as the Hanta virus, which was first identified in the Far East. More recently 'epidemic nephropathy', caused by different strains of the same virus, has been described in Continental Europe, with the vole identified as the probable vector.

### 5.2.2 Pathogenesis of ascending infection

Table 5.2 lists the bacteria known to infect the urinary tract by the ascending route. With few exceptions they are commensal in sites adjacent to the urethral orifice – the bowel, distal urethra and perineum – and the factors that determine their ability to gain access to the urinary tract will be considered later. Ascent of infection from bladder to kidneys occurs in only a small minority of patients. Some of the determining factors are well understood, others less so. At present there is no definitive test of renal infection other than culture of urine collected by ureteric catheter – an invasive procedure which is not undertaken lightly. Indirect evidence derives from the clinical features of acute renal infection, non-specific tests such as for C-reactive protein in the blood and the results of renal imaging. In the past, the latter has usually been confined to retrospective findings of the consequences of infection. However, the advent of computerized tomographic (CT) scanning, ultrasonography and gallium scanning have facilitated earlier accurate diagnosis, in particular of renal and perinephric abscesses.

There seems little doubt that the most important determinant of

**Table 5.2** Organisms that infect the urinary tract via the ascending route

| | |
|---|---|
| **Gram negative bacilli** | *Escherichia coli*<br>*Proteus* spp<br>*Klebsiella* spp<br>Other members of the Enterobacteriaceae<br>*Pseudomonas* spp<br>*Haemophilus influenzae*<br>*Acinetobacter* spp |
| **Gram positive bacilli** | *Lactobacillus* spp<br>*Corynebacterium* spp |
| **Gram positive cocci** | *Staphylococcus aureus*<br>*Staphylococcus epidermidis*<br>*Staphylococcus saprophyticus*<br>*Enterococcus faecalis*<br>*Enterococcus faecium*<br>Group B streptococcus<br>*Streptococcus milleri*<br>Other fastidious streptococci |
| **Others** | *Gardnerella vaginalis*<br>*Neisseria gonorrhoeae*<br>*Candida* spp<br>*Chlamydia trachomatis*<br>Ureaplasmas and mycoplasmas |

ascending renal infection is mechanical – the presence of VUR (Figure 5.1). This may be primary, as occurs in some babies or young children, or in the ureter draining the lower moiety of a duplex kidney. Alternatively, it may be secondary to hormonal relaxation of ureteric muscle during pregnancy; to obstruction of the bladder outlet; or to oedema around the ureteric orifices, such as occurs in patients with severe or long-standing cystitis, indwelling catheters or neuropathic bladders. VUR may also occur in the ureters of transplanted kidneys. The usual cause of primary VUR is a short intramural course of the ureter giving rise to incompetence of the 'valve' mechanism during micturition.

Minor and moderate degrees of reflux correct themselves as the child matures [5]. As yet, there is no reliable non-invasive method of diagnosing the presence of VUR, and its incidence in children is not known. It comes to light either on investigation of children with UTI or as a chance finding on ultrasonographic scanning during pregnancy. Several studies of ultrasonic screening of newborn babies for detection of reflux have been reported, and there have been conflicting reports as

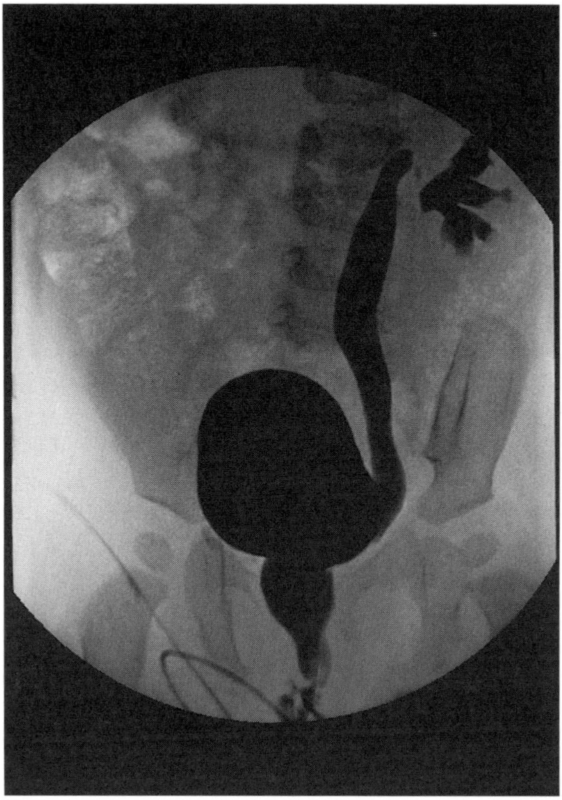

**Figure 5.1** Micturating cystourethrogram showing unilateral grade IV vesicoureteric reflux

to its usefulness. Hiroaka *et al.* [6] have recently reported a new sign – ballooning of the renal pelvis during voiding – which they suggest may be more specific than dilatation of the pelvis as an indicator of reflux. However, validation of any ultrasonic screening method necessitates the use of micturating cystourethrography, and the justification for this on the basis of antenatal findings is not clear. There is no convincing evidence that VUR in itself is harmful to kidneys. It is the combination of reflux and UTI which presents the threat, and this threat is greatest in children, because infection has greater potential for damaging the growing kidney.

It seems unlikely that factors other than mechanical ones are relevant to the ascent of organisms from bladder to kidney. Once there, however, whether or not such organisms initiate pathological changes is probably determined by several factors. Intra-renal reflux into areas drained by compound papillae may occur in the immature kidney [7]. Pyelotubular backflow resulting from increased pressure in the renal pelvis may also occur in patients with outflow obstruction. Apart from these mechanical factors, some bacterial properties are thought to be associated with damage to renal tissue. It is often difficult, however, to distinguish between the relevance of these factors to initial invasion of the urinary tract and a particular ability to cause renal damage. Such factors include the possession of P-fimbriae and of K (capsular) antigens. Whether the possession of P-fimbriae, which facilitate adherence to the urothelium of the lower urinary tract, may also facilitate adhesion to epithelium in the kidney is unknown. Carriage of P-fimbriated *Escherichia coli* is associated with the P blood group, and it has been reported that persons with blood group $P_1$ have a relative risk of recurrent pyelonephritis that is 11 times higher than that of the population as a whole [8]. The role of other bacterial virulence factors has been reviewed by Stamm and colleagues [9]. At present the relevance of these factors to clinical practice is unclear.

Certain chemical factors affect the ability of particular organisms to multiply in the kidney. Those which require an oxygen concentration below that of urine are unlikely to survive in the renal pelvis but may do so in the reduced oxygen tension of previously damaged and fibrotic renal parenchyma. The likely natural history, therefore, of infective renal damage is that the initial changes occur as a result of invasion by aerobic Gram negative bowel organisms. Once inflammatory changes are established in the renal parenchyma, infection with secondary pathogens with different chemical requirements may then supervene. Organisms that have been isolated from the urine of patients with advanced renal inflammatory change include *Haemophilus influenzae* [10] and various species of fastidious streptococci. The presence of infection-related magnesium ammonium phosphate (MAP) stones is of considerable importance in harbouring microbes and leading to persistent infection and renal parenchymal damage (Section 5.2.5).

There are two important difficulties in assessing the role of particular organisms as renal pathogens. First, there is the problem of determining whether organisms isolated from urine are actually in the kidney; much of the literature has rested on indirect, and therefore inconclusive, evidence. Second, most studies of urine from patients with renal damage have used conventional aerobic urine culture techniques and only aerobic pathogens have been isolated. In the few studies in which techniques capable of detecting fastidious and anaerobic organisms have been used [11, 12] a much wider variety of organisms has been isolated. Furthermore, when pus from renal or perinephric abscesses has been cultured, not only have anaerobes and fastidious organisms been isolated, but many infections have been shown to be polymicrobial, aerobes and fastidious organisms or anaerobes being isolated from a single specimen [4]. It must be concluded that current information about the causes of renal infection is incomplete and that the possibility of the presence of organisms not detected by standard culture methods must be borne in mind. Failure to seek and detect such organisms may account for the prevalent view that progressive changes in infection-damaged kidneys is due to causes other than persistent infection [13].

In summary, therefore, infecting organisms in the early stages of renal infection are likely to be the common Gram negative bowel pathogens, in particular *Escherichia coli.* As the disease progresses other Gram negative bowel organisms, for example *Proteus* spp, *Klebsiella* spp or *Pseudomonas* spp, or aerobic cocci such as enterococci or staphylococci, may become involved. These may be selected as secondary pathogens as a result of imbalance in the commensal flora of the bowel and elsewhere, consequent upon administration of antibiotics. This applies particularly to ascending infection from the chronically infected bladders of patients with long-term indwelling catheters or with neurological impairment of bladder function. When no aerobic pathogens can be isolated from the urine, and when there is clear evidence of previous infection and of progressive damage, especially if there is persistent pyuria, the possibility of infection with organisms other than the aerobic pathogens should be considered.

Once organisms have reached the kidney from below, a variety of clinical and pathological consequences may ensue. Hitherto it has not always been possible to differentiate clearly between one consequence and another. The account which follows, therefore, will inevitably be oversimplified. The use of modern imaging techniques may make it possible in the future to define each process more accurately, and to clarify the extent to which they are separate or form part of a single natural history.

### 5.2.3 Acute pyelonephritis

This condition is characterized by the symptoms and clinical signs of acute infection – fever, rigors and vomiting – loin pain and tenderness, leucocytosis, pyuria and urinary infection with an acute pathogen such as *Escherichia coli* or *Staphylococcus saprophyticus*. On the rare occasions when renal biopsy is justified, for example in the differential diagnosis of fever after renal transplantation or of rapidly progressive renal failure, diffuse infiltration with neutrophils and formation of micro-abscesses is observed. Rarely, there may be widespread parenchymal destruction. In most patients with acute pyelonephritis, however, these changes are likely to be of lesser degree, and they may be localized to one or more areas of the kidney (Figure 5.2), for example in young

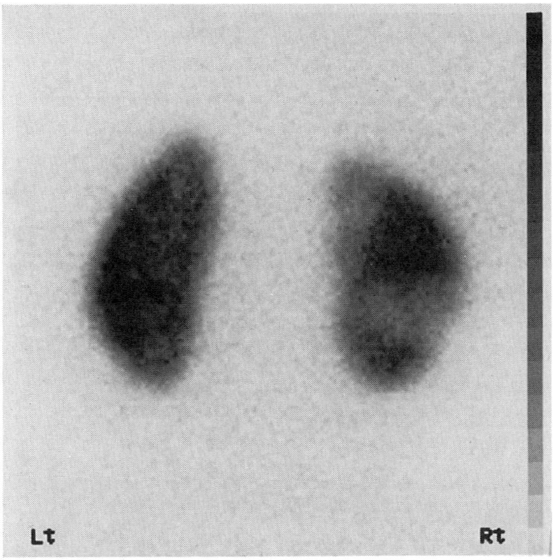


**Figure 5.2** DMSA renogram showing focal scarring of the right kidney.

children with intra-renal reflux. A rare consequence of localized infection is acute focal bacterial nephritis [14], which can mimic renal abscess or other non-inflammatory renal masses.

Acute pyelonephritis occurs in children and young adults with VUR, in pregnant women and others with secondary reflux and sometimes in adults with apparently normal urinary tracts. In the latter there may be a precipitating factor such as the use of a non-steroidal anti-inflammatory drug [15]. Rarely, acute renal failure may ensue. Acute pyelonephritis may also occur as an acute episode in the natural history of patients with chronic atrophic pyelonephritis (renal scarring) or of infection stone disease.

It seems possible that acute infection may sometimes be confined to the renal pelvis and that pyelitis and pyelonephritis may be two distinct entities. This distinction might apply to those patients in whom imaging of the urinary tract after clinical recovery from an attack of acute renal infection reveals no structural or functional abnormality. In this context, infection with *Staphylococcus saprophyticus* is of particular interest. These infections are virtually confined to young, sexually active women [16] and in a high proportion there is clinical and other evidence of renal involvement [17]. Structural or functional abnormalities of the urinary tract, however, are rarely found. Possible explanations include the fact that this is a very rare pathogen in children, in whom the likelihood of

VUR is greatest. Alternatively, the fact that it is a very acute pathogen with an incidence of pyuria of 94% [16] could mean that bladder inflammation is so intense as to cause secondary reflux due to oedema around the urethral orifices. Mechanical or other factors necessary for damage to the renal parenchyma are absent and the infection resolves completely with antibacterial treatment.

### 5.2.4 Chronic pyelonephritis

It is likely that the changes of chronic atrophic pyelonephritis are preceded by at least one episode of acute pyelonephritis. However, a history of such an attack is often lacking. It may have gone unrecognized in feverish babies or children; in patients with secondary reflux it may have contributed to a feverish episode thought to be due to other causes. Chronic pyelonephritis develops when the focal inflammation of the acute attack fails to resolve, and scarring and fibrosis develop. The reason for this progression is difficult to establish because the diagnosis rests upon imaging. Before three-dimensional techniques were available some renal scars were thought to be newly formed, when they may have represented progressive fibrosis in existing scars not detected on previous imaging. Hence some disagreement has arisen as to the cause of the progression of scarring initiated by infection.

When there has been no apparent recurrence of infection, but scarring has progressed, another explanation has been sought. It has been suggested that progression could be due to the development of a glomerulopathy resulting from hyperfiltration by the intact glomeruli in unscarred areas of the kidney. Another possible explanation is that secondary fastidious pathogens perpetuating the infective process have not been detected. This explanation seems particularly likely when there is persistent pyuria. Yet another possibility is that the hypertension known to occur as a consequence of renal scarring may be responsible for progressive renal damage, in particular the bilateral loss of function which can occur in patients with unilateral scarring. There may also be immunological mechanisms, responsible for renal damage, which might be augmented by bacterial determinants [18].

Many patients with radiological evidence of chronic atrophic pyelonephritis, especially those in whom the disease is unilateral, show no evidence of progressive renal damage and do not develop hypertension. In others, however, the disease pursues a less benign course. The risk of repeated infection may still be present, for example in patients with persistent primary or secondary reflux, and further tissue destruction may occur on each occasion. Even in the absence of reflux, infection may have become established in the renal substance, causing progressive changes.

### 5.2.5 Infection stones

One of the most important of these changes is the formation of infection stones. These stones comprise about 10% of all renal calculi [19] and they are formed as a consequence of multiplication of bacteria in the renal substance (Figure 5.3). Organisms particularly associated with such stones are those which metabolize urea in the urine – *Proteus* spp, staphylococci, some *Klebsiellae* and, probably rarely, *Ureaplasma urealyticum* [20]. Multiplication of these organisms results in deposition of carbonate-apatite and struvite in a friable matrix – the so-called mixed phosphatic or MAP stones. Living bacteria persist in the substance of this matrix [21] which calcifies and grows, sometimes with alarming rapidity, until it eventually fills the renal pelvis, forming a staghorn calculus. The presenting features differ from those associated with

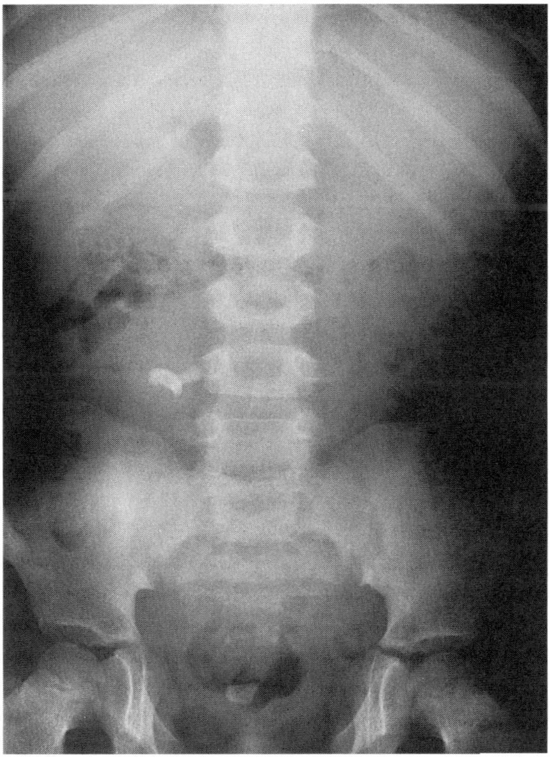

**Figure 5.3** Plain abdominal radiograph showing renal and bladder 'infection stones' in a five-year-old boy who had previously undergone surgery for ectopic bladder.

metabolic stones. There may be a dull ache in the loin, sometimes with haematuria, and urinary infection which either fails to respond to appropriate antibacterial treatment or recurs rapidly after it.

The infecting organisms may be *Proteus* or other urea-splitting organism, but superinfection with other commoner organisms such as *E. coli* may occur. Colic is rare. Patients at an advanced stage of the disease may be apparently symptom-free and they seldom complain of lower tract symptoms related to their bacteriuria. If the presence of such stones remains undetected the gradual loss of renal tissue may result in renal failure if the condition is bilateral. Perhaps the greater risk is posed, even in unilateral disease, by the combination of infection and obstruction of the renal pelvis. Pyonephrosis, perinephric abscess (which may track down the psoas muscle) and septicaemia may ensue. Infection stones are, in fact, the only type of renal stone that may become life-threatening.

### 5.2.6 Xanthogranulomatous pyelonephritis

This is a progressive granulomatous reaction to chronic renal inflammation. It is characterized by the accumulation of large numbers of lipid-laden macrophages in inflamed and often suppurating areas of renal tissue. It is probably not as rare as was previously believed and occurs most often in association with infection stone disease. The patient usually presents with severe toxaemia and a tender mass in the loin.

### 5.2.7 Emphysematous pyelonephritis

This is a rare condition characterized by gas formation in infarcted renal tissue, essentially a gas gangrene which requires a necrotic substrate with secondary infection by gas-forming organisms. The gas is made up of hydrogen and carbon dioxide, generated by common urinary pathogens, usually *E. coli*, although the condition has been reported in association with *Candida albicans*, when the gas is probably carbon dioxide. It is most often seen in elderly female diabetics with chronic urinary sepsis and renal vascular disease. It is a potentially lethal condition and presents as a severe toxaemic illness.

## 5.3 LOWER TRACT INFECTION

Infection of the lower urinary tract – the bladder, urethra and its communicating structures – is much more common than upper tract infection. It presents a considerable problem to patients, in terms of unpleasant symptoms and loss of time from work or school, and to doctors. Furthermore, the importance of distinguishing those patients in whom the upper tract is involved from the majority in whom it is not, cannot be over-emphasized. Traditionally, the latter has involved imaging procedures and instrumental examination of the bladder; there are now sufficient data to suggest that this approach should be used much more selectively than hitherto. There is also evidence that infection of the bladder, urethra and its communicating structures, the prostate in men and paraurethral glands in women, are stages in a dynamic process and that they should not be considered as separate entities. The sexually transmitted infections do not often present to nephrologists and will not be discussed here.

### 5.3.1 Pathogenesis

As mentioned earlier, the distal third of the urethra is colonized by commensal flora consisting of several bacterial species which differ in the sexes and at different stages of life. The normal constituents are Gram positive organisms – streptococci, staphylococci, corynebacteria and lactobacilli; Gram negative bowel organisms are absent. The two principal influences upon the composition of this flora are hormonal status and the administration of antibacterial agents. The primary pathological process in the development of infection of the lower urinary tract is the ascent of bowel organisms, usually Gram negative, but occasionally Gram positive, such as *Staphylococcus saprophyticus*, to the bladder, where they multiply in urine, giving rise to an acute inflammatory process. The natural defence mechanisms against such ascent are the mechanical washout effect of micturition and the competitive inhibition mechanisms of the distal urethral flora. Thus, anything that diminishes the efficacy of these mechanisms, or that directly introduces pathogenic organisms via the urethra, will predispose to such infection. The principal predisposing factors are listed in Table 5.3.

These factors are relevant to a greater or lesser extent in patients of different ages and in different clinical circumstances. For example, whilst a good fluid intake and regular complete micturition are of great importance in children, other factors such as sexual intercourse, instrumentation and impairment of bladder function may come into play in older patients. The role of antibacterial agents is complex and often unrecognized. If broad-spectrum antibiotics are administered for longer than a few days, sensitive Gram negative organisms in the bowel are eradicated and replaced by resistant ones, which may then invade the urinary tract if the predisposing factors persist. In addition, sensitive Gram positive organisms in the distal urethral flora will be destroyed, allowing excessive multiplication of resistant ones, which may then assume a pathogenic role, invading the proximal urethra, the paraurethral glands and, eventually, in a minority of patients, the bladder.

**Table 5.3** Factors that predispose to infection of the lower urinary tract

| | |
|---|---|
| **Inefficient washout mechanism** | Low fluid intake, low urinary output, infrequent or incomplete micturition |
| **Poor bladder emptying** | Neuropathic bladder, bladder diverticulum, post-micturition residue (VUR, chronic cystitis) |
| **Bladder outlet obstruction** | Congenital urethral valves, constipation, urethral stricture, prostatic hypertrophy, bladder stone, periurethral inflammation |
| **Direct introduction of organisms per urethram and trauma to urethral epithelium** | Catheterization, instrumentation, sexual intercourse |
| **Direct spread of organisms from the bowel** | Diverticular disease, appendix abscess |

These latter changes are rare, or possibly do not occur at all, in children, in whom the urethral commensal flora consists mainly of sensitive organisms. However, in the adult, when colonization with more resistant organisms such as lactobacilli and *Gardnerella vaginalis* has occurred, they are frequently encountered in clinical practice. The clinico-pathological conditions resulting from all these processes are acute cystitis, chronic or persistent cystitis, so-called interstitial cystitis, urethritis and paraurethritis (so-called urethral syndrome) in the female and prostatitis in the male.

### 5.3.2 Acute cystitis

Acute infection within the bladder occurs when Gram negative bowel organisms, most commonly *E. coli*, gain access to the bladder and multiply in urine. It presents with onset of dysuria and frequency, sometimes with haematuria, and malaise but no fever. It responds rapidly to treatment with an appropriate antibacterial agent. Scanning electron microscopy has shown that there is minimal disruption of the cells of the bladder wall [22]. Unless the predisposing factors are corrected by appropriate management the condition tends to be recurrent. Recurrences, however, are unusual within three months of successful treatment of an attack. This is useful clinically for distinguishing between reinfection (the commonest cause of recurrence) and relapse, which occurs earlier and is indicative of structural or functional abnormality.

### 5.3.3 Chronic (persistent) cystitis

This condition is much less common than acute cystitis. The pathological inflammatory process involves the superficial and deep layers of the bladder wall. It occurs characteristically in the situations listed below.

1. Long-term indwelling catheterization
2. Long standing, inadequately treated cystitis
3. Bladder calculi
4. Bladder diverticulum
5. Neuropathic bladder (diabetes, multiple sclerosis, congenital or post-traumatic abnormalities of the spinal cord)
6. Urinary diversions

Whilst antibacterial treatment may sterilize the urine temporarily, infection either recurs on cessation of treatment or the original organism is replaced by a more resistant one. An understanding of this pathogenesis is essential to the correct management of the condition.

### 5.3.4 'Abacterial' and 'interstitial' cystitis

These diagnostic labels have been applied to situations in which there is clinical and pathological evidence of inflammatory change in the bladder but no bacteria are isolated from the urine. Careful examination of the literature leads to the conclusion that they may not be genuine entities but rather that such patients have acute or chronic cystitis of infective cause which has remained undetected by the culture methods employed. Some patients with urethral syndrome (see below) are mistakenly believed to have abacterial cystitis. There are others, however, in whom acute bladder infection, usually accompanied by pyuria, is caused by fastidious bacteria such as *Gardnerella vaginalis*.

So-called 'interstitial' cystitis is a chronic, disabling condition in which the patient has crippling frequency of micturition and persistent pyuria. There are inflammatory changes extending into the deep layers of the bladder wall, and the bladder capacity is eventually reduced as a result of fibrosis. Examination of bladder tissue by scanning electron microscopy has demonstrated that bacteria may be seen embedded in the bladder wall at times when conventional aerobic culture of the urine is negative [22, 23]. This finding seems to invalidate the widely held view that the inflammation is due to causes other than infection. Even when urine culture is negative, culture of bladder biopsy tissue may yield aerobic pathogens such as *E. coli* [22]. Furthermore, when urine and bladder biopsies from these patients are cultured by methods capable of detecting fastidious organisms, bacteria including fastidious species of streptococci, *Gardnerella vaginalis* and lactobacilli may be isolated [23]. This suggests that the condition could be the end-point of a natural history that begins as acute cystitis and urethral syndrome.

### 5.3.5 Urethral and paraurethral infection in women

Until recently this has been considered only as the consequence of infection with sexually transmitted pathogens and to be the province of the genitourinary physician. Limited urine culture methods led to the view that the urinary symptoms of which so many women complain at times when urine culture is apparently negative were not due to infection. Indeed they were often dismissed as of psychological origin. The microbiological advances of recent years have offered an explanation and hope to those who suffer from so-called urethral syndrome.

In adult women the first attack of urinary tract infection is usually acute cystitis due to the common organisms, and the onset of sexual activity is often the predisposing factor. This responds rapidly to appropriate antibacterial treatment, but unless an attempt is made to identify the predisposing factors, and to take appropriate measures to correct them, infection is likely to recur. Further antibiotic treatment, often given in longer courses, may then set up a vicious cycle of infection. One of the unwanted side effects of administration of antibiotics is distortion of the composition and balance of the commensal flora of the distal urethra and vagina.

The effect will differ according to the sensitivities of the constituent bacteria. For example, if ampicillin is given, most vaginal bacteria will be killed and yeasts, which are normally present in small numbers, will multiply and cause thrush. If trimethoprim, cotrimoxazole or a fluoroquinolone, to which lactobacilli are intrinsically resistant, is given, the lactobacilli remain to balance the yeasts and thrush is uncommon. However, most of the bacterial species in the distal urethra are killed, leaving the lactobacilli to multiply disproportionately. There is evidence [24] that they migrate into the proximal urethra, paraurethral glandular tissue, and, rarely, the bladder [23]. They may assume a pathogenic role (analogous to the pathogenicity in the bladder of bowel commensals such as *E. coli*) and give rise to symptoms. These differ qualitatively from those of acute cystitis. As well as dysuria and frequency there is often urgency of micturition, sometimes with urge incontinence, post-micturition dribble, a feeling of pressure in the perineum, nocturia and dyspareunia. Such symptoms are readily understood if urethral and periurethral inflammation is postulated. The most common causative organism is *Lactobacillus* spp [24]; other fastidious organisms sometimes isolated from the urine are *Gardnerella vaginalis*, some species of streptococci and corynebacteria.

There is some evidence that urethral infection may also be caused by Gram negative pathogens, probably during the process of invasion of the bladder [25]. Once it is recognized that urethral and paraurethral infection occurs as a consequence of distortion of commensal flora by antibacterial agents, the natural history of the condition is readily understood. Some women continue to have episodes of cystitis alternating with 'urethral syndrome'; others develop chronic and persistent urethral symptoms; a very small minority may progress to bladder involvement and 'interstitial cystitis'.

Long standing infection and inflammation of the paraurethral glands causes constriction of the urethral canal, usually diagnosed on cystoscopy as stenosis. Development of a diverticulum in chronically inflamed tissue [26] is probably rare, but may go unrecognized. It can be a source of very unpleasant symptoms, the most characteristic of which is post-micturition dribble.

### 5.3.6 Prostatitis

The pathogenesis of prostatic infection is ascending, the organisms reaching the prostate via the urethra and prostatic ducts. It may occur in the intact urogenital tract but is also precipitated by instrumentation or the presence of an indwelling catheter. It may be acute or chronic. With the advent of effective antibacterial treatment *Neisseria gonorrhoeae* has been virtually eliminated as a cause.

Acute prostatitis is usually due to infection with common Gram negative bowel pathogens and occurs more commonly in clinical practice than is generally realized. It is characterized by sudden chills and fever, often with rigors, frequency and dysuria, and occasionally retention of urine. Prostatitis occurring in the instrumented or catheterized patient is commonly caused by resistant Gram negative bacteria or urethral Gram positive commensals such as *Staphylococcus epidermidis*, which have multiplied disproportionately as a result of the selective effects of antibacterial agents given to these patients.

The non-acute conditions – chronic bacterial and 'non-bacterial' prostatitis – are caused either by persistence of Gram negative infection after inadequately treated acute prostatitis or by infection with fastidious bacteria such as *Gardnerella vaginalis* or with chlamydia or mycoplasma [27]. Pyuria is often present, although when there is chronic inflammatory change and fibrosis in the prostatic tissue the cells do not always appear in the urine. In some patients with the characteristic clinical picture of chronic prostatitis there is no pyuria and no organisms are found either in urine or prostatic secretion. In the past, such patients have been thought to have a non-infective condition – so-called prostatodynia – but it is equally possible that the culture methods used have failed to detect the pathogen. Microbiological knowledge in this field is progressing rapidly and thorough investigation may yield a more satisfactory answer for these patients.

Patients with non-acute infection of the prostate often have disturbances of bladder function such as increased frequency and urgency of micturition, dysuria and a watery urethral discharge. A dull suprapubic pain may radiate to the perineal area, the loins, testes and penis. Calculi may form as a long-term consequence of infection in the prostate. They are of the mixed phosphatic type and the pathogenesis is similar to that of renal infection stones.

## 5.4 INVESTIGATIONS

### 5.4.1 Laboratory investigations

Urine microscopy and culture are the essential tools in the diagnosis of urinary tract infection. Clinicians should ensure that urine specimens are collected by the method appropriate to the patient and clinical situation, refrigerated immediately and transported to the laboratory as soon as possible. Symptoms and antibacterial treatment should be accurately documented. In the light of what is now known about the pathogenesis of various infective conditions in the urinary tract, laboratory investigation should not be limited to overnight aerobic culture. Interpretation of the findings should not be left to inexperienced staff using a rigid numerical criterion of significance. Clinicians anxious to diagnose and manage urinary tract infection correctly should at least be aware of the protocols used in the laboratory to which they send urine specimens.

Techniques for obtaining urine specimens include suprapubic aspiration in babies (most reliably and easily performed under ultrasound control [28]), clean catch collection from young children, midstream collection from the great majority of patients and catheterization (in the course of an investigation such as micturating cystourethrography, in patients such as some elderly women with poor bladder control, or in those with indwelling catheters).

At present there are no serological tests in general use for the diagnosis of urinary tract infection or for the differentiation of upper tract from lower tract infection.

A white blood cell count provides important contributory evidence in the diagnosis of acute upper tract and septicaemic infections. The biochemical findings are normal in most patients with UTI, and, once found to be so, there is no justification for repeated measurements unless there has been some clinical event, such as an episode of acute pyelonephritis, that might have affected renal function.

### 5.4.2 Imaging

Advances in imaging techniques in recent years, and the need to avoid unnecessary exposure to radiation, have resulted in the modification of hitherto accepted protocols. The usefulness of some of the techniques in current use has been reviewed elsewhere [29]. Since that time further advances in radionuclide imaging have prompted suggestions that radionuclide scintigraphy and cystography should replace intravenous urography and micturating cystourethrography in the identification of VUR and pyelonephritic scarring in children [30]. The limitations of ultrasonography in detecting these abnormalities should be recognized [31].

Imaging of the urinary tract in adults for the investigation of urinary tract infection should be restricted to those patients in whom upper tract infection is suspected, and the techniques employed should be those appropriate to the elucidation of the problem in the individual patient. Routine imaging of those with lower tract infection has a low yield of abnormalities and is neither indicated nor justified [32]. Factors which suggest the possibility of upper tract infection are listed below.

1. Persistent or rapidly recurring UTI
2. UTI with fever
3. An attack of acute pyelonephritis
4. Haematuria persisting after eradication of infection
5. Infection with unusual or resistant organisms
6. Recurrent or persistent *Proteus* infection

These provide guidelines for the selection of patients who should undergo imaging. Advances in CT scanning that enable the identification of intra-renal inflammatory disease [33] may have a place in the investigation of patients with pyelonephritis.

### 5.4.3 Invasive investigations

Because of the patchy nature of infective disease of the kidneys renal biopsy has no place in the investigation of urinary infection. However, when undertaken for other reasons, for example to determine the cause of deteriorating renal function after renal transplantation, it may show the infiltration with polymorphonuclear leucocytes characteristic of infection.

Pus from renal or perinephric abscesses can be obtained by direct needle aspiration for culture.

Urine for culture can be collected directly from each kidney by ureteric catheterization under general anaesthesia. At present this is the only way in which the presence of infection in one or both kidneys can be confirmed. It does not, of course, rule out previous infection and the use of this procedure is limited. It may, however, have a place in determining the advisability or otherwise of unilateral nephrectomy, for example in a patient with extensive infection stone disease in one kidney and no radiological evidence of disease in the other.

Cystoscopy is seldom indicated for the investigation of urinary tract infection and has been widely overused in surgical practice in the past. Exceptions include patients with haematuria persisting after successful treatment of UTI and those with such severely damaged bladders that the possibility of urinary diversion is being considered.

## 5.5 MANAGEMENT AND PREVENTION

The four principal planks upon which effective management and prevention of urinary tract infection rest are:

1. accurate diagnosis;
2. explanation of the condition to the patient (or parent);
3. imaging, if indicated; and
4. appropriate use of antibacterial agents.

Although clinical history and examination may strongly suggest UTI, diagnosis ultimately rests on microscopy and culture of urine. A finding of UTI should always prompt an explanation of the pathogenesis of the condition to the patient. In this way, important predisposing factors such as infrequent or incomplete micturition, inadequate fluid intake, or relationship to sexual intercourse are elicited and discussed; efforts can be made to correct them and further infections prevented. The indications and contraindications for imaging will be discussed in relation to individual conditions. Antibacterial treatment should be guided by an up-to-date knowledge of the available agents. In general, those used should be known to be effective against the likely pathogens; should be well absorbed after oral administration, thus minimizing the selection of a resistant flora in the lower bowel; should attain a high concentration in the urine and, when tissue is involved (kidney or prostate), in the appropriate tissue.

Agents used for long-term low-dose prophylaxis should be widely effective against the likely pathogens; they should be excreted in effective concentration in the urine whilst having a minimum effect on the commensal flora of the bowel and other neighbouring sites. Agents such as the penicillins, to which resistance develops rapidly in Gram negative organisms, are unsuitable for this use. Suitable agents include nitrofurantoin (or its macrocrystalline preparation Macrodantin), cotrimoxazole and cefaclor. Ciprofloxacin or other fluoroquinolones may be used for refractory cases, in particular in men, in whom the choice of agents that penetrate the prostate is limited. The dosage for prophylaxis is one quarter to one third of the treatment dose, given at night. The duration of treatment will be discussed in relation to the different clinical conditions.

### 5.5.1 Vesico-ureteric reflux and reflux nephropathy (See also Chapter 14)

The earlier in life that VUR is detected and appropriate management instituted, the less likely that the patient will develop chronic pyelonephritic changes of reflux nephropathy. Ureteric dilatation seen on antenatal ultrasonography should always be followed up by a repeat investigation soon after delivery, and by micturating cystourethrography if the dilatation persists or if there is a history of VUR or pyelonephritis in parents or siblings. VUR may still be present even when no abnormality is noted on antenatal scanning. It then comes to light as a result of investigations undertaken after an episode of UTI. The diagnosis of UTI should be considered in all children who present with fever of no obvious other cause, or with recurrent fevers. Ideally, all children with UTI should undergo imaging to determine the presence or absence of VUR and of renal scarring.

It is recognized that all but the most severe degrees of VUR disappear as the child matures [5], and usually before the age of six years. It can be argued, therefore, that cystography is unnecessary after that age in a child in whom imaging has demonstrated no abnormality of the kidneys. However, the limitations of all imaging techniques with respect to an individual patient should be remembered, and persistence or recurrence of UTI should prompt a review of the advisability of further imaging. When the diagnosis is missed in early childhood renal damage may occur and progress. Such patients present in adolescence or early adult life or early pregnancy with UTI, sometimes with hypertension and occasionally in renal failure. This situation can be prevented by appropriate clinical management in the early stages of the disease.

Management consists of careful explanation to the parent, and the child when old enough, that a good fluid intake, two-hourly double micturition, regular bowel action (to avoid obstruction of bladder emptying by a loaded colon), and regular urine cultures are essential. The latter should be undertaken, additionally, at any time of fever or unexplained illness. Antibacterial treatment should not be delayed until laboratory confirmation of infection has been obtained, but should be started immediately after the urine specimen has been collected. A five-day course of an appropriate agent should be instituted and changed if necessary in the light of the reported sensitivity of the organism isolated. On completion of the course, if the child is under six years of age, has had a previous episode of UTI or has had a fever, a low-dose antibacterial prophylactic regimen should be instituted and arrangements made for imaging. If the latter shows either VUR or any evidence of renal scarring the prophylaxis should be continued, with regular urine culture checks.

If infection persists or recurs on prophylaxis, and this is rare (provided the regimen is reliably adhered to) except in children with severe degrees of reflux, treatment should be repeated and prophylaxis reinstated. If still unsuccessful, an explanation (for example the presence of an infection stone) should be sought and managed appropriately. Surgical correction of reflux may be considered. Open operation has now been supplanted in some centres by submucosal injection of Teflon – the so-called Sting operation [34]. Neither of these procedures should be considered an alternative to antibiotic management; careful prevention of further infection is still necessary and the long-term care of such children should ideally be in the hands of a paediatric nephrologist [35]. It should be understood that, if renal infection has become established, cure or improvement of reflux does not necessarily prevent progressive renal damage, although it may facilitate prevention of further infection in conjunction with careful antibacterial management. The duration of prophylaxis must be determined for individual children. Sometimes it is necessary to continue it until maximum renal growth is achieved, probably by the time of puberty. If renal damage is absent or minimal and the child is over the age of five years with no infection for two years, a trial without prophylaxis may be justified. It is essential, however, that the parent and general practitioner should understand the need for careful follow-up and the need to monitor for UTI and react appropriately to any recurrence. Blood pressure should be monitored regularly in all children with reflux nephropathy.

Because of the familial incidence of VUR the parent should be alerted to the possibility of UTI in siblings. Screening of siblings for reflux by micturating cystourethrography (MCU) is rarely indicated in the absence of proven UTI, but may be considered in the neonatal period if there is a family history of severe disease.

In summary, the purpose of good management of VUR is to identify it as early as possible before renal damage has occurred and to protect the kidneys from initiation or extension of pyelonephritic scarring by appropriate antibacterial management.

### 5.5.2 Acute pyelonephritis and its sequelae

Although a clinical diagnosis may be made from the characteristic combination of fever, rigors, loin tenderness and lower urinary tract symptoms (although these are not always present) the diagnosis should be confirmed by urine microscopy and culture. Antibacterial treatment with an agent that achieves effective tissue concentration should be initiated immediately. Parenteral administration, together with general measures to combat fever and maintain hydration, may be necessary for the first 48 hours if the patient is vomiting. Treatment should be amended if necessary in the light of the sensitivity of the isolate and should be continued for seven days, during which time an explanation for the attack should be sought.

The possibility of VUR, whether primary in children or young adults, or secondary due to pregnancy or in patients with indwelling catheters or neuropathic bladders, should be considered. Any relevant drug history, for example treatment with non-steroidal anti-inflammatory agents [15], should be elicited and renal function checked by appropriate biochemical tests. Blood pressure should be checked. Surgical intervention may be required if the rare complications of renal or perinephric abscess develop or if there is obstruction of kidney or ureter by an infection stone. A decision about imaging and whether to institute a low-dose antibacterial regimen should be made in the light of the individual clinical circumstances and past history. Most patients who have an attack of acute pyelonephritis should undergo appropriate renal imaging; the likelihood of finding an abnormality requiring long-term management is high. Pregnant women who develop acute pyelonephritis in the second trimester should be investigated after the puerperium. In general, antibacterial prophylaxis should be used when there is a possibility of success and avoided in patients with inevitable bacteriuria (see below).

### 5.5.3 Chronic pyelonephritis

The diagnosis is made by imaging, either following an attack of acute pyelonephritis or to seek a cause for recurrent or persistent urinary tract infections. The objectives of management must be to elicit and remedy, if possible, the cause of the condition, to prevent further renal damage and preserve renal function, and to treat hypertension if present. Although factors other than UTI or hypertension may be responsible for progression of renal scarring initiated by infection, they are not, at present, amenable to treatment. Infection can, however, be treated and recurrence prevented in many patients by long-term low-dose antibacterial prophylaxis [36]. Patients should remain under expert supervision until they have been free of UTI for at least two years, when a carefully monitored trial without prophylaxis may be attempted. It should be re-established if infection recurs or if the patient becomes pregnant.

Failure to control infection with an appropriate antibacterial regimen, or rapid relapse after stopping treatment, should prompt a search for possible causes of persistent infection, in particular infection stone formation. There is evidence that control of infection becomes more difficult once a moderate degree of renal impairment is present, but that function can be preserved, and even improved, in patients with mild degrees of renal failure by appropriate antibacterial management [36].

### 5.5.4 Infection stones

Effective management requires good cooperation between nephrologist, microbiologist and surgeon. The earlier in the natural history of the disease that these patients are identified the better the chance that the stones will be amenable to treatment and that renal function can be preserved. It is important, therefore, that all those, including general practitioners, who treat patients with UTI should be alert to the clinical and microbiological pointers to stone formation. It is a recognized complication of reflux nephropathy and chronic pyelonephritis. Occasionally patients, both adults and children, with these conditions are found to have stones at the time of initial presentation. Renal infection occurring in patients with VUR secondary to a neuropathic bladder or long-term indwelling catheter is often associated with stone formation. The microbiological indicators which are suggestive of infection stones are UTI which persists or recurs rapidly after appropriate treatment, and recurrent or persistent infection with bacteria which metabolize urea in urine, in particular *Proteus* spp and staphylococci.

Because these stones are bound to and embedded in renal tissue, extracorporeal shock wave lithotripsy cannot be a definitive treatment. It carries the risk, not only of dissemination of organisms further into the renal substance and thence into the bloodstream, but also of the formation of new niduses of infected material and further stone formation around them. Percutaneous nephrolithotomy can be more effective in removing most of the friable calculous material, but the risk of further stone formation remains.

Open operation is used infrequently nowadays, for large obstructing stones or for recurrence. Both these situations can be avoided by early diagnosis. Any surgical technique should be combined with careful antibiotic management. An appropriate antibiotic should be given in therapeutic dosage perioperatively to prevent bacteraemia, and this should be followed by a prolonged period of low-dose prophylaxis to prevent further stone formation [37]. Nitrofurantoin should not be used because *Proteus* spp are almost invariably resistant. After one year free of UTI a trial off prophylaxis with regular monitoring of urine cultures is justified. This management protocol is only possible if there is a clear understanding of the pathology of the condition, not only by the physician, surgeon and general practitioner, but also by the patient.

Regular monitoring for infection stones by annual plain abdominal radiography, and appropriate surgical management, can help to preserve renal function in patients with neuropathic bladders and other conditions in which bacteriuria is inevitable.

### 5.5.5 Neuropathic bladders or urinary diversions (inevitable bacteriuria)

If impairment of bladder function is mild, for example in the early stages of diabetic neuropathy, it may be possible to sterilize the urine by appropriate treatment followed by low-dose prophylaxis. The patient should endeavour to empty the bladder as completely as possible by double or triple micturition using suprapubic pressure.

If a careful attempt at treatment and low-dose prophylaxis fails it should be stopped. Continuation will result in selection of resistant organisms, making prompt treatment of episodes of clinical infection difficult. The urine should be cultured only at times when there is a clinical indication for treatment, such as fever. If antibiotics have been withheld, the infecting organisms are likely to be sensitive, and treatment should be started as soon as the urine specimen has been collected. In this way damage to renal tissue and function can be minimized.

Renal function should be monitored regularly by appropriate biochemical tests, and infection stone formation should be detected at an early stage by plain film radiography at intervals appropriate to the age and clinical condition of the patient.

Clean intermittent self-catheterization is useful in well-motivated patients. The urine is likely to remain infected, but the incidence of fever and ascending infection is reduced. Antibacterial treatment should be reserved for episodes of clinical infection. Urine from collection bags should never be sent for culture. In patients with urinary diversions urine should be collected from the stoma by catheter.

### 5.5.6 Cystitis and urethral syndrome

A concept of lower UTI that takes account of the possible involvement of the urethra and tissues below the bladder, and an understanding of the role of antibacterial treatment as an aetiological factor, is fundamental to the correct management of the condition. The earlier in the natural history that management is based on these considerations the more likely that the advanced, and possibly intractable, stages such as severe paraurethral inflammation leading to urethral stenosis, or 'interstitial cystitis', can be prevented. Episodes of acute cystitis should be treated for three days with an appropriate antibacterial agent. An explanation of the pathogenesis should be given to the patient, who should be instructed to drink well and empty the bladder completely every two hours and after sexual intercourse. A diagnosis of cystitis, whilst it can justifiably be made from the history and symptoms on one or two occasions without bacteriological confirmation, should never be made repeatedly without culture of a mid-stream urine (MSU). If repeated attacks of infection with aerobic pathogens are confirmed, or there are any indications suggesting upper tract abnormality (Section 5.4.2), a cause should be sought by appropriate investigations.

Prevention of further infections in such patients – including those in whom there is no indication for imaging or other investigations – by a low-dose prophylactic regimen will spare them repeated courses of treatment in therapeutic dosage, and unwanted side effects such as thrush and urethral syndrome. Should aerobic MSU cultures from women with symptoms be negative, fastidious organisms should be sought. If the laboratory does not provide this service, the likelihood of urethral or paraurethral infection should be explained to the patient, who may then understand that antibacterial treatment is contraindicated. An alkalinizing agent such as effervescent potassium citrate may be given for symptomatic relief. The patient should be told that the symptoms will resolve only slowly as the normal balance of commensal urethral flora is restored [24]. Such reassurance that the symptoms are real and have a logical explanation will encourage patients to pursue an expectant policy and to refrain from requesting repeated courses of antibiotics from their doctors. Laboratory confirmation of the presence of urethral organisms, usually lactobacilli, in large numbers will, of course, add to the conviction of the doctor in making the diagnosis.

A few patients will fail to respond to this management and it is then necessary to consider the possibility of infection with less common fastidious organisms such as *Gardnerella vaginalis*. In view of the fact that this organism is known to invade the bladder, it is probably advisable to attempt antibacterial treatment in the early stages before chronic inflammatory changes have occurred. Metronidazole has not been found to be effective, but some success has been seen with a 14-day course of doxycycline. There is no effective treatment for the established chronic inflammatory changes of 'interstitial cystitis', which emphasizes the importance of appropriate management of the earlier stages of the condition.

### 5.5.7 Prostatitis

Nephrologists are only infrequently called upon to treat prostatitis, but they may encounter it in patients under their care for other reasons. It is important to be aware that the bacterial count in urine may be low. If infection extends to the bladder high bacterial counts may be obtained, but this does not always occur. The two important principles of management are that antibiotic treatment should be given for at least 14 days in order to treat tissue infection adequately, and that the agent used should achieve a therapeutic concentration in prostatic tissue. Appropriate agents include cotrimoxazole and trimethoprim, the tetracyclines, of which doxycycline is usually preferred, and the fluoroquinolones. Low-dose prophylaxis with one of these agents may be required for the management of patients with persistent or frequent attacks.

## REFERENCES

1. Wing, A.J., Brunner, F.P., Brynger, H. *et al.* (1978) Combined report on regular dialysis and transplantation in Europe, viii, 1977. *Proc. Europ. Dialysis Transplant. Assoc.*, **15**, 3–77.
2. Esbjörner, E., Aronson, S., Berg, U. *et al.* (1990) Children with chronic renal failure in Sweden 1978–1985. *Pediatr. Nephrol.*, **4**, 249–52.
3. Green, L.F., Weed, L.A. and Albers, D.D. (1952) Brucellosis of the urinary tract. *J. Urol.*, **67**, 765–72.
4. Edelstein, H. and McCabe, R.E. (1988) Perinephric abscess. Modern diagnosis and treatment in 47 cases. *Medicine*, **67**, 118–31.
5. Edwards, D., Normand, I.C.S., Prescod, N. and Smellie, J.M. (1977) Disappearance of vesicoureteric reflux during long-term prophylaxis of urinary tract infection in children. *Br. Med. J.*, **ii**, 285–8.
6. Hiroaka, M., Kasuga, K., Hori, C. and Sudo, M. (1994) Ultrasonic indicators of ureteric reflux in the newborn. *Lancet*, **343**, 519–20.
7. Rolleston, G.L., Maling, T.M.J. and Hodson, C.J. (1974) Intra-renal reflux and the scarred kidney. *Arch. Dis. Child.* **49**, 531–9.
8. Lomberg, H., Jodal, U., Svanborg-Edén, C. *et al.* (1981) Blood group and urinary tract infection. *Lancet*, **i**, 551–2.
9. Stamm, W.E., Hooton, T.M., Johnson, J.R. *et al.* (1989) Urinary tract infections: from pathogenesis to treatment. *J. Infect. Dis.*, **159**, 400–6.
10. Granoff, D.M. and Roskes, S. (1974) Urinary tract infection due to *Hemophilus influenzae* type B. *J. Pediatr.*, **84**, 414–6.
11. McDowall, D.R.M., Buchanan, J.D., Fairley, K.F. and Gilbert, G.L. (1981) Anaerobic and other fastidious micro-organisms in asymptomatic bacteriuria in pregnant women. *J. Infect. Dis.*, **144**, 114–22.
12. Birch, D.F., D'Apice, A.J.F. and Fairley, K.F. (1981) *Ureaplasma urealyticum* in the upper renal tracts of renal allograft recipients. *J. Infect. Dis.*, **144**, 123–7.
13. Arze, R.S., Ramos, J.M., Owen, J.P. *et al.* (1982) The natural history of chronic pyelonephritis in the adult. *Q. J. Med.*, New Series L1, No 204, 396–410.
14. Zanontz, M.R., Pahira, J.J., Wolfman, M. *et al.* (1985) Acute focal bacterial nephritis: a systematic approach to diagnosis and treatment. *J. Urol.*, **133**, 752–7.
15. Atkinson, L.K., Goodship, T.H.J. and Ward, M.K. (1986) Acute renal failure associated with acute pyelonephritis and consumption of non-steroidal anti-inflammatory drugs. *Br. Med. J.*, **292**, 97–98.
16. Pead, L., Maskell, R. and Morris, J. (1985) *Staphylococcus saprophyticus* as a urinary pathogen: a six year prospective survey. *Br. Med. J.*, **291**, 1157–9.

17. Hedman, P. and Ringertz, O. (1991) Urinary tract infections caused by *Staphylococcus saprophyticus*. A matched case control study. *J. Infect.*, **23**, 145–53.
18. Andriole, V.T. (1987) Urinary tract infections: recent developments. *J. Infect. Dis.*, **156**, 865–9.
19. Rose, G.A. and Harrison, R. (1974) The incidence, investigation and treatment of idiopathic hypercalciuria. *Br. J. Urol.*, **46**, 261–74.
20. Hedelin, H., Brorson, J.-E., Grenard, L. and Pettersson, S. (1984) *Ureaplasma urealyticum* and upper urinary tract stones. *Br. J. Urol.*, **56**, 244–9.
21. Nemoy, N.J. and Stamey, T.A. (1971) Surgical, bacteriological and biochemical management of 'infection stones'. *J. Am. Med. Assoc.*, **215**, 1470–6.
22. Elliott, T.S.J., Reed, L., Slack, R.C.B. and Bishop, M.C. (1985) Bacteriology and ultrastructure of the bladder in patients with urinary tract infections. *J. Infect.*, **11**, 191–9.
23. Wilkins, E.G.L., Payne, S.R., Pead, P.J. *et al.* (1989) Interstitial cystitis and urethral syndrome: a possible answer. *Br. J. Urol.*, **64**, 39–44.
24. Maskell, R., Pead, L. and Sanderson, R.A. (1983) Fastidious bacteria and the urethral syndrome: a 2 year clinical and bacteriological study of 51 women. *Lancet*, **ii**, 1277–80.
25. Fihn, S.D., Johnson, C. and Stamm, W.E. (1988) *Escherichia coli* urethritis in women with symptoms of acute urinary infection. *J. Infect. Dis.*, **157**, 196–9.
26. Woodhouse, C.R.J., Flynn, J.T., Molland, E.A. and Blandy, J.P. (1980) Urethral diverticulum in females. *Br. J. Urol.*, **52**, 305–10.
27. Lipsky, B.A. (1989) Urinary tract infections in men. Epidemiology, pathophysiology, diagnosis and treatment. *Ann. Intern. Med.*, **110**, 138–50.
28. Buys, H., Pead, L., Hallett, R. and Maskell, R. (1984) Suprapubic aspiration under ultrasound guidance in children with fever of undiagnosed cause. *Br. Med. J.*, **308**, 690–92.
29. Maskell, R. (1988) *Urinary Tract Infection in Clinical and Laboratory Practice.* Edward Arnold, London, pp. 234–45.
30. Conway, J.J. and Cohn, R.A. (1994) Evolving role of nuclear medicine for the diagnosis and management of urinary tract infection. *J. Pediatr.*, **124**, 87–90.
31. Stokland, E., Hellström, M., Hansson, S. *et al.* (1994) Reliability of ultrasonography in identification of reflux nephropathy in children. *Br. Med. J.*, **309**, 235–9.
32. Fowler, J.E. and Pulaski, E.T. (1981) Excretory urography, cystography, and cystoscopy in the evaluation of women with urinary tract infection. *N. Engl. J. Med.*, **304**, 462–5.
33. June, C.H., Browning, M.D., Smith, P. *et al.* (1985) Ultrasonography and computed tomography in severe urinary tract infection. *Arch. Intern. Med.*, **145**, 841–5.
34. O'Donnell, B. and Puri, P. (1986) Endoscopic correction of primary vesicoureteric reflux: results in 94 ureters. *Br. Med. J.*, **293**, 1404–6.
35. Maskell, R., Vinnicombe, J., Abercrombie, G.F.A. and Walmsley, B.H. (1991) Correction of vesicoureteric reflux by endoscopic injection. *Lancet*, **338**, 1460.
36. Mihindukulasuriya, J.C.L., Maskell, R. and Polak, A. (1980) A study of fifty eight patients with renal scarring associated with urinary tract infection. *Q. J. Med.*, **49**, 165–78.
37. Chinn, R.H., Maskell, R., Mead, J.A. and Polak, A. (1976) Renal stones and urinary infection: a study of antibiotic treatment. *Br. Med. J.*, **ii**, 1411–3.

# 6

# Diabetic nephropathy

*G. F. Watts and K. M. Shaw*

This chapter deals with overt diabetic nephropathy, the early renal changes in the diabetic kidney, microalbuminuria, and with practical aspects of the detection, treatment and prevention of diabetic renal disease.

Diabetic nephropathy is still a serious and life-threatening complication of diabetes. Once overt nephropathy is established, life expectancy is substantially reduced and the quality of life impaired by other microvascular complications, including retinopathy and neuropathy, as well as by a significant increase in the risk of cardiovascular disease, especially coronary heart disease. Of those diabetic patients developing persistent macroproteinuria, up to 50% will die within a 10-year period compared with only 2% of those without macroproteinuria.

## 6.1 OVERT DIABETIC NEPHROPATHY

### 6.1.1 Diagnosis

The hallmark of overt diabetic nephropathy is persistent proteinuria in excess of 0.5 g/24 h [1]. This degree of urinary protein loss is referred to as macroproteinuria, detectable by indicator dye-binding methods, such as Albustix (Miles Ltd, Stoke Poges, Bucks, UK); a positive Albustix dipstix test is equivalent to a concentration of urinary protein (predominantly albumin) of at least 300 mg/l. The syndrome of overt nephropathy in insulin-dependent patients also typically includes systemic hypertension, retinopathy and an elevation in serum creatinine concentration [2, 3].

*Renal Disease.* Edited by G. Venkat Raman. Published in 1998 by Chapman & Hall, London. ISBN 0 412 45700 8.

The link between diabetes mellitus and proteinuria was first recognized in 1770 by Cotunnius, who reported that the urine from a diabetic patient coagulated on heating [1]. This association was repeatedly confirmed by several early workers, and the introduction of percutaneous renal biopsy established that proteinuria was an indicator of the glomerular lesions seen in diabetic patients [4]. Typical renal lesions include glomerular basement membrane thickening, mesangial expansion, hyalinosis of afferent and efferent arterioles, and increased localization of albumin and other plasma proteins within the glomerular basement membrane. Nodular and diffuse glomerulosclerosis is positively associated with the duration of diabetes. Advanced diabetic glomerulosclerosis may, however, occur in a proportion of insulin-dependent patients without clinical evidence of renal disease.

### 6.1.2 Natural history

Diabetics with persistent proteinuria have a markedly reduced survival compared to those without proteinuria [5]. Persistent proteinuria is a strong predictor of mortality not only from uraemia, but also from cardiovascular disease [6]. The mean duration of diabetes in insulin-dependent patients at the onset of proteinuria is 18 years, and end stage renal failure (ESRF) and death follow approximately seven years thereafter [3].

The natural history of established diabetic nephropathy has been best described in insulin-dependent patients. Intermittent proteinuria heralds persistent proteinuria by a variable period of up to several years. Persistent proteinuria is followed by progressive loss of renal function, manifesting as a steady increase in urinary protein loss and as an unremitting decline in the glomerular filtration rate (GFR). Once serum creatinine concentration reaches 200 μmol/l, the GFR falls evenly with time at a mean rate of 1 ml/min/month, acceleration of other long-term complications in diabetes occurring simultaneously. The major clinical determinant of the fall in GFR and rise in proteinuria is systemic blood pressure [7]. The influence of dietary protein and glycaemic control on the course of the disease, however, has not been fully resolved. By the time ESRF is reached, insulin-dependent patients are typically aged less than 50 years, with duration of diabetes between 20 and 25 years and manifest advanced proliferative retinopathy, severe peripheral neuropathy and widespread macrovascular disease. The natural history of overt nephropathy in a patient with non-insulin-dependent diabetes mellitus (NIDDM) is probably similar to that of insulin-dependent diabetes mellitus (IDDM) [8,9]. The greater proportion of non-insulin dependent patients, however, die from cardiovascular disease before reaching end stage renal failure.

### 6.1.3 Epidemiology

Clinical and epidemiological studies of diabetic populations have reported a prevalence of clinical proteinuria ranging between 4.4 and 33% [2,3]. In IDDM the prevalence of persistent proteinuria increases with the duration of diabetes. The cumulative incidence of persistent proteinuria is 40 to 50% after 40 years of diabetes, the highest incidence (*c.* 3% per year) has been found between 16 and 20 years' duration. Up to 70% of insulin-dependent diabetic patients, however, never develop overt diabetic nephropathy, the reasons for which are unknown. Projected estimates from the incidence of overt nephropathy in insulin-dependent patients suggest that in the UK approximately 600 relatively young patients develop renal failure each year [10]. The frequency of diabetic renal disease appears to be greater in certain US populations than in Europe [11].

The mortality rate of insulin-dependent diabetic patients is 20 times greater than the general population, the excess being chiefly due to cardiovascular and renal disease. In the UK renal disease accounts for up to 15% of deaths in diabetics aged less than 50 years and is particularly common in young males [10]. Studies from Denmark have demonstrated that the relative mortality in IDDM patients aged 20–40 years and with persistent proteinuria is 25–100 times greater than in patients without proteinuria, and that a significant proportion of the excess is due to macrovascular disease [5].

In the USA the percentage of all new cases accepted for the treatment of ESRF due to diabetic nephropathy increased from 7% in 1974 to 25% in 1980 [12]. In the UK 1.4% of patients with ESRF admitted to renal units for treatment in 1974 were diabetics, but by 1980 the figure had risen to 11.1% [10]. In Europe the highest acceptance rate (19%) is in Scandinavian countries, suggesting that there is probably still a shortfall of diabetics receiving treatment for ESRF in the UK. The high rate of coronary heart disease, peripheral vascular disease, neuropathy, and proliferative retinopathy in diabetic patients with ESRF collectively account for their increased morbidity and mortality compared with non-diabetics receiving similar treatment [2].

### 6.1.4 Therapy

Several therapies may be employed to retard the increase in proteinuria and fall in GFR in diabetics with overt nephropathy [7,13]. Of these the most important is the control of elevated arterial blood pressure. The diagnosis and treatment of hypertension is, therefore, essential and the most promising drugs appear to be angiotensin-converting enzyme inhibitors [14]. The benefits from very tight glycaemic control and a low-protein diet have not been fully established. A recent meta-analysis has indicated that dietary protein restriction effectively slows progression of both diabetic and non-diabetic renal disease [15]. Once a diabetic reaches ESRF the two options are dialysis treatment or renal transplantation (preferably from a living related donor). The outcome of renal replacement therapy in diabetics remains worse than in non-diabetics and this is likely to be related to associated vascular, neuropathic and infective co-complications.

Diabetic nephropathy is a serious and common long-term complication of diabetes mellitus. It threatens the health and life of up to half of the patients who develop IDDM in youth and a smaller but significant number of those with NIDDM. The cumulative risk in non-insulin-dependent diabetics varies with ethnic origin, being higher in the UK among Asian patients. Available medical therapy has little impact on the decline of established nephropathy to ESRF. Management of patients is severely hampered by coexistent atherosclerosis, retinopathy and neuropathy. The financial burdens imposed by treatment and care of diabetic patients in ESRF are colossal [12]; in the USA the annual cost in 1989 was estimated at greater than $2 000 000 000. There is clearly a major demand to identify and treat patients at the earliest possible stage of diabetic renal involvement [16, 17]. This introductory section therefore provides the rationale for preventative programmes involving the screening and monitoring of patients with early diabetic nephropathy.

## 6.2 THE STAGES OF DIABETIC RENAL DISEASE

Diabetic nephropathy is a chronic renal disease which takes several years to become clinically manifest [2,3]. A wide spectrum of functional morphological and biochemical changes occur in the diabetic kidney and will be described in detail later [18]. To assist research and clinical practice Mogensen *et al.*, have proposed a classification system for the stages of diabetic nephropathy [19] as follows:

- Stage I. Glomerular hypertrophy and hyperfunction with normal glomerular histology, which is invariably present at the onset of insulin-dependent diabetes. These abnormalities tend to disappear after commencing insulin therapy.
- Stage II. Glomerular basement membrane thickening and mesangial expansion with normal urinary albumin excretion and unmasking of microalbuminuria by moderate physical exercise and poor metabolic control.
- Stage III. Persistently elevated urinary albumin excretion (microalbuminuria), heralding the progression to clinically overt renal disease. The GFR is normal or elevated and hypertension often present.
- Stage IV. Overt diabetic nephropathy characterized by clinical protei-

nuria, hypertension, declining GFR and the development of advanced glomerular lesions.
- Stage V. Generalized glomerular sclerosis leading to ESRF (GFR less than 10 ml/min), requiring renal replacement therapy for patient survival.

The later stages of this classification are associated with increasing duration of diabetes. The classification, which is to some extent arbitrary, applies only to insulin-dependent patients since there are few data on the spectrum of renal abnormalities in NIDDM [9]. At all stages it is important to emphasize that any type of renal disease may affect the diabetic in the same way as non-diabetics. Typically, deteriorating renal function in a diabetic patient without retinopathy or neuropathy should lead to the suspicion of non-diabetic renal disease which will need to be investigated in its own right.

## 6.3 EARLY CHANGES IN THE DIABETIC KIDNEY

Several early renal abnormalities have been described in diabetes mellitus and these are summarized in Table 6.1 and discussed below.

**Table 6.1** Early renal abnormalities in diabetes mellitus

| | |
|---|---|
| | *Functional* |
| Haemodynamics | ↑ Glomerular filtration rate<br>↑ Renal blood flow<br>↑ Transglomerular capillary pressure |
| Microproteinuria | ↑ Albuminuria<br>↑ Immunoglobulinuria<br>↑ Transferrinuria |
| | *Morphological* |
| Ultrastructure | ↑ Glomerular basement membrane<br>↑ Mesangial expansion<br>Widening of the foot processes<br>Glomerular occlusion |
| Macrostructure | ↑ Kidney size<br>Glomerular hypertrophy<br>Tubular hypertrophy |
| | *Glomerular barrier biochemistry* |
| | ↓ Anionic membrane charge<br>↓ Heparan sulphate proteoglycans<br>↑ Deposition of albumin and immunoglobulin G4<br>↑ Collagen |

↑ = Increased. ↓ = Decreased.

### 6.3.1 Renal haemodynamics

The concept of elevated GFR leading to hyperfiltration in diabetes was conceived several years ago by Cambier [1]. The GFR is often increased by 20–40% in insulin-dependent patients on conventional treatment. The exact mechanism for this is unknown, but probably involves alterations in renal plasma flow, trans-capillary hydraulic pressure, renal morphology, and metabolic and endocrine factors [9, 18]. The increased renal plasma flow only explains approximately 50% of the increase in GFR. The contributory role of raised intracapillary pressure has been suggested by animal experiments and by findings of an increased filtration fraction in insulin-dependent patients. In experimental animals, Hostetter *et al.* [20] have shown that a reduction in total arteriolar vascular resistance, more marked in afferent than efferent arterioles may account for the increase in intraglomerular pressure, and this has been indirectly confirmed in human subjects. In insulin-dependent patients a close association has been reported between hyperfiltration and kidney size. Renal structural changes are, however, unlikely to be the sole determinant of hyperfiltration, since significant changes can occur in GFR under conditions of good metabolic control without major influence on filtration surface area or renal size [18]. Hyperfiltration is more likely to be due to alterations in several vasoactive control mechanisms consequent on changes in metabolic control.

Both short and long-term correction of hyperglycaemia are known to lower renal plasma flow and GFR significantly. The reduction in GFR is more closely associated with blood glucose control than with insulin levels [9, 18]. The effect of hyperglycaemia may be mediated by renal vasodilatation and increased glucose coupled sodium reabsorption in the proximal tubules. Ketones in supraphysiological levels result in a marked increase in GFR. By contrast modest effects have been recognized with glucagon, growth hormone and insulin-like growth factor-1 (IGF-1). Glomerular hyperfiltration may additionally depend on increased renal prostaglandin production and depressed renin levels, increased atrial natriuretic peptide and endothelium-derived relaxation factor (nitric oxide), and hyperactivity of the polyol pathway [21]. The importance of these metabolic and hormonal changes *in vivo*, however, remains to be established [18].

Several workers have proposed that haemodynamic factors may determine the onset of progression of diabetic glomerulopathy [20]. Thus Hostetter *et al.* have employed the remnant kidney hypothesis to propose that a reduction in nephron number leads to compensatory renal haemodynamic changes which in turn disrupt the structure and function of the kidney. This view is compatible with that of Mauer *et al.* who have suggested that a critical degree of mesangial expansion by reducing capillary luminal space and filtration surface area results in renal hyperfiltration and the perpetuation of diabetic glomerulopathy [18].

The hyperfiltration hypothesis, however, needs to be reconciled with the finding that all long-term insulin-dependent patients have elevated GFR and increased glomerular basement membrane thickening with mesangial expansion, but only approximately 30% develop clinically significant nephropathy [2, 3]. Mogensen *et al.* have shown that in patients with microalbuminuria, hyperfiltration accelerates the deterioration of renal function [9]. The haemodynamic changes have been discussed in detail in Chapter 1.

### 6.3.2 Renal morphology

*Ultrastructural changes*

Using percutaneous renal biopsy and electron microscopy, several workers have concurred that the histological hallmark of early diabetic renal disease is a glomerulopathy characterized by thickening of the glomerular basement membrane and proliferation of mesangial tissue [22]. Osterby showed that thickening of the glomerular basement membrane was established two and a half years after the onset of diabetes and mesangial expansion after a further three years. The dependence of glomerular ultrastructural alterations on metabolic control and haemodynamic changes has been shown in experimental animals. In humans, regression of glomerular basement membrane thickening and mesangial expansion was shown when cadaveric kidneys with typical diabetic glomerulopathy were transplanted into non-diabetic recipients. Successful pancreatic transplantation has also been shown to prevent the progression of glomerulopathy in kidneys transplanted into diabetic patients [23].

Although a direct correlation between the degree of glomerulopathy and the degree of albuminuria has been reported in diabetic patients, there is uncertainty concerning the role of structural changes in the initiation of diabetic nephropathy [22]. An association between various ultrastructural parameters and microalbuminuria has not been confirmed. Moreover advanced glomerular sclerosis is known to occur in many diabetic patients who never develop significant nephropathy. The pathogenetic significance of altered glomerular ultrastructure in diabetes therefore remains open to question.

*Gross structural changes*

Intravenous urography and ultrasonography have convincingly demonstrated that whole kidney size is increased in diabetic patients, consistent with data on experimental diabetes. Nephromegaly of human and experimental diabetes is due to an increase in both glomerular and tubular size with enlargement in glomerular filtration surface area [22]. This is due to both cellular hypertrophy and hyperplasia. The mechanism for increase in renal size is unknown but may be due to direct or indirect effects of glucose, glucagon, insulin and IGF-1 [18]. Strict metabolic control in experimental animals can prevent nephromegaly and an increase in glomerular volume.

### 6.3.3 Glomerular barrier biochemistry

The glomerular filtration barrier has an electrical charge (due to anionic glycosaminoglycans) and size (pores of mean diameter 550 nm), permselectivity properties that restrict the transglomerular passage of plasma proteins. A large body of data has indicated that in early diabetic renal disease there is a marked reduction in the anionic charge of the glomerular basement membrane, though the glomerular pore size remains unaltered [1, 18, 22]. Reduced electrical permselectivity may account for the accumulation of anionically charged macromolecules within the membrane, which increases its thickness and leads to mesangial proliferation. Increased quantities of plasma proteins, chiefly albumin and immunoglobulins (IgG subclass 4), have been identified in the glomerular basement membranes within two years of onset of diabetes and after transplantation of normal kidneys into diabetic recipients. The increased thickness of the glomerular basement membrane may also be related to altered collagen metabolism and increased activity of the polyol pathway [21].

## 6.4 MICROALBUMINURIA

### 6.4.1 Historical background

In 1963 Keen and Chlouverakis developed a new radioimmunoassay for human albumin in urine and used it to measure 'microalbuminuria' or 'subclinical increases in albuminuria' in the Bedford Study [1]. Newly diagnosed non-insulin-dependent patients were found to have a 3–4 fold higher urinary albumin excretion rate than non-diabetics, and positive associations were reported with glycaemia and arterial blood pressure. Microalbuminuria was confirmed in patients with established diabetes by Balodimos *et al.* in 1971 [1]. Extensive work followed over the next decade from the Danish and Guy's Hospital Groups, but focused almost exclusively on insulin-dependent patients. The most interesting of these early findings was that improvement of glycaemic control with insulin could reverse microalbuminuria in insulin-dependent diabetes, consistent with data from experimental animals.

However, the modest elevation of urinary albumin excretion was not considered to be of major clinical importance until 1982 when Viberti *et al.* [24] and Parving *et al.* [25] independently published longitudinal evidence showing that microalbuminuria was a powerful predictor of future overt nephropathy in insulin-dependent patients. It was probably these seminal reports that spawned the vast body of research now aimed at the detection and prevention of diabetic renal disease.

### 6.4.2 Prognostic value

Four well-known longitudinal studies [24–27] collectively showed that microalbuminuria is a powerful predictor of clinical nephropathy in insulin-dependent diabetic patients (see Table 6.2). The different thresholds of albumin excretion rate were arbitrarily selected to maximize the detection of patients at risk of developing clinical nephropathy (risk 75–100%), and those not at risk of this complication (0–13%). Progressive or persistent microalbuminuria, particularly greater than 70 μg/min, is likely to have the worst prognosis [28, 29]. Mogensen proposed the term 'incipient diabetic nephropathy' to describe microalbuminuria present on two out of three occasions over a period of six months, and seen in association with elevated GFR (>150 ml/min), diastolic hypertension (>90 mm Hg) and duration of diabetes between 7 and 20 years [9, 19]. Microalbuminuria tends to lose its prognostic value for diabetic nephropathy with duration of IDDM greater than 15 years. Moreover, since elevated urinary albumin excretion rate is rare in patients with duration less than five years, microalbuminuria may be regarded as a sign of renal disease rather than a marker of susceptibility.

Although the thresholds of albumin excretion rate given in Table 6.2 are useful in clinical practice, microalbuminuria could be considered as a continuum of subclinical albuminuria representing a varying degree of risk of nephropathy. The risk factors for the development of microalbuminuria in insulin-dependent patients have recently been identified as being poor long-term glycaemic control, hypertension and possibly smoking and dyslipoproteinaemia [30–36]. These and other factors, such as parental history of hypertension, glomerular hyperfiltration, ultrastructural changes and elevated urinary excretion of low-molecular-weight proteins have not been hitherto shown to be as sensitive in predicting clinical diabetic nephropathy as microalbuminuria [37, 38].

Longitudinal studies have also demonstrated that microalbuminuria markedly increased the risk of death due to cardiovascular disease in NIDDM patients (see Table 6.2) [39–43]. This applies to both clinic-based and geographically defined populations. In these patients microalbuminuria is also associated with the development of clinical proteinuria, but its prognostic power appears to be less for this complication

**Table 6.2** Prognostic value of microalbuminuria and diabetes mellitus

| Study | Viberti *et al.* (24) | Parving *et al.* (25) | Mogensen and Christensen (26) | Mathiesen *et al.* (27) | Jarrett *et al.* (39) | Mogensen (40) |
|---|---|---|---|---|---|---|
| Type of diabetes | IDDM | IDDM | IDDM | IDDM | NIDDM | NIDDM |
| No. of patients | 87 | 26 | 44 | 71 | 44 | 232 |
| No. of males/females | 54/33 | 9/17 | 44/0 | 29/42 | 27/17 | 127/105 |
| Initial age (y) | 40(17–60) | 29(16–40) | 25(18–31) | 30(13–50) | 52(33–60) | 67(50–75) |
| Duration DM (y) | 10(1–41) | 17(13–24) | 12(7–20) | 12(2–36) | 6(1–20) | 9(1–28) |
| Follow-up (y) | 14 | 5 | 10 | 6 | 14 | 10 |
| No. followed up | 63 | 24 | 43 | 71 | 42 | 204 |
| Proposed DV | 30 μg/min | 28 μg/min | 15 μg/min | 70 μg/min | 10 μg/min | 30 mg/l |
| No. with DN above DV | 7/8 | 6/8 | 12/14 | 7/7 | ? | 17/76 |
| No. with DN below DV | 2/55 | 2/15 | 0/29 | 3/64 | ? | 7/128 |
| No. died above DV | 3/8 | 1/8 | 2/14 | 0 | 10/17 | 59/76 |
| No. died below DV | 5/55 | 0/15 | 0/29 | 0 | 7/25 | 62/128 |
| Urine sample | Overnight | 24 h | Resting | 24 h | Overnight | Early morning |
| No. of urine samples | ⩾ 1 | ⩾ 1 | ⩾ 3 | ⩾ 3 | ⩾ 1 | ⩾ 1 |

DV = discrimination value; DN = diabetic nephropathy (clinical proteinuria).

than in insulin-dependent patients. Surveys in epidemiologically defined populations have also shown that microalbuminuria predicts cardiovascular disease and mortality in non-diabetic subjects [6]. Endothelial dysfunction and coexistent cardiovascular risk factors, such as hyperinsulinaemia, dyslipidaemia and hypertension, may partly account for this very important association of microalbuminuria [6,44,45]. Microalbuminuria is, however, a better short-term predictor of cardiovascular mortality than conventional risk factors.

### 6.4.3 Definition

Microalbuminuria may be defined as a level of urinary albumin excretion in excess of the upper limit of the reference range for non-diabetic subjects, and which is undetectable by Albustix test [1]. Urinary albumin concentration should be measured by an immunochemical method sensitive to at least 5 mg/l [46]. Albumin excretion should be expressed as an excretion rate or as an albumin/creatinine ratio and not as concentration. Reference ranges for urinary albumin excretion depend on several factors of which the most important are probably posture and exercise [46]. The method of urine sampling must, therefore, be specified. For example, the upper limits of albumin excretion rate in an overnight and a 24 hour collection are, approximately 10 and 20 μg/min, respectively. Patients with urine positive to Albustix usually have a total protein excretion greater than 300 μg/min, of which approximately 50% is albumin. Microalbuminuria, therefore, describes a hyperexcretion of albumin across a wide range from approximately 10 to 300 μg/min. Within this range microalbuminuria may be subclassified according to the various prognostic thresholds of albumin excretion shown in Table 6.2. This then allows further descriptions of the intermittent and persistent subtypes of microalbuminuria [28]. Because of the differences in the thresholds employed to define microalbuminuria a consensus group has proposed that it should be defined at an albumin excretion rate between 20 and 200 μg/min [47], but this requires qualification as indicated above.

Since one is interested in defining microalbuminuria with reference to diabetic glomerulopathy, non-diabetic renal disease (pyelonephritis, renal papillary necrosis) must be excluded, as must also the other risk factors leading to transitory increases in urinary albumin, e.g. severe acute deterioration in glycaemic control, congestive cardiac failure, strenuous exercise, acute water loading and essential hypertension.

### 6.4.4 Pathogenesis

Although tubular dysfunction cannot be totally excluded, albuminuria in diabetic patients without clinical nephropathy is probably predominantly glomerular in origin [1,48]. The pathogenesis of microalbuminuria must be considered in relation to the ultrastructural, haemodynamic and permselectivity changes seen in the diabetic glomerulus.

### *Glomerular ultrastructure*

Mild glomerulopathy may be seen in patients with microalbuminuria [22]. Correlations between certain ultrastructural abnormalities (e.g. glomerular basement membrane and matrix thickness, mesangial and matrix volume fractions) of the diabetic kidney and subclinical albuminuria have been reported, but not all the findings had been consistent. Moreover, the associations cannot be assumed to be causal in nature. Since 90% of insulin-dependent patients develop pronounced glomerular sclerosis but only 30–40% exhibit clinically significant renal disease, the significance of ultrastructural changes must be questioned [22]. Morphological abnormalities alone cannot, therefore, be sufficient for the development of microalbuminuria. The degree of glomerular basement membrane thickening and mesangial expansion may, however, identify a subset of patients with microalbuminuria who have the worst prognosis.

### *Glomerular haemodynamics*

The role of renal hypertension and hyperfiltration in the aetiology of diabetic nephropathy was referred to earlier [20]. Urinary albumin excretion may be determined by glomerular haemodynamics, but experimental evidence suggests that elevated glomerular pressure does not initiate diabetic nephropathy. In laboratory animals high-protein feeding increases single nephron glomerular filtration rate, glomerular plasma flow and trans-capillary hydraulic pressure, events which precede the development of proteinuria and severe glomerular lesions. Not all the studies are consistent with this chain of events. In diabetic patients moderate exercise is well known to increase filtration fraction and arterial blood pressure, but these changes are poorly correlated with the increase in urinary albumin. Acute and long-term studies of antihypertensive agents and low-protein diets have suggested that haemodynamic factors may be important in the pathogenesis of microalbuminuria. Thus, renal hyperfiltration may aggravate the prognosis of patients with established microalbuminuria, but there is at present little clinical evidence that it is responsible for initiating microalbuminuria. Moreover, while it is widely accepted that an elevation in arterial blood pressure is a concomitant of microalbuminuria, there is continuing dispute as to whether an elevation in blood pressure is a prelude to the development of microalbuminuria [30,31,34,35].

*Glomerular permselectivity*

The glomerular capillary wall has size and charge permselectivity properties that restrict the transfer of plasma proteins into the urinary space. The basement membrane consists of an anionic layer of non-collagen glycoproteins and proteoglycans rich in heparan sulphate. The transglomerular passage of negatively charged molecules such as albumin is therefore restricted relative to molecules of positive or neutral charge [1]. Studies of the renal clearance of neutral dextrans have indicated that pore size is unaltered in diabetic patients with normal and slightly elevated albumin excretion. The selectivity index (clearance ratio of neutral IgG to anionic albumin) is, however, reduced in diabetic patients with urinary albumin excretion rates between 30 and 90 μg/min. This suggests loss of anionic membrane charge in microalbuminuria. Supportive evidence for this is derived from a decrease in the urinary IgG/IgG4 ratio in patients with incipient nephropathy. Compelling data show that the diabetic state reduces the anionic charge of heparan sulphate proteoglycan of the glomerular wall by complex mechanisms involving the increase of synthesis and glycation of both collagen IV and fibronectin and decreased activity of *N*-deacetylase, the key enzyme in the sulphation of proteoglycans [6]. The net effect is increased transfer of macromolecules such as albumin into the basement membrane and the glomerular ultrafiltrate. Loss of heparan sulphate has been shown to stimulate mesangial expansion. Impaired metabolic control may additionally contribute to microalbuminuria by facilitating the transfer of glycated albumin across the glomerular basement membrane, but this remains controversial. Abnormal polyol and myoinositol metabolism [21] has been incriminated in the pathogenesis of experimental diabetic nephropathy and may also influence glomerular permselectivity, but further work is required.

*Conclusion: a hypothetical model for the pathogenesis of microalbuminuria*

The pathogenesis of diabetic microalbuminuria is multifactorial and a hypothetical model is proposed in Figure 6.1. The most convincing primary event at present is the loss of anionic charge of heparan sulphate proteoglycan within the glomerular basement membrane. The determinants of the activity of the enzyme glucosaminyl-*N*-deacetylase may be fundamental. Hyperglycaemia is a major factor and may also act through additional mechanisms [49], such as increased polyol activity, non-enzymatic glycation, glucose autoxidation and activation of protein kinase C. The accumulation of albumin and other macromolecules within the glomerular basement membrane leads to mesangial

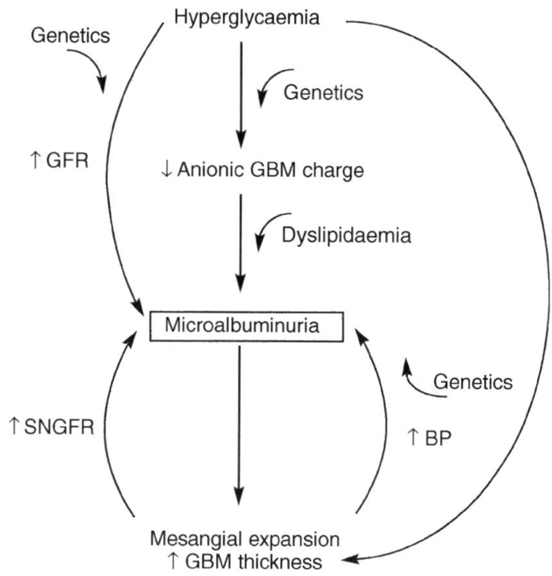


**Figure 6.1** Potential pathogenetic mechanisms resulting in microalbuminuria. GBM = glomerular basement membrane; GFR = glomerular filtration rate; SNGFR = single nephron glomerular filtration rate; BP = blood pressure.

proliferation and compensatory renal haemodynamic changes. The latter promote the transfer of proteins across the glomerular wall and accelerate progression of microalbuminuria to overt nephropathy. Microalbuminuria may actively damage mesangial tissue. Reports of the familial aggregation of diabetic nephropathy [50] and the well-known finding that only 30–40% of insulin-dependent patients develop clinically significant renal disease [2, 3] suggest that some or all of the aforementioned processes must be genetically determined. The role of essential hypertension and increased erythrocyte sodium–lithium counter-transport has not been fully established in this context. Dyslipidaemia may be causally related to microalbuminuria [36].

There is no definitive evidence that endocrine or haemorrheological factors are responsible for initiating microalbuminuria [18]. Finally, although microalbuminuria is considered to be almost exclusively of glomerular origin, studies based on the excretion of retinol-binding protein, lysozyme and *N*-acetyl-β-D-glucosaminidase suggest that there may also be a renal tubular component [46]. This hypothesis warrants further study, but preliminary evidence suggests that albuminuria is the most significant independent predictor of the development of diabetic renal disease [38].

### 6.4.5 Prevalence, incidence and associations

Cross-sectional studies have reported a prevalence of microalbuminuria ranging from 6 to 59% [37, 46]. The prevalence clearly depends on the threshold of albumin excretion employed to define microalbuminuria and on several other factors, such as the methods and number of urine collections and the clinical features of the population. For example, urinary albumin excretion is higher in 24 hour and random urine collections than overnight or early morning collections, and in insulin-dependent diabetics the presence of microalbuminuria is almost restricted to patients with duration of diabetes between 5 and 15 years. Ethnic factors may be important, particularly in non-insulin-dependent patients in whom microalbuminuria has been reported to be more common in those of Asian than of European extraction [51].

Cross-sectional and case-control studies in insulin-dependent patients have shown that microalbuminuria has a wide spectrum of clinical associations, including the following: early age at onset and long duration of diabetes, male sex, high body mass index, cigarette smoking, family history of cardiovascular disease, family history of hypertension and increased erythrocyte sodium–lithium counter-transport, family history of renal disease, poor short and long-term glycaemic control, arterial hypertension, high dietary fat and protein intake, dyslipoproteinaemia including elevation of lipoprotein (a), presence of retinopathy and neuropathy [6, 46, 52]. Not all the findings have been consistent and this is probably due to differences in the selection of patients. The associations of microalbuminuria may differ between insulin-dependent and non-insulin-dependent patients [53, 54]. Microalbuminuria may be part of the insulin-resistance syndrome or prediabetic state and appears to be a good predictor of cardiovascular disease. In both IDDM and NIDDM microalbuminuria has recently been shown to be associated with elevated serum concentrations of sialic acid, a marker of vascular damage [55, 56]. Microalbuminuria may appear for the first time during gestational diabetes and in insulin-dependent patients it may be associated with elevated blood pressure and poor fetal outcome. Despite the many associations of microalbuminuria, a large proportion of the variation between subjects remains unexplained, suggesting that in practical terms there are little grounds for a selective screening programme [57].

The association between microalbuminuria and macrovascular disease was referred to earlier, especially in relation to NIDDM [6]. Dyslipoproteinaemia, increased vascular permeability to albumin and a prothrombotic state have been described in patients with microalbuminuria. Generalized vasculopathy is also suggested by increased serum levels of von Willebrand factor antigen and sialic acid. The common plasma lipid and lipoprotein disturbances are an increase in low-density-lipoprotein cholesterol, apolipoprotein B and lipoprotein (a), and low levels of high-density-lipoprotein cholesterol and apolipoprotein Al [33, 52, 58]. Hyper-apobetalipoproteinaemia may antedate the development of microalbuminuria in IDDM [36]. Hypertriglyceridaemia is typically seen in non-insulin-dependent patients. The aforementioned factors may collectively account for the premature atherosclerosis seen in early diabetic nephropathy. Insulin-dependent patients with persistent microalbuminuria have been shown to have cardiac dysfunction and reduced aerobic working capacity [6]. 'Silent cardiac ischaemia' has also been recently described in non-insulin-dependent patients with microalbuminuria.

Compared with the several cross-sectional reports, few studies have examined the progression of urinary albumin excretion and its determinants. In a seven-year longitudinal study Cooper *et al.* [32] found that in patients with an initial albumin excretion rate less than 30 μg/min the annual incidence of persistent microalbuminuria above this threshold was 2% for IDDM patients and 4% for NIDDM patients; insulin-dependent patients who progressed tended to have retinopathy and a longer duration of diabetes, and the transition to microalbuminuria was associated with reduction in glomerular filtration rate and increasing blood pressure. Mathiesen *et al.* [27] found that normoalbuminuric IDDM patients (less than 20 μg/min) had a mean annual increase in urinary albumin excretion rate of 0.7 μg/min; those with microalbuminuria greater than 20 μg/min had a mean annual increase of 12 μg/min. A phase of highly variable albuminuria, referred to as intermittent microalbuminuria, precedes the emergence of persistent microalbuminuria [28]. Our own studies have shown that intermittent microalbuminuria is most closely associated with changes in glomerular filtration rate alone [28]. The Microalbuminuria Collaborative Study [30] in the UK reported that in patients with an albumin excretion rate of less than 30 μg/min, persistent microalbuminuria developed at the rate of 2% per year, and this was dependent on the initial level of albuminuria, blood pressure and glycated haemoglobin.

Our own 10-year follow-up study of insulin-dependent patients in Portsmouth, UK, showed that the most powerful determinant of the progression from normoalbuminuria to persistent microalbuminuria (after adjusting for initial level of albuminuria) was the initial level of glycated haemoglobin [34], consistent with another recent report [35]. Once microalbuminuria becomes established the average annual increase in albumin excretion rate tends to rise and ranges from 7 to 20%, but the rate differs widely among patients [9]. Increases in albumin excretion rate are then more closely associated with arterial blood pressure, long-term glycaemic control and hyperfiltration. In summary, the rate of progression of subclinical albuminuria involves a multifactorial process. It accelerates directly with the initial level of albumin excretion, poor long-term glycaemic control being the major clinical determinant of the development of microalbuminuria. The combination of hypertension, hyperfiltration and poor diabetic control influences the progression of microalbuminuria to established nephropathy. Variation in the rate of progression at all levels of urinary albumin excretion also depends on genetic factors, such as family history of hypertension, polymorphisms in *N*-deacetylase and histocompatibility antigen status [6, 18, 59].

### 6.4.6 Intervention studies

*Insulin-dependent diabetes*

*Glycaemic control*

Preliminary reports showed that a continuous subcutaneous insulin infusion (CSII) could significantly reduce resting microalbuminuria and abolish microalbuminuria provoked by exercise [1]. The Steno I Study carried out over six months and the eight-month KROC Study concurred that very tight glycaemic control could diminish subclinical albuminuria [60]. The Steno II Study showed that near-normoglycaemia for two years prevented the progression of persistent microalbuminuria to clinical proteinuria, a combined analysis of both Steno Studies demonstrating that the most pronounced benefit was in patients with higher levels of albuminuria. By contrast to trials in patients with established microalbuminuria, the Oslo Study examined the impact of tight glycaemic control on a level of urinary albumin excretion around the upper limit of the reference range: four years of treatment with CSII achieved a significant reduction in albuminuria compared with no reduction on conventional insulin treatment. The association between improved glycaemic control, as measured by $HbA_1$, and albuminuria was confirmed in the seven-year results from this study. The findings of these earlier small studies [60] have recently been confirmed by eight-year data from the Stockholm Study [61] and from the large Diabetes Control and Complications Trial (DCCT) [62]. In the DCCT, 1441 insulin-dependent patients were randomly assigned to intensive therapy administered by either CSII or multiple insulin injections or to conventional therapy. Six and a half years of intensive therapy that achieved a mean $HbA_{1C}$ of 7% reduced the development of microalbuminuria (>40 mg/24 h) by 39% and clinical albuminuria (>330 mg/24 h) by 54%. The effects of treatment on the cumulative incidence of microalbuminuria and clinical albuminuria in the primary-prevention cohort (IDDM for one to five years, no retinopathy, albumin excretion

<40 mg/24 h) and secondary-prevention cohort (IDDM for one to 15 years, mild–moderate retinopathy, albumin excretion <200 mg/24 h) are shown in Figures 6.2 (a) and (b), respectively. In the DCCT, parallel improvements were seen in the incidence of retinopathy and neuro-

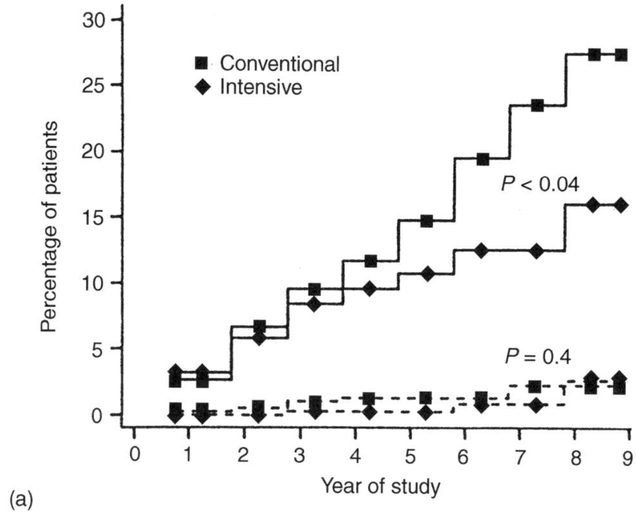


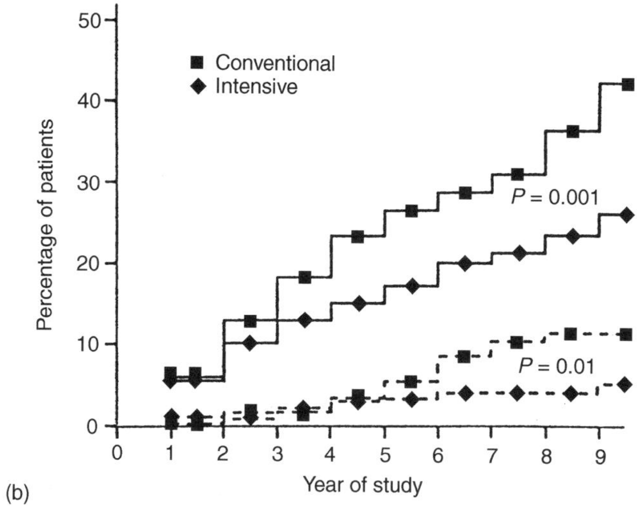


**Figure 6.2** Cumulative incidence of microalbuminuria (⩾ 40 mg/24 h; solid line) and macroalbuminuria (⩾ 300 mg/24 h; dashed line) in patients with IDDM in the DCCT. (a) primary-prevention cohort; (b) secondary-prevention cohort; see text for further details. Intensive treatment reduced the risk of microalbuminuria in (a) by 34% and in (b) by 43%.

pathy. This important trial, therefore, showed that intensive glycaemic control is effective in reducing both the development of microalbuminuria and its progression to clinical diabetic nephropathy.

*Blood pressure*

Subclinical elevation in blood pressure is a feature of insulin-dependent patients with incipient nephropathy. In a five-year open study of six patients with progressive microalbuminuria and mild hypertension, Mogensen reported that sustained reduction of blood pressure with metoprolol and bendrofluazide achieved marked regression of microalbuminuria [13]. Similar treatment reduced microalbuminuria provoked by exercise. Because activation of the renin–angiotensin–aldosterone system (RAAS) is well known to induce hyperfiltration and to increase intraglomerular pressure, the major focus on antihypertensive agents has been on the angiotensin-converting enzyme (ACE) inhibitors. In a one-year, randomized placebo-controlled trial involving normotensive patients with persistent microalbuminuria, Marre *et al.* [63] reported that enalapril diminished elevated urinary albumin excretion and prevented progression to clinical proteinuria; mean arterial blood pressure was reduced in this study to an average of 85 mm Hg. ACE inhibition may reduce microalbuminuria by specific modulation of intra-renal haemodynamics. In a randomized control trial of four years' duration, Mathiesen *et al.* [64] showed that captopril delayed the development of clinically overt diabetic nephropathy in normotensive insulin-dependent patients. This has now been confirmed by other trials. Agents that inhibit the RAAS appear to be better than drugs that stimulate this endocrine pathway, such as thiazide diuretics [65]. There is some dispute, however, as to whether calcium channel blockers are as effective as ACE inhibitors in treating microalbuminuria [18, 57, 66]. Experimental evidence favours ACE inhibitors, since besides improving intra-renal haemodynamics they appear to have a direct benefit on the properties of the glomerular filtration barrier that reduces the permeability to plasma protein. The issue is discussed in greater detail in Chapter 3.

*Dietary protein restriction*

The 'nephrotoxicity' of high protein intake has been well recognized for several years and is now considered to be due to increased renal blood flow and intraglomerular pressure. The role of low-protein diets in treating microalbuminuria has not been as well tested as the control of blood glucose and blood pressure. In a six-week randomized crossover trial of six insulin-dependent patients with persistent microalbuminuria, Viberti's group reported that a reduction in dietary protein from 92 to 47 g/day resulted in a significant decrease in microalbuminuria and in hyperfiltration independent of changes in glycaemia and blood pressure [67]. In younger patients these effects may be most pronounced in those with elevated GFR. The findings are consistent with the effects of dietary manipulation on glomerular morphology and function in experimental animals. Reductions in animal protein instead of vegetable protein may be better in preserving renal function in patients [67]. A recent meta-analysis concluded that protein restriction may benefit the course of established diabetic and non-diabetic renal disease [15].

*Non-insulin-dependent diabetes*

In contrast to IDDM, fewer trials have been carried out in patients with NIDDM [68]. Short-term studies have shown that microalbuminuria may be diminished in patients with newly diagnosed or established NIDDM treated with diet alone or by diet and oral agents. In the UK Prospective Diabetes Survey (UKPDS) in Oxford, 585 newly diagnosed patients receiving diet alone showed improvement in albumin excretion rate within three months, but no further improvement over three years [69]. Over this period urinary albumin excretion was independently associated with fasting plasma glucose, triglyceride and systolic blood pressure, but these only explained 10% of the total variance. It is possible that the effect of hypocaloric diets in improving microalbuminuria may be due to the concomitant restriction of dietary protein. That improvement in glycaemic control in non-insulin-dependent patients reduces the incidence and progression of microalbuminuria may be indirectly inferred from the results of DCCT [62], although these data need to be supplemented by further reports from UKPDS [68]. The relationship between hypertension and nephropathy in NIDDM is less clear than in IDDM [9]. Many patients with NIDDM are hypertensive and a few short-term trials have shown a reduction in microalbuminuria with ACE inhibitors [68]. Long-acting calcium antagonists may, however, be as effective as ACE inhibitors in treating normotensive patients with microalbuminuria and are probably better than the combination of a beta-blocker and loop diuretic. The issues are addressed in greater detail in Chapter 3. There is a need for more long-term studies of the effects of conventional treatment on the incidence and progression of microalbuminuria in non-insulin-dependent patients. A recent randomized controlled study of seven years' duration has affirmed that angiotensin-converting enzyme inhibition has a renoprotective effect in NIDDM with microalbuminuria [70].

*Other interventions*

Since the pathogenesis of diabetic nephropathy is multifactorial, the effectiveness of several therapies other than the above should also be studied [68]. These include prostaglandin synthesis inhibitors to improve intra-renal haemodynamics, aldose reductase inhibitors to correct the tissue ratios of sorbitol/myoinositol, aminoguanidine to reduce advanced glycosylation end-products, and growth factor inhibitors or ornithine decarboxylase to diminish glomerular enlargement and hyperfiltration. There is good experimental evidence to support clinical trials of these agents in patients. Antiplatelet aggregators, such as thromboxane synthesis inhibitors, have been shown to improve microalbuminuria and renal haemodynamics, but further studies are required. Initial reports of the potential benefits of omega-3 fatty acids on microalbuminuria have not been confirmed. The efficacy of all forms of interventions is probably subject to the effects of genetic determinants, e.g. histocompatibility antigen status and ACE genotype[34, 59]. This field needs further research.

It must be noted that microalbuminuria is only a surrogate end-point for diabetic nephropathy and cardiovascular disease. Although the above studies suggest that it may be amenable to various forms of treatment, no trial has hitherto shown that end stage renal failure or cardiovascular mortality can be prevented.

## 6.5 SCREENING AND PREVENTION OF DIABETIC NEPHROPATHY

### 6.5.1 Criteria for screening

To justify screening for a particular condition, whether in the community or in the clinic, certain classical criteria must be fulfilled [71]. These are briefly discussed below as they apply to a screening programme for early diabetic renal disease/microalbuminuria:

1. The disease should be common and clinically important. Diabetic renal disease is a major long-term complication of both types of diabetes, associated with high morbidity, mortality and financial costs [12].
2. The disease should have an early presymptomatic or latent phase. Unassailable evidence shows that the earliest indication of diabetic renal disease is microalbuminuria [37], a major risk factor for renal and macrovascular disease [6].
3. Effective treatment should be available for patients who screen positive. Tight glycaemic control, lowering of blood pressure and dietary protein restriction may arrest or reverse the progression of microalbuminuria to clinical proteinuria [68] in both types of diabetes. There is therefore clear evidence then that medical intervention may benefit the natural history of patients with a positive test.
4. The natural history of the latent phase should be characterized. Several studies have now indicated that microalbuminuria passes through an intermittent phase prior to becoming persistent and

progressing to clinical proteinuria [9, 46, 57]. The onset of microalbuminuria appears to be closely related to poor long-term glycaemic control and its course to overt nephropathy is accelerated by systemic and intra-renal hypertension. All these factors tend to influence the wide variation among patients in the natural history of the latent phase of diabetic nephropathy.

5. A reliable and acceptable test should be available for the latent disease. Considerable advances have been made in the development of laboratory and clinical methods for the detection of microalbuminuria and these are referred to later [46].
6. Facilities should be available for the follow-up of patients. The monitoring of microalbuminuria and the efficacy of treatment may be undertaken in diabetic or renal clinic and possibly in specialized clinics in general practice [57]. Planning of follow-up is referred to later.
7. The cost-to-benefit ratio of screening should be favourable. This depends on the balance between the costs of the diagnostic services and the costs of effective medical treatment. The economic burden of screening programmes for microalbuminuria will be lessened by the design of effective and practicable methodologies (see later). A recent analysis concluded that screening for microalbuminuria and intervention with antihypertensive drugs would have life-saving effects and considerable economic savings [72]. This analysis was based on a programme of 30 years with annual screening for microalbuminuria starting five years after the onset of diabetes; it employed computerized simulation of a cohort of 8 000 insulin-dependent diabetic patients with main outcome measures being mortality, incidence of diabetic nephropathy, incidence of end stage renal failure and associated costs versus savings. Further economic analyses would be required in relation to other forms of intervention and the efficacy of multiple therapies.

Screening for early diabetic renal disease by the detection and treatment of microalbuminuria clearly meets most of the above criteria. Accordingly, the World Health Organization (WHO) and International Diabetes Federation (IDF) have recommended annual screening for microalbuminuria in all patients with insulin-dependent diabetes over the age of 12 years with diabetes duration in excess of five years.

### 6.5.2 Methods of screening

*Measurement of microalbuminuria*

The methods must be specific for albumin, have an imprecision of less than 10% and a sensitivity down to a concentration of at least 3 mg/l

[46]. These criteria require the use of immunochemical assays. Immunoturbidimetry using a centrifugal analyser may be the most convenient assay because of its high-speed, high-precision, inexpensive running costs and requirement for low technical skills. Small analysers are particularly suited for on-line measurements in the diabetic clinic. Urine samples may be stored at $-20°C$ for up to three months. Assay performance may vary widely and it is therefore recommended that all laboratories belong to a national quality control scheme [46].

*Urine collection and expression of albumin excretion*

Timed collections are not recommended in clinical practice [46]. The most precise and accurate test is the urine albumin/creatinine ratio ($U_A/U_C$) in an early morning sample; a random $U_A/U_C$ may be more convenient initially but is less specific owing to the effects of posture and exercise. Initially the programme should aim to detect those with a $U_A/U_C$ of $>3.5$ mg/mmol (equivalent to an albumin excretion rate of $>30$ μg/min) [57]. Thresholds may be regulated according to workload and resources. Measurement of $U_A$ followed by $U_A/U_C$ may be used in combination as a screening test, particularly if there is reason to limit the measurement of $U_C$. To facilitate follow-up and treatment strategies we recommend that real-time measurements should ideally be carried out during consultations in the clinic.

*Side-room testing*

Immunochemical tests such as the latex bead-immunoagglutination test and Micral test [46] only measure urinary albumin concentration and may fail to detect patients with microalbuminuria and high urine flow rates. We recommend that patients who screen negative by side-room tests should be retested in the laboratory with accurate measurement of $U_A/U_C$ particularly when there is evidence that the urine is very dilute. In general practice this would require sending additional samples to the biochemistry laboratory. Brief training of personnel undertaking side-room tests is recommended.

### 6.5.3 Strategies for screening for microalbuminuria

*Selective screening*

Since clinical variables commonly recorded or measured in the diabetic clinic cannot confidently predict microalbuminuria, an effective selective screening programme cannot be recommended [57]. However, if screening has to be rationed for any reason it should focus on insulin-dependent patients with early age at onset of diabetes, duration of diabetes between five and 20 years, retinopathy, neuropathy, clinical hypertension (BP > 160/95 mm Hg) and persistent hyperglycaemia ($HbA_1 > 12\%$). It must be emphasized that these criteria will not sufficiently increase the sensitivity and specificity of screening to fully justify a selective strategy.

### *Monitoring microalbuminuria and planning follow-up*

Once screening has been initiated, there is a commitment to the follow-up of patients. The most reproducible and convenient test should be used to monitor microalbuminuria [57]. The test of choice is the urinary albumin/creatinine ratio in an early morning (first void) sample. As with first-stage screening, the availability of on-line analyses with the results available at consultation will increase the efficiency of follow-up and treatment. Timed collections, random samples and measurement of urinary albumin concentration alone are not recommended for monitoring purposes. It is not necessary to test the urine for infection in patients who screen positive, unless urinary symptoms are reported or blood is detected on dipstick urinanalysis [73].

When patients are repeatedly tested for microalbuminuria, many are only found to be intermittently positive. Re-testing should aim to identify patients with microalbuminuria present on three consecutive occasions, i.e. persistent microalbuminuria [28, 57]. The re-testing interval will depend on the threshold employed in the screening programme to define microalbuminuria and on the level of albuminuria at initial screening. Use of the threshold to define microalbuminuria is recommended since this will assist clinical decisions. It is suggested that $U_A/U_C$ of 3.5 mg/mmol be adopted to decide whom to follow-up with a view to treatment when screening is first introduced in the clinic.

The algorithm in Figure 6.3a is based on our own data of the natural history of microalbuminuria in insulin-dependent patients [28, 31, 57]. The figure gives re-testing intervals based on the level of $U_A/U_C$ in an early morning urine sample at initial screening and a policy to treat patients with microalbuminuria of >3.5 mg/mmol on three consecutive occasions. The principle of the algorithm is that the higher the initial value of $U_A/U_C$ the more frequently should re-testing be carried out with a view to expediting treatment. Information on the level of glycaemic control and blood pressure should be taken into account. For example, if the $U_A/U_C$ is <2.5 mg/mmol with an $HbA_1$ of > 12% and/or a BP of > 160/95 mm Hg, the patient should be re-tested every six months. The $HbA_1$ and blood pressure should be recorded on each occasion that a patient is re-tested for microalbuminuria since this information will not only be useful for deciding further follow-up but will also be important for therapy.

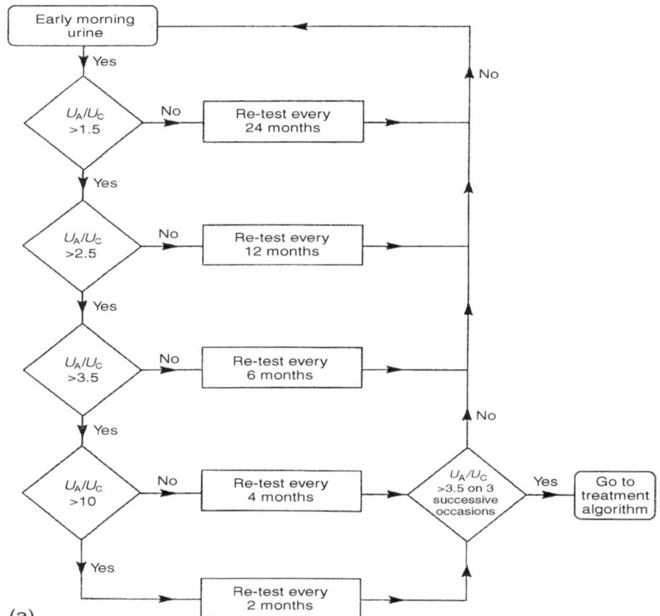


(a)

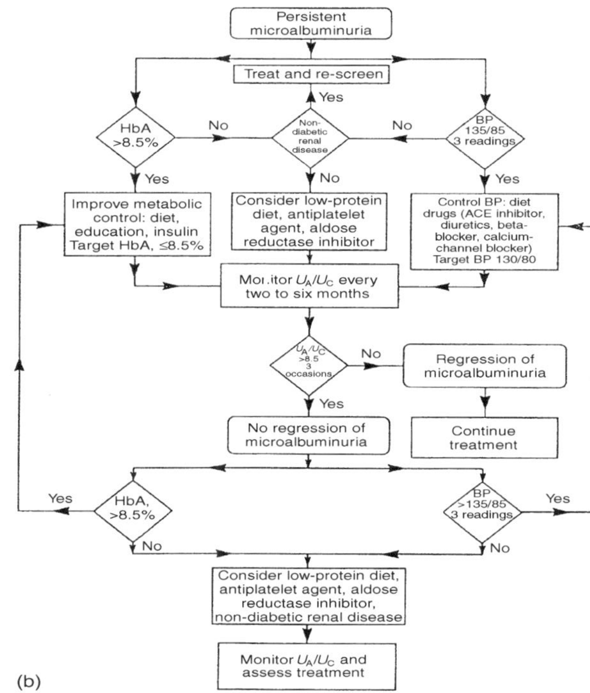


(b)

**Figure 6.3** (a) Algorithm for screening and monitoring microalbuminuria based on the measurement of the urinary albumin/creatinine ratio ($U_A/U_C$, mg/mmol) in an early morning sample and a policy to treat those patients found to have a $U_A/U_C > 3.5$ mg/mmol on three successive occasions. If the policy is to treat at a lower level of $U_A/U_C$, re-testing intervals should be shorter. The algorithm excludes patients with persistent clinical proteinuria (Albustix > +ve) and elevated serum creatinine. (b) Algorithm for treating persistent microalbuminuria (present on three successive occasions). Therapeutic response is based on the measurement of the urinary albumin/creatinine ratio ($U_A/U_C$, mg/mmol) in an early morning sample.

The above recommendations are only provisional and must be validated in a clinical environment. Simpler recommendations have been provided elsewhere, but we consider that these have not been adequately qualified to take account of variation in the individual risk of nephropathy attributable to a given level of microalbuminuria. The role of exercise testing is a long-term predictor of the development of microalbuminuria in normoalbuminuric patients looks promising [74], but this needs further validation.

*Screening type II diabetic (NIDDM) patients*

The clinical associations and natural history of microalbuminuria in type II patients have not been as well studied as in type I patients. Moreover the significance of microalbuminuria and the benefits of treatment need to be further established. We consider therefore that the routine screening of type II patients for microalbuminuria should only be implemented once such information is available from studies currently in progress [69]. It is possible that microalbuminuria may be more specifically and clinically useful as a marker of cardiovascular disease than of nephropathy in type II diabetes [6].

## 6.6 TREATMENT

Treatment should focus on patients with persistent microalbuminuria (present on three successive occasions) particularly when the $U_A/U_C$ is rising rapidly. It will need to be individualized, acknowledging that more than one therapeutic option may have to be tried and that the responses among patients may differ. Close monitoring of the efficacy of treatment is required by measuring the $U_A/U_C$ at regular intervals. Ideally the $U_A/U_C$ (early morning sample) should be lowered to within the reference range of non-diabetic subjects, i.e. $< 1.5$ mg/mmol. The principal aims of therapy are improved glycaemic control, lowering of blood pressure and low-protein diets [13]. Use of these in relation to the measurement of microalbuminuria is summarized in the algorithm shown in Figure 3b. Alternative therapies such as antiplatelet agents and aldose reductors inhibitors are still at the experimental stage. The recommendations for treatment refer specifically to type I diabetic patients.

### 6.6.1 Glycaemic control

Measurement of glycated haemoglobin is important to identify at risk patients and assess therapeutic outcome. Treatment should aim to achieve values below one standard deviation above the mean for non-diabetic subjects, e.g. $HbA_1 < 7.5\%$ (equivalent $HbA_{1C} < 6.5\%$) [13]. Control may be improved by conventional insulin treatment or multiple insulin injections. Insulin pump therapy may be considered in selected patients who are highly motivated and well disciplined and for whom the clinic can provide adequate support. Very tight glycaemic control may have drawbacks such as weight gain and unacceptable hypoglycaemia. Attention to regular home glucose monitoring and contact with specialist nurses is important. Given the adequate information from their carers, patients will ultimately need to make the choice between the effort and risk of intensified glycaemic control and the risks of developing progressive microalbuminuria and diabetic nephropathy.

### 6.6.2 Blood pressure

Conventional levels of blood pressure used to define hypertension are probably too high for patients with microalbuminuria [13, 68]. Both the WHO and IDF have recommended early antihypertensive treatment of patients with microalbuminuria at blood pressures $\geqslant 140$ mm Hg systolic or $\geqslant 90$ mm Hg diastolic. It may be useful to employ age–sex matched centile blood pressure charts to define hypertension. We consider that blood pressure should be reduced to $< 135/85$ mm Hg (equivalent mean arterial blood pressure 100 mm Hg), with due consideration to age and other complications such as coronary artery disease. A reasonable target would be a blood pressure of 130/80 mm Hg, with avoidance of hypotension. A conventional sphygmomanometer with diastolic blood pressure readings being recorded at Korotkov phase V is recommended for clinical purposes. Three measurements of blood pressure should be made in the sitting or supine position, with careful attention paid to identifying postural hypotension, particularly in patients with autonomic neuropathy or ischaemic heart disease.

Treatment should initially be dietary, with restriction of salt and alcohol, and weight loss wherever appropriate. If drugs are required various options include low-dose diuretics (with occasional potassium supplementation), alpha-blockers, calcium antagonists and ACE inhibitors. Dual or triple therapy may be necessary [13, 68] and plasma electrolyte concentrations should be checked regularly. The efficacy of ACE inhibitors has been well demonstrated in clinical trials and we consider them the agent of first choice. Use of ACE inhibitors requires regular checks on electrolytes, particularly for hyperkalaemia, and renal function, which should be undertaken until treatment is stabilized. Dual therapy may take the form of the addition of a small dose of a loop diuretic to an ACE inhibitor to achieve good blood pressure control. Use of beta-blockers and thiazide diuretics need to take account of the symptoms of hypoglycaemic unawareness, dyslipidaemia and peripheral vascular disease.

Blood pressure is discussed in detail in Chapter 3.

### 6.6.3 Dietary protein restriction

We recommend that patients with microalbuminuria should have specialist dietary assessment to check that protein intake is appropriate but not excessive. A reasonable compromise may be a protein intake of between 12 and 15% of total calories per day or approximately 1 g of protein/kg body weight per day [57, 67]. Reduction in protein intake should ensure that the patient is receiving an adequate supply of proteins with high biological value and the diet is not deficient in other essential nutrients. When other therapeutic options have not influenced the course of microalbuminuria and serum creatinine rises progressively, further restriction of dietary protein or a switch from animal to vegetable-type protein may be considered. The above dietary changes can be unpalatable and consequently there may be problems with compliance.

## 6.7 CONCLUSIONS AND PERSPECTIVES

A joint survey by the Royal College of Physicians and British Diabetic Association in 1979 assessed the factors contributing to premature mortality of the diabetic patient under 50 years of age [75]. Diabetic renal disease accounted for 19% of the total deaths, and the risk was greatest for those with age at onset of diabetes especially under 10 years of age and those with long duration of disease. The report noted that of those dying prematurely of nephropathy, only 13% of patients had been offered active management of end stage renal failure. This situation has now changed considerably, as diabetic patients are increasingly accepted for renal replacement, and indeed may now account for between 20 and 25% of a specialist renal centre workload [76]. Despite this improvement, the cost and resource implications are considerable, and the prognosis, even with dialysis or transplantation, is still less favourable than that of other non-diabetic causes of end stage renal failure.

Although more patients with diabetic nephropathy are being offered specialist renal management, it should be noted that the numbers of such patients needing renal replacement may actually be diminishing [77]. The cause for this is somewhat uncertain. It may well reflect trends towards better treatment strategies for diabetes, particularly insulin regimens and more definitive monitoring of control, leading to improved blood glucose control, as well as more effective treatment of hypertension.

It would, therefore, seem that we are already witnessing an alteration in the natural history of diabetic nephropathy. Nonetheless substantial numbers are still at risk of developing serious renal disease and continued efforts in terms of prevention need to be made. The recent increase in knowledge and understanding of the early stages of diabetic nephropathy and underlying pathogenesis now offer the opportunity of assessing the development of nephropathy at a time when the process may be potentially influenced by therapeutic intervention.

The full natural history of early diabetic nephropathy, as characterized by the detection of microalbuminuria, progressing to macroproteinuria and advanced nephropathy, still remains to be determined. However, it is probable that microalbuminuria over a period of time will progress in the vast majority of patients, where it has been detected, to overt nephropathy, although the rate of progression will vary from one individual to another. The period of microalbuminuria is a critical time, for it is evident that reversibility is still possible and the process is potentially contained by measures such as strict diabetic control and antihypertensive drug intervention. Conversely, patients in whom microalbuminuria has not been detected even after a few years from diagnosis may still progress to significant microalbuminuria, especially if diabetic control has been poor over intervening years [34]. The risk of developing nephropathy if microalbuminuria has not presented after 20 years from diagnosis of diabetes is relatively small.

Screening for microalbuminuria offers the opportunity of identifying those individuals at greatest risk of progressing to overt diabetic nephropathy and end stage renal failure, as well as identifying those with a greater risk of developing other complications of diabetes and those liable to suffer premature mortality from coronary heart disease. Although the detection of microalbuminuria is associated with at least a ten-fold increase in the likelihood of progression to overt diabetic nephropathy, a proportion of those with microalbuminuria will not progress with time, and a significant number with initial microalbuminuria may, in fact, return to normo-albuminuria. Equally, some with initial normo albuminuria may progress in due course to significant microalbuminuria and future risk of nephropathy. Guidelines for the management of insulin-dependent diabetes must therefore include routine monitoring for microalbuminuria in all IDDM cases. The requirements for non-insulin-dependent diabetes have yet to be established, though there is no doubt that the detection of microalbuminuria in these patients identifies a substantial increase in risk of cardiovascular disease. It is quite possible it also determines those at risk of developing renal failure, although evidence is not as clear as in IDDM patients.

It is apparent that of those IDDM patients under regular clinic supervision, the patients most likely to develop microalbuminuria and subsequent nephropathy are those of young onset diabetes, relatively long duration of diabetes, those who are hypertensive and above all poorly controlled. Those who fail to maintain supervision (clinic defaulters) are considerably more at risk of long-term complications, including nephropathy. It is likely that these clinic non-attenders (at least 10% of all IDD) take less responsibility for their diabetes care and therefore blood glucose control may be less than optimal. An effective initiative to retrieve clinic defaulters and review their management could make a substantial impact on the numbers of diabetic patients progressing to renal failure.

It is now evident that screening protocols should be established routinely by those involved in the care of insulin-dependent diabetics to determine those with significant microalbuminuria and individuals who are considered at potential risk of long-term life-threatening complications, including nephropathy. Equally, there is now convincing evidence that treatment intervention strategies during the stage of microalbuminuria can be very effective. Intensified glycaemic control, as illustrated in the Diabetes Control and Complications Trial [62], has shown that intensified glucose control significantly reduces the incidence and progression of microalbuminuria. Although observations on long-term outcome in terms of prevention of end stage renal failure are still awaited, it would seem reasonable to presume that reduction in microalbuminuria during the early stages of nephropathy will be reflected in either a delay or indeed arrest of more advanced renal change, thus leading to both prolongation and improvement of the quality of life.

Despite the wish to obtain as near optimal glycaemic control as possible, there will always be individuals in whom it cannot be achieved for various reasons. Intensified diabetic control itself will, therefore, not result in the prevention or reversal of microalbuminuria in many instances. Under such circumstances it is encouraging that many studies of drug intervention, particularly using antihypertensive agents, have shown that significant benefit can be obtained from such means. ACE inhibitors seem to have a particularly beneficial role, with evidence of sustained reduction of microalbuminuria [78], and, more recently, observation that long-term outcome measures such as mortality risk and progression to end stage renal failure may be substantially improved [14]. The role of dietary protein restriction is significant [67], but it should be recognized that initiation of a protein-reduced diet for a diabetic patient does pose extra difficulties when the diet has already been modified for the diabetes itself. If protein restriction is recommended, a specialist dietitian should be involved in ensuring a correct balance is obtained.

The present trend in the delivery of diabetes care is towards a more integrated, structured service with general practitioners undertaking much more involvement as health centre mini-clinics are established. Many health districts have now established shared protocols for the management of diabetes, such that hospital diabetes centres can focus more directly on those patients with more complicated and specialized problems of diabetes management, and particularly those considered at greatest risk. Insulin-dependent diabetics with microalbuminuria should be regarded as individuals at risk and come under the supervision of a hospital diabetes centre so that optimum treatment strategies can be established and maintained, both for diabetic control and the institution and monitoring of drug intervention. In view of the potentially very large numbers of patients with microalbuminuria, responsibility for the management of early nephropathy must remain with the specialist diabetes unit. Close liaison and common protocols should, however, be established with the local renal unit so that there is common understanding and awareness, and that patients in whom renal function continues to deteriorate despite treatment are anticipated and long-term plans for end stage renal management put into operation.

## REFERENCES

1. Viberti, G.C. and Keen, H. (1984) The patterns of proteinuria in diabetes mellitus. *Diabetes*, **33**, 686–92.
2. Andersen, A.R., Christensen, J.S., Andersen, J.K. *et al.* (1983) Diabetic nephropathy in type I (insulin dependent) diabetes: an epidemiological study. *Diabetologia*, **25**, 496–501.
3. Krowlewski, A.S., Warram, S.H., Christlieb, A.R. *et al.* (1985) The changing natural history of nephropathy in type I diabetes. *Am. J. Med.*, **78**, 785–94.
4. Grenfell, A. (1986) Diabetic nephropathy: historical aspects. *Clin. Endocrinol. Metab.*, **15**, 727–31.
5. Borch-Johnsen, K. and Kreiner, S. (1987) Proteinuria-value as a predictor of cardiovascular mortality in insulin-dependent diabetes mellitus. *Br. Med. J.*, **294**, 1651–4.
6. Deckert, T., Kofoed-Enevoldsen, A., Noregaard, K. *et al.* (1992) Microalbuminuria. Implications for micro and macrovascular disease. *Diabetes Care*, **15**, 1181–91.
7. Parving, H.H. and Hominel, E. (1989) Prognosis in diabetic nephropathy. *Br. Med. J.*, **299**, 230–4.
8. Fabre, J., Balant, L.P., Dayer, P.G. *et al.* (1982) The kidney in maturity onset diabetes mellitus. A clinical study of 510 patients. *Kidney Int.*, **21**, 730–8.
9. Mogensen, C.E., Schmitz, A. and Christensen, C.K. (1988) Comparative renal pathophysiology relevant to IDDM and NIDDM patients. *Diabetes Metab. Rev.*, **4**, 453–83.
10. Joint Working Party. (1985) Renal failure in diabetics in the United Kingdom: deficient provision of care in 1985. *Diabetic Med.*, **5**, 79–84.
11. Lloyd, C.E., Stephenson, J., Fuller, J.H. and Orchard, T. (1996) A comparison of renal disease across two continents. *Diabetic Care*, **19**, 219–25.
12. Narins, B.E. and Narins, R.G. (1988) Clinical features and health-care costs of diabetic nephropathy. *Diabetes Care*, **11**, 833–9.
13. Mogensen, C.E. (1988) Management of diabetic renal involvement and disease. *Lancet*, **i**, 867–70.

14. Lewis, E.J., Hunsicker, L.G., Bain, R.P. and Rohde, R.D. (1993) The effect of angiotensin-converting-enzyme inhibition on diabetic nephropathy. *N. Engl. J. Med.*, **329**, 1456–62.
15. Pedrini, M.T., Levey, A.S., Lau, J. *et al.* (1996) The effect of dietary protein restriction on the progression of diabetic and non-diabetic renal disease: a meta-analysis. *Ann. Intern. Med.*, **124**, 627–32.
16. Herman, W., Hawthorne, V., Hamman, R. *et al.* (1989) Consensus statement on preventing the kidney disease of diabetes mellitus. *Am. J. Kidney Dis.*, **13**, 2–6.
17. Diabetes care and research in Europe: The St Vincent Declaration. (1990) *Diabetic Med.*, **7**, 360.
18. Mauer, M., Mogensen, C.E. and Viberti, G.C. (eds) (1992) Symposium on Diabetic Nephropathy. *Kidney Int.*, **41**, 717–929.
19. Mogensen, C.E., Christensen, C.K. and Vittinghus, E. (1983) The stages in diabetic renal disease with emphasis on the stage of incipient nephropathy. *Diabetes*, **32**, suppl 2, 64–78.
20. Hostetter, T.H. (1992) Diabetic nephropathy. Metabolic versus haemodynamic considerations. *Diabetes Care*, **15**, 1205–15.
21. Tomlinson, D.R. (1993) Aldose reductase inhibitors and the complications of diabetes mellitus. *Diabetic Med.*, **10**, 214–30.
22. Osterby, R. (1992) Glomerular structural changes in Type I (insulin-dependent) diabetes mellitus causes, consequences, and prevention. *Diabetologia*, **35**, 803–12.
23. Tydeng, A., Mellgren, A., Brattstrom, C. *et al.* (1986) Stockholm experience with 32 combined renal and segmental pancreatic transplants. *Transplant. Proc.*, **18**, 1114–7.
24. Viberti, G.C., Jarrett, R.J., Mahmud, U. *et al.* (1982) Microalbuminuria as a predictor of clinical nephropathy in insulin-dependent diabetes mellitus. *Lancet*, **i**, 430–4.
25. Parving, H.H., Oxenboll, B., Johansen, K. *et al.* (1982) Early detection of patients at risk of developing diabetic nephropathy: a longitudinal study of urinary albumin excfretion. *Acta Endocrinol*, **100**, 550–5.
26. Mogensen, C.E. and Christensen, C.K. (1984) Predicting diabetic nephropathy in insulin-dependent patients. *N. Engl. J. Med.*, **311**, 89–93.
27. Mathiesen, E.R., Oxenboll, B., Johansen, K. *et al.* (1984) Incipient nephropathy in type I (insulin-dependent) diabetes. *Diabetologia*, **26**, 406–10.
28. Watts, G.F., Taub, N., Mazurkiewicz, J. and Shaw, K.M. (1993) An examination of the covariability of subclinical albuminuria in insulin-dependent diabetes mellitus: implications for monitoring microalbuminuria. *Diabetes Res. Clin. Pract.*, **21**, 177–85.
29. Almdal, T., Feldt-Rasmussen, B., Norgaard, K. and Deckert, T. (1994) The predictive value of microalbuminuria in IDDM. *Diabetes Care*, **17**, 120–5.
30. Microalbuminuria Collaborative Study Group. (1993) Risk factors for development of microalbuminuria in insulin-dependent diabetes mellitus: a cohort study. *Br. Med. J.*, **306**, 1235–9.
31. Watts, G.F., Harris, R. and Shaw, K.M. (1991) The determinants of early nephropathy in type I (insulin-dependent diabetes mellitus: a prospective study based on the urinary excretion of albumin. *Q. J. Med.*, **79**, 365–78.
32. Cooper, M.E., Frauman, A., O'Brien, R.C. *et al.* (1988) Progression of proteinuria in type 1 and type 2 diabetes. *Diabetic Med.*, **5**, 361–8.
33. Watts, G.F., Naumova, R., Slavin, B.M. *et al.* (1989) Serum lipids and

lipoproteins in insulin-dependent diabetics with persistent microalbuminuria. *Diabetic Med.*, **6**, 25–30.

34. Powrie, J.K., Watts, G.F., Taub, N. *et al.* (1994) Role of gycaemic control in development of microalbuminuria in patients with insulin dependent diabetes. *Br. Med. J.*, **309**, 1608–12.
35. Mathiesen, E.R., Rønn, B., Storm, B. *et al.* (1995) The natural course of microalbuminuria in insulin-dependent diabetes: a 10-year prospective study. *Diabetic Med.*, **12**, 482–7.
36. Watts, G.F., Powrie, J.K., O'Brien, S.F. and Shaw, K.M. (1996) Apolipoprotein B independently predicts progression of very-low-level albuminuria in insulin-dependent diabetes mellitus. *Metabolism*, **44**, 1052–7.
37. Mogensen, C.E. (1990) Prediction of clinical diabetic nephropathy in IDDM patients. Alternatives to microalbuminuria? *Diabetes*, **39**, 761–7.
38. O'Brien, S.F., Powrie, J.K. and Watts, G.F. (1997) Comparison of urinary albumin, retinol binding protein and NAG in predicting the development of diabetic microalbuminuria. *Ann. Clin. Biochem.*, **34**, 202–4.
39. Jarrett, R.J., Viberti, G.C., Arygropoulos, A. *et al.* (1984) Microalbuminuria predicts mortality in non-insulin-dependent diabetes. *Diabetic Med.*, **1**, 17–9.
40. Mogensen, C.E. (1984) Microalbuminuria predicts clinical proteinuria and early mortality in maturity-onset diabetes. *N. Eng. J. Med.*, **310**, 356–60.
41. Deckert, T., Yokoyama, H., Mathiesen, E. *et al.* (1996) Cohort study of predictive value of urinary albumin excretion for atherosclerotic vascular disease in patients with insulin dependent diabetes. *Br. Med. J.*, **312**, 871–4.
42. MacLoed, J.M., Lutale, J. and Marshall, S.M. (1995) Albumin excretion and vascular deaths in NIDDM. *Diabetologia*, **38**, 610–6.
43. Mattock, M.B., Morrish, N.J., Viberti, G.C. *et al.* (1992) Prospective study of microalbuminuria as a predictor of mortality in NIDDM. *Diabetes*, **41**, 736–41.
44. Haffner, S.M., Stern, M.P., Kozlowski-Gruber, M.K. *et al.* (1990) Microalbuminuria – potential marker for increased cardiovascular risk factors in non-diabetic subjects. *Arteriosclerosis*, **10**, 727–31.
45. Niskaney, L.K., Peuttilä, A., Parviaimen, M. and Unsitupa, M.I.J. (1996) Evolution, risk factors, and prognostic implications of albuminuria in NIDDM. *Diabetes Care*, **19**, 486–93.
46. Rowe, D.J.F., Dawnay, A. and Watts, G.F. (1990) Microalbuminuria in diabetes mellitus: review and recommendations for the measurement of albumin in urine. *Ann. Clin. Biochem.*, **27**, 297–312.
47. Mogensen, C.E., Chachati, A., Christensen, C.K. *et al.* (1985/6) Microalbuminuria: an early marker of renal involvement in diabetes. *Uremia Invest.*, **9**, 85–95.
48. Abrass, C.K. (1984) Diabetic proteinuria. Glomerular or tubular in origin? *Am. J. Nephrol.*, **44**, 337–46.
49. Larkins, R.G. and Dunlop, M.E. (1992) The link between hyperglycaemia and diabetic nephropathy. *Diabetologia*, **35**, 499–504.
50. Seaquist, E.R., Goetz, F.C., Rich, S. and Barbosa, J. (1989) Familial clustering of diabetic kidney disease. Evidence of genetic susceptibility to diabetic nephropathy. *N. Engl. J. Med.*, **320**, 1161–5.
51. Allawi, J., Rao, P.V., Gilbert, R. *et al.* (1988) Microalbuminuria in non-insulin-dependent diabetes: its prevalence in Indian compared with European patients. *Br. Med. J.*, **296**, 462–4.
52. Kapelreed, H., Bangstad, H.J., Dahl-Jorgensen, K. *et al.* (1991) Serum Lp(a) lipoprotein concentrations in insulin-dependent patients with microalbuminuria. *Br. Med. J.*, **303**, 675–8.

53. Marshall, S.M. and Alberti, K.G.M.M. (1989) Comparison of the prevalence and associated features of abnormal albumin excretion in insulin-dependent and non-insulin-dependent diabetes. *Q. J. Med.*, **261**, 61–71.
54. Watts, G.F., Jasik, M. and Cooper, M.E. (1995) The implications of the detection of proteinuria and microalbuminuria in insulin-dependent and non-insulin dependent diabetic mellitus. *Aus. NZ J. Med.*, **25**, 157–61.
55. Powrie, J.K., Watts, G.F., Crook, M.A. *et al.* (1996) Serum sialic acid and the long-term complications of insulin-dependent diabetes mellitus. *Diabetes Care*, **13**, 238–43.
56. Chen, J.W., Gall, M.A., Yokoyama, H. *et al.* (1996) Raised serum sialic acid concentration in NIDDM patients with and without diabetic nephropathy. *Diabetic Care*, **19**, 130–4.
57. Watts, G.F., Lowy, C., Sonksen, P.H. and Shaw, K.M. (1992) Setting the standard for diabetes care microalbuminuria. *Pract. Diabetes*, **9**, 84–6.
58. Haaber, A.B., Kofoed-Enevoldsen, A. and Jensen, T. (1992) The prevalence of hypercholesterolaemia and its relationship with albuminuria in insulin-dependent diabetic patients: an epidemiological study. *Diabetic Med.*, **9**, 557–61.
59. Watts, G.F., Taub, N., Wilson, P. and Shaw, K.M. (1992) The immunogenetics of early nephropathy in insulin-dependent diabetes mellitus: association between the HLA-A2 antigen and albuminuria. *Q. J. Med.*, **83**, 461–71.
60. Hansen, K.F., Bangstad, H.J., Brinchmann-Hansen, O. and Dahl-Jorgensen, K. (1992) Blood glucose control and diabetic microvascular complications: long-term effects of near-normoglycaemia. *Diabetic Med.*, **9**, 697–705.
61. Reichard, P., Nilsson, B.Y. and Rosenquevist, M.D. (1993) The effect of long-term, intensified treatment on the development of microvascular complications of diabetes mellitus. *N. Engl. J. Med.*, **329**, 304–9.
62. The Diabetes Control and Complications Research Group. (1993) The effect of intensive treatment of diabetes on the development and progression of long-term complications in insulin-dependent diabetes mellitus. *N. Engl. J. Med.*, **329**, 977–86.
63. Marre, M., Chatellier, G., Leblanc, M. *et al.* (1988) Prevention of diabetic nephropathy with enalapril in normotensive diabetics with microalbuminuria. *Br. Med. J.*, **297**, 1092–5.
64. Mathiesen, E.R., Hommel, E., Giese, J. and Parving, H.H. (1991) Efficacy of captopril in postponing nephorpathy in normotensive insulin-dependent diabetic patients with microalbuminuria. *Br. Med. J.*, **303**, 81–7.
65. Hallab, M., Gallois, Y., Chatellier, G. *et al.* (1993) Comparison of reduction in microalbuminuria by enalapril and hydrochlorothiazide in normotensive patients with insulin-dependent diabetes. *Br. Med. J.*, **306**, 175–82.
66. Melbourne Diabetic Nephropathy Study Group. (1991) Comparison between perindopril and nifedipine in normotensive diabetic patients with microalbuminuria. *Br. Med. J.*, **302**, 210–6.
67. Viberti, G.C., Dodds, R.A., Bending, J.J. *et al.* (1988) Non-glycaemic intervention in diabetic nephropathy: the role of dietary protein intake, in *The Kidney and Hypertension in Diabetes* (ed. C.E. Mogensen), Martinus Nijhoff Boston, pp. 205–15.
68. Marshall, S.M. (1993) therapeutic options in early diabetic nephropathy. *Diabetes Rev.*, **2**, 6–9.
69. UK Prospective Diabetes Study Group. (1993) Urinary albumin excretion over 3 years in diet-treated Type 2 (non-insulin-dependent) diabetic

patients, and association with hypertension, hyperglycaemia and hypertriglyceridaemia. *Diabetologia*, **36**, 1021–9.

70. Ravid, M., Lang, R., Rachmani, R. and Lishner, M. (1996) Long-term renoprotective effect of angiotensin converting enzyme inhibition in non-insulin-dependent diabetes mellitus. *Arch. Intern. Med.*, **156**, 286–9.
71. Burr, M.L. and Elwood, P.C. (1985) Research and development of health promotions services – screening, in *Oxford Textbook of Public Health* Vol. 3 (eds. W.W. Holland, R. Detels and G. Knox), Oxford University Press, Oxford, pp. 373–84.
72. Borch-Johnsen, K., Wenzel, H., Viberti, G.C. and Mogensen, C.E. (1993) Is screening and intervention for microalbuminuria worthwhile in patients with insulin dependent diabetes? *Br. Med. J.*, **306**, 1722–3.
73. Watts, G.F., O'Brien, S.F. and Shaw, K.M. (1996) Urinary infection and albumin excretion in insulin-dependent diabetes mellitus: implications for the measurement of microalbuminuria. *Diabetic Med.*, **13**, 520–4.
74. O'Brien, S.F., Watts, G.F., Powrie, J.K. and Shaw, K.M. (1995) Exercise testing as a long-term predictor of the development of microalbuminuria in normoalbuminuric IDDM patients. *Diabetes Care*, **18**, 1602–5.
75. Tunbridge, W.M.G. (1981) Factors contributing to deaths of diabetics under 50 years of age. *Lancet*, **11**, 569–72.
76. Catalano, C., Goodship, T.H.J., Tapson, J.S. *et al.* (1990) Renal replacement treatment for diabetic patients in Newcastle upon Tyne and the Northern Region, 1964–88. *Br. Med. J.*, **301**, 535–40.
77. Bojestig, M., Arnovist, H., Hermansson, G. *et al.* (1994) Declining incidence of nephropathy in insulin-dependent diabetes mellitus. *N. Engl. J. Med.*, **330**, 15–8.
78. European Microalbuminuria Captopril Study Group. (1994) Effect of captopril on progression to clinical proteinuria in patients with insulin-dependent diabetes mellitus and microalbuminuria. *J. Am. Med. Assoc.*, **271**, 275–9.

# 7

# Urinary stone disease

*P. Jungers*

Stone disease is now the most common renal disorder. Nearly 10% of men and 5% of women will experience renal colic at least once in their lifetimes, and these episodes will recur within five years in more than 50% of affected subjects [1]. The incidence of urolithiasis has markedly increased in all industrialized countries since the end of World War II, especially with respect to calcium oxalate stones, which presently account for more than 65% of cases. This increase in calcium oxalate urolithiasis parallels the profound changes in dietary habits encountered in industrialized countries during the past few decades, and suggests a role for such environmental factors superimposed on endogenous factors [1, 2].

Obviously, major advances have been made in the treatment of urinary stones by means of extracorporeal shock wave lithotripsy (ESWL), and percutaneous and endoscopic surgery [3]. However, such methods do not prevent stone recurrence and entail the risk of neglecting etiological investigation and prophylaxis of stone recurrence. Severe forms of urolithiasis still too often lead to loss of renal function and the need for supportive therapy. Such an outcome can now be largely prevented by proper evaluation and treatment adapted to the diverse chemical forms of stone disease [4–6].

## 7.1 PATHOGENESIS AND CLASSIFICATION

### 7.1.1 Classification of kidney stones

Renal stones may be classified according to both chemical composition and etiology. The relative prevalence of stones according to the main

*Renal Disease.* Edited by G. Venkat Raman. Published in 1998 by Chapman & Hall, London. ISBN 0 412 45700 8.

**Table 7.1** Respective prevalence of renal stones according to the main component among 10 000 stones analyzed at Necker Hospital during the past decade

| *Main component (> 50% of stone content)* | *Per cent frequency* | | |
|---|---|---|---|
| | *Total* | *Males* | *Females* |
| Calcium oxalate | 65 | 72 | 52 |
| Calcium phosphate | 17.4 | 10 | 31 |
| Uric acid | 10 | 12 | 6 |
| Struvite (MAP) | 2.8 | 1.8 | 5 |
| Cystine | 1.2 | 0.8 | 3 |
| Other | 3.6 | 3.4 | 4 |

component (i.e. accounting for 50% or more of the stone content) as presently observed in France is indicated in Table 7.1. The most frequent types (calcium and uric acid stones) present either as secondary to an underlying pathological condition, or as idiopathic. This indicates the need for proper identification of the chemical nature of stones and of the etiopathogenic factors involved in their formation.

### 7.1.2 Mechanisms of lithogenesis

The mechanism of lithogenesis in specific forms of stone disease such as urate, cystine, 2,8-dihydroxyadenine (2,8-DHA) or magnesium ammonium phosphate (MAP) stones is monofactorial, involving the excessive concentration of the respective compounds in urine, and leading to supersaturation and crystal formation. The mechanism is more complex and multifactorial in calcium oxalate and calcium phosphate stones, which together account for more than 80% of stones. Stone formation here depends on an imbalance between promoters and inhibitors of crystallization [6]. When urine is supersaturated with a stone constituent (calcium oxalate), the formation of crystals by homogeneous nucleation occurs. In addition, the presence of particles such as cell debris or other crystals such as uric acid or calcium phosphate may induce heterogeneous nucleation of calcium oxalate crystals at even lower saturation levels [7]. Urinary pH has little influence on calcium oxalate crystallization, but markedly influences uric acid crystallization (favored by a pH under 5.5) and calcium phosphate precipitation (which occurs at a urine pH over 6.2). Once formed, crystal nuclei grow and aggregate. Crystal aggregation is an important process that may lead, within as little as one minute, to the formation of particles of 100 nm or more, which can attach to the wall of the collecting duct or the tip of the papilla. In the absence of rapid aggregation, the crystals may easily pass through the entire length of the tubule during the urine transit time, 5–7 min [1,7].

Normal urine contains natural inhibitors of stone formation, including small ion inhibitors (such as citrate, magnesium and pyrophosphate) which are especially active in inhibiting calcium phosphate crystallization and calcium oxalate crystal aggregation, and macromolecular polyanions (such as nephrocalcin, glycosaminoglycans and non-polymerized Tamm–Horsfall protein) which especially inhibit calcium oxalate crystallization. In addition, citrate also acts by complexing calcium [8]. Thus, hypocitraturia is an important risk factor in calcium oxalate lithiasis [9]. The role of macromolecular inhibitors is not fully established, and in any case they are not presently available for therapeutic use.

The main steps of crystal formation and the sites of action of the main inhibitors are depicted in Figure 7.1. The main mechanisms involved in lithogenesis in the various types of urolithiasis are summarized in Table 7.2. An issue under debate is whether hypercalciuria or hyperoxaluria is the more important in inducing calcium oxalate (CaOx) crystal formation. A widely accepted view is that a small increase in oxalate concentration is more potent than a similar increase in calcium concentration in inducing CaOx supersaturation [10]. However, both are important and one has to consider both the CaOx molar product, which correlates with the incidence of CaOx crystals, and the Ca to Ox molar ratio, which determines the type of CaOx crystals [8]. We have observed that a low Ca/Ox ratio induces the formation of CaOx monohydrate crystals, whereas a high Ca/Ox ratio favors CaOx dihydrate crystallization [11].

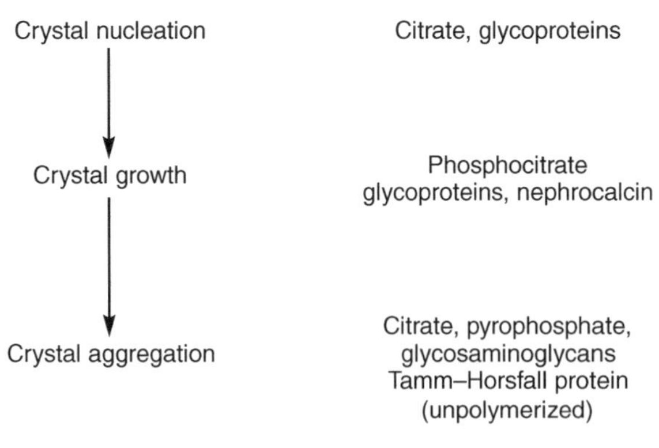


**Figure 7.1** The steps of crystalluria and stone formation with indication of the site of action of the main crystallization inhibitors in calcium oxalate urolithiasis.

**Table 7.2** Urinary risk factors of lithogenesis involved in the various types of urinary stones

| Stone type | Urinary risk factor | Chemical effect |
|---|---|---|
| Calcium oxalate | ↓ Volume<br>↑ Oxalate<br>↑ Calcium | ↑ CaOx supersaturation |
| | ↓ Citrate<br>↓ Macromolecules | ↓ Inhibitory activity |
| | ↑ Uricosuria | Epitaxial nucleation |
| Calcium phosphate | ↑ pH | ↑ CaP supersaturation |
| Struvite (infection stones)<br>supersaturation | ↑↑ pH | ↑ MAP and calcium<br>phosphate |
| Uric acid | ↓ pH<br>↑ Uricosuria<br>↓ Volume | ↑ Undissociated uric acid<br>↑ Uric acid supersaturation |
| Cystine | ↑ Cystine | ↑ Cystine supersaturation |
| 2,8-DHA | ↑ 2,8-DHA | ↑ 2,8-DHA supersaturation |

## 7.2 CLINICAL PRESENTATION AND SURGICAL MANAGEMENT

### 7.2.1 Clinical presentation

The most common revealing symptom is renal colic, an extremely intense pain starting in the costovertebral angle and radiating downward to the inguinal ligament, often associated with nausea, vomiting and abdominal distention. Urinary frequency and dysuria occur when the stone is located in the ureterovesical junction, thus possibly resembling and mistaken for cystitis or prostatitis. Gross or microscopic hematuria may be associated with any of these patterns of pain, or may occur as the sole symptom [7]. Urinary stones may also be discovered on incidental abdominal echography or radiography. Silent, painless stones may rarely cause undiagnosed obstructive uropathy and lead to parenchymal destruction.

Renal colic is the consequence of the distension of the renal capsule due to increased backpressure above the obstructive stone, with increased intra-renal generation of prostaglandin E2 and increased glomerular filtration pressure. This explains why non-steroidal anti-inflammatory drugs (NSAIDs) are effective (in association with antispasmodics and analgesics) in relieving the pain of acute urinary obstruction [1]. Of note, NSAIDs should be used only in the presence of a normal contralateral kidney and in the absence of infection. More than 80% of stones are passed spontaneously. The probability of spontaneous passage is greater than 90% if the stone diameter is <6 mm but virtually nil if it exceeds 10 mm. Intervention of a urologist is needed to relieve ureteric obstruction in the case of untractable pain, superimposed urinary tract infection or significant pyelocaliceal distension [1,7]. It is worth noting that the most common metabolic stones, calcium oxalate, do not produce renal failure, whereas infection related stones do (see below).

### 7.2.2 Surgical management

The need for conventional surgery has been virtually eliminated since the introduction of ESWL, percutaneous nephrolithotomy and endoscopic lithotripsy [3]. ESWL (using either shock waves or piezoelectric waves) allows successful, non-invasive treatment of stones less than 2 cm in diameter when lodged in the renal pelvis or calices. Stones lodged in the upper extremity of the ureter may be pushed upward into the renal pelvis prior to being disrupted by ESWL. Usually a double-J stent is then placed in the ureter in order to allow passage of stone fragments without inducing the risk of ureteric obstruction. Calculi lodged in the middle or lower part of the ureter may also be disrupted *in situ* with ESWL, or extracted by ureteroscopy [12]. Larger kidney stones and especially staghorn calculi preferably require percutaneous nephrolithotomy (PCNL) or a combination of PCNL and complementary ESWL [13]. The success rate (i.e. stone-free state) of PCNL is nearly 100%, whereas a stone-free state at three months after ESWL is about 80% for stones less than 2 cm in diameter situated in the kidney pelvis or upper calices, and only about 60% for stones lodged in the lower calices. Repeated ESWL procedure may produce deleterious side effects such as renal hematoma and scarring, as well as possibly favoring systemic hypertension [14]. Clearly, new techniques to destroy calculi do not in any way preclude the need for proper etiologic evaluation of the stone former and prophylactic treatment aimed at preventing stone recurrence.

## 7.3 ETIOLOGICAL INVESTIGATION

Careful history, together with pertinent radiology and laboratory examination, is the only way to identify an underlying disease or risk factors responsible for stone formation.

### 7.3.1 History and clinical examination

History is of greater interest than physical examination in the etiological evaluation of stone formers. To be considered are the patient's age at onset of stone disease and the total number of stones produced, the latter being an index of stone disease activity. A stone index higher than 0.6 stones/year is indicative of a metabolically active disease, as well as the presence of multiple stones at presentation. Attention should be paid to possible history of bowel disease or occult diarrhea, and all drugs taken by the patient, such as vitamin D or calcium supplements, antacids, triamterene, diuretics, carbonic anhydrase inhibitors or cadmium exposure [1].

Taking a dietary history is essential in stone formers, with the assistance of a skilled dietitian whenever possible, to assess fluid, protein, purine, carbohydrate, fiber and salt intake, as well as daily consumption of dairy products and of oxalate-rich foods [15]. Family history is often positive in patients with idiopathic hypercalciuria, cystinuria, gout, renal tubular acidosis, or other genetically transmitted disorders. Familial transmission should be analyzed as extensively as possible, as significant advances are expected from molecular genetics in the near future.

### 7.3.2 Radiological examination

Although ultrasonography is now widely used and is able to recognize any chemical type of calculus provided it is at least 2 mm in size, a plain X-ray is still needed to distinguish radio-opaque stones (made of calcium oxalate, calcium phosphate, struvite or cystine) from radiolucent calculi (pure uric acid, 2,8-DHA and xanthine). An excretory urogram will usually identify anatomical abnormalities (such as hydronephrosis) that predispose to urine stasis and is essential to the diagnosis of medullary sponge kidneys (MSK), a frequent cause of recurrent calcium nephrolithiasis. A peculiar aspect of this disease is medullary nephrocalcinosis, characterized by multiple calcium-dense deposits at the corticomedullary junction. MSK is the most frequent cause of nephrocalcinosis in recurrent stone formers, with renal tubular acidosis, hypercalcemic primary hyperparathyroidism or calcified papillary necrosis being other common causes [16].

### 7.3.3 Stone analysis

Stone identification should never be neglected whenever a calculus (or fragments extracted by PCNL or passed after ESWL) is available for analysis. Pure chemical methods are inaccurate and often misleading. X-ray diffraction, or, better, infrared spectrography, allows recognition and quantification of all the stone components [1]. Careful morphological examination of the calculus using binocular lenses, coupled with infrared spectroscopic analysis, provides the most complete information and is our preferred method [17]. In addition to accurate identification of the chemical nature of stones, this 'morphoconstitutional' approach offers many useful correlations between composition and morphology of stones, and the corresponding etiological conditions that led to their formation.

A complete description of our proposed classification of stones is given in ref. 17. Among calcium oxalate stones, calculi predominantly made of whewellite (CaOx monohydrate, or COM) are dark brown, smooth and spherical, with an umbilication, whereas those made of weddellite (CaOx dihydrate or COD) are usually light brown and spiculated like small gypsum flowers. The former are mainly associated with mild hyperoxaluria, whereas the latter are essentially associated with hypercalciuria. A peculiar morphology of some COM calculi (termed Ic) is, in our experience, virtually pathognomonic of massive hyperoxaluria as encountered in primary hyperoxaluria type I; they are smooth and white, in contrast to the usual dark-brown umbilicated appearance of the standard COM calculi. In other types of stone disease, stone analysis *per se* immediately solves the etiologic problem when revealing specific types of calculi such as those made of cystine, 2,8-DHA, xanthine, MAP (pathognomonic of urinary tract infection with urease-producing microorganisms), ammonium acid urate (suggestive of chronic diarrhea or laxative abuse) or a peculiar morphology of calcium phosphate stones (type IVa2) which strongly correlates with renal distal tubular acidosis. It is worthy of note that examination of urinary crystals (coupled with infrared spectroscopy) provides essentially the same information as stone analysis and may often allow identification of the type of urolithiasis when no calculus is available.

### 7.3.4 Blood and urine biochemistry

*Why, and whom to investigate?*

Laboratory investigation is aimed at identifying the etiology of stone disease and risk factors of lithogenesis. Therefore, the patient's initial evaluation, without being unduly extended, must cover all usually encountered types of urolithiasis [1,4]. Whether full evaluation should be reserved to patients with recurrent stone formation or should be performed at first stone episode is debatable. In our opinion, all patients should undergo metabolic evaluation, as the cost of such laboratory investigation is far lower than the direct cost of urological interventions or the indirect cost of worktime loss during renal colic episodes.

*When to investigate?*

Metabolic investigation (especially 24 hour urine analysis) should be best deferred for at least one month after a stone episode or PCNL, or three months after ESWL, because transient tubular alterations result from obstruction, use of NSAIDs, or the ESWL procedure itself. Initial laboratory testing should be performed in an ambulatory patient having normal physical activity and usual diet.

*How to investigate?*

Table 7.3 shows urine and blood parameters that may be recommended as a minimal initial approach to etiologic diagnosis. Although many authors still ask for two or three 24 hour urine collections, we instruct our patients to collect carefully 24 hour urine only once, usually during the weekend, because when using two 24 hour collections we found that the first one exhibited more marked abnormalities than the second one in more than 90% of cases. In addition to 24 hour collection, patients separately collect first voided morning urine (for study of crystalluria, pH and specific gravity) and keep it at room temperature. At 8 am, in the fasting state after an overnight fast, blood is drawn and a second urine sample is collected for determination of the fasting calcium to creatinine (fCa/Cr) ratio. In addition, urine analysis with culture is performed.

**Table 7.3** Basal laboratory investigation in the stone-former patient

| |
|---|
| Blood chemistry (serum) |
| Calcium, phosphate, uric acid |
| Total proteins and albumin, glucose |
| Creatinine, urea |
| Sodium, potassium, chloride, bicarbonate |
| 24 hour urine (on usual food intake) |
| Volume, specific gravity |
| Calcium, phosphate, uric acid |
| Oxalate, citrate, magnesium |
| Creatinine, urea, sodium |
| First-voided morning urine |
| Specific gravity, pH |
| Crystalluria |
| Second morning urine (in the fasting state) |
| Urinalysis, culture |
| Fasting calcium to creatinine ratio |

Combining data from history, radiology, stone analysis, and blood and urine biochemistry allows us to identify specific forms of urolithiasis, secondary forms of calcium or uric acid stone disease, and lithogenic risk factors in idiopathic calcium urolithiasis, in order to define an adapted and individualized basis for prophylactic treatment. Proper etiological diagnosis is of obvious clinical relevance, because only etiological therapy is able to prevent stone recurrence in specific and secondary forms of stone disease.

## 7.4 SECONDARY FORMS OF CALCIUM STONE DISEASE

A number of specific pathological conditions are associated with the formation of calcium stones. The main factors are listed in Table 7.4. Only the most frequent or more severe will be briefly described here.

**Table 7.4** Main causes of calcium urolithiasis

| Metabolic factor | Etiological conditions | |
|---|---|---|
| Hypercalcemia with hypercalciuria | Primary hyperparathyroidism<br>Sarcoidosis<br>Immobilization<br>Malignancy-associated osteolysis | Vitamin D intoxication<br>Paget's disease<br>Hyperthyroidism |
| Hypercalciuria without hypercalcemia | High calcium intake<br>Phosphate depletion (phosphate-binding antacids)<br>Hereditary distal renal tubular acidosis*<br>Acquired distal renal tubular acidosis*<br>(Sjögren's syndrome, hypergammaglobulinemia, chronic active hepatitis)<br>Acetazolamide*, loop diuretics, lithium salts<br>Cushing's syndrome, primary aldosteronism*<br>Glucocorticoid therapy<br>Medullary sponge kidney<br>Idiopathic hypercalciuria | |
| Massive hyperoxaluria ($>0.9$ mmol/day) | Primary hyperoxaluria | Enteric hyperoxaluria |
| Moderate hyperoxaluria (0.5–0.9 mmol/day) | Oxalate-rich foods gluttony<br>Pyridoxine deficiency<br>Low dietary calcium intake<br>Idiopathic hyperoxaluria | Ascorbic acid abuse<br>Piridoxilate abuse<br>Mild metabolic hyperoxaluria |
| Moderate hypocitraturia | Chronic diarrheal states<br>Chronic potassium depletion (laxatives, diuretics)<br>Idiopathic hypocitraturia | High animal protein intake |

* associated with marked hypocitraturia.

One can distinguish calcium stones associated with hypercalciuria (with or without hypercalcemia), hyperoxaluria, or renal tubular acidosis with hypocitraturia.

### 7.4.1 Hypercalcemia and/or hypercalciuria

Primary hyperparathyroidism is found in about 3–5% of calcium stone formers. The lithogenic factors are hypercalciuria and alkaline urine, leading to a stone composition that is a mixture of COD and calcium phosphate (carbapatite and/or brushite) [1, 17]. Parathyroid hormone (PTH) enhances the synthesis of calcitriol, resulting in increased intestinal calcium absorption, hypercalcemia and hypercalciuria, because the increase in the filtered calcium load exceeds the PTH-stimulated tubular reabsorption of calcium [18]. PTH also diminishes tubular reabsorption of phosphate and may result in hyperphosphaturia, hypophosphatemia and inhibition of proximal tubular reabsorption of bicarbonate, the latter resulting in alkaline urine [6]. Hyperparathyroidism induces stone formation preferentially in young subjects with preserved renal parenchymal mass, able to respond to PTH oversecretion by increased calcitriol synthesis [19].

The diagnosis is made on the combination of a slightly raised total calcium (usually between 2.6 and 2.8 mmol/l) and ionized calcium, and of an inappropriately high level of intact PTH (normal range: 1–6.5 pmol/l or 10–65 pg/ml) which does not decrease following an oral calcium load [7]. The source of PTH hypersecretion is a solitary adenoma in about 95% of cases, or diffuse hyperplasia of the parathyroid glands in some patients (especially in familial cases). Localization or hyperactive parathyroid gland(s) may be made by echography, tomodensitometry and/or magnetic resonance imaging. In a symptomatic patient with recurrent stones, surgical excision of the adenoma (or subtotal parathyroidectomy in the case of diffuse hyperplasia) is required to stop stone formation and bone demineralization. In some cases hypercalciuria persists, suggesting that underlying idiopathic hypercalciuria was probably the initial stimulus for parathyroid cell hyperactivity [1].

An important differential diagnosis of hyperparathyroidism is familial hypocalciuric hypercalcemia (rarely responsible for stones), a benign autosomal dominant disorder in which parathyroidectomy would be ineffective and even deleterious [20]. Lithium therapy also can mimic parathyroid hyperplasia. Sarcoidosis is often associated with mild hypercalcemia and hypercalciuria and may result in urolithiasis and nephrocalcinosis. Calcitriol level is usually elevated (due to ectopic synthesis), thus resulting in low or normal PTH level. The disease responds well to moderate doses of corticosteroids. Other causes of hypercalcemia-associated stones, such as malignancies, immobilization (in a growing adolescent or in subjects with active Paget's disease) or hypervitaminosis D, are less frequent [2].

### 7.4.2 Hypercalciuria without hypercalcemia

High dietary or supplemental calcium intake (in excess of 1.5 g/day) may induce reversible 'dietary' hypercalciuria [21]. Prolonged antacid use induces phosphate depletion and may result in hypophosphatemia and hypercalciuria. Acetazolamide (or other carboanhydrase inhibitors) used for glaucoma treatment may induce hypercalciuria, hypocitraturia and alkaline urine, leading to formation of calcium phosphate stones [22]. Furosemide increases both sodium and calcium urinary excretion. Endogenous or iatrogenic glucocorticoid excess, through increased bone resorption, favors hypercalciuria.

MSK is a frequent cause of recurrent stone disease associated with hypercalciuria. Calculi form in ectatic tubules, due to the combined effect of slowed flux, hypercalciuria and local tubular acidification defects. Stones have a mixed composition, being made of carbapatite, COM and COD in variable proportions [23]. On X-ray, multiple small calculi are disposed just behind the tips of papillae. Tubular ectasiae appear as linear striations in the concavity of calices and, in florid cases, appear like 'bunches of grapes'.

### 7.4.3 Hyperoxaluria

The upper limit of oxalate excretion in healthy adults is about 0.5 mmol/day [24] (1 mmol = 90 mg of oxalate). In our patients, the incidence of calcium oxalate crystalluria was found to rise sharply when urinary oxalate concentration exceeded 0.3 mmol/l. Mild hyperoxaluria (ranging from 0.5 to 0.9 mmol/day) may result from a high intake of oxalate-rich foods (spinach, rhubarb, sorrel, chocolate), ascorbic acid abuse (consumption of 4 g per day or more), or prolonged therapy with piridoxilate. However, more than 90% of oxalate production comes from endogenous metabolism [24].

Marked acquired hyperoxaluria (up to 1 mmol/day or more) complicates chronic inflammatory ileal disease, ileal resection, or jejuno-ileal bypass for obesity, in the presence of an intact colon [25]. Lithogenic risk factors in such 'enteric hyperoxaluria' are hyperoxaluria, reduced urine volume, hypomagnesuria and hypocitraturia, resulting in stones mainly made of COM. Hyperoxaluria results from both increased free oxalate content in the intestinal lumen (due to malabsorption of fatty acids which bind calcium and magnesium and thus reduce the formation of insoluble oxalate complexes) and enhanced colonic permeability to oxalate due to the increased content of bile acids. Treatment is based on calcium and magnesium supplementation (the latter ideally in the form of potassium magnesium citrate), oxalate-poor diet, medium-chain triglycerides, increased diuresis and cholestyramine to bind oxalate [7, 25].

The most massive urine oxalate excretion, together with the most severe clinical course, is observed in primary hyperoxaluria type I, an autosomal recessive disease. The metabolic defect is a deficiency in the hepatic peroxisomal enzyme alanine glyoxylate aminotransferase which utilizes pyridoxine (vitamin B6) as a coenzyme [26]. Massive hyperoxaluria (up to 3 mmol/day or more) associated with increased glycolate excretion is the hallmark of the disease [27]. Hyperoxaluria results in active, recurrent formation of COM stones (with the peculiar type IIIc aspect as mentioned above) associated with parenchymal calcium oxalate deposits and nephrocalcinosis. Renal failure often develops in childhood, leading to increased plasma oxalate concentration and tissue accumulation (oxalosis). A proportion of patients respond to pharmacological pyridoxine supplementation which enhances the metabolic pathway from glyoxylate to glycine [28], but about half of patients do not respond. In any case, the symptomatic treatment is based on high urine flow rates (at least 3 l/day), thiazide diuretics to decrease urinary calcium concentration and inorganic phosphate (neutral salts) to inhibit CaOx crystal growth. When end stage renal failure occurs, even high-efficiency haemodialysis fails to remove oxalate efficiently. The ideal treatment is now combined hepatic (to restore normal enzyme production) and renal transplantation [26, 29].

Primary hyperoxaluria type II is due to D-glycerate dehydrogenase deficiency and results in hyperoxaluria and L-glyceric aciduria. The condition is less frequent and less severe than type I [30]. Mild metabolic hyperoxaluria, possibly a variant of the preceding conditions, has been reported as a cause of stones [24], as well as a hyperabsorptive form of primary hyperoxaluria (type III).

### 7.4.4 Hypocitraturia and renal tubular acidosis

Renal distal tubular acidification (RDTA) defects, either complete (with systemic acidosis) or incomplete, result in marked hypocitraturia, hypercalciuria and alkaline urine, together with potassium loss, all the conditions favoring intratubular precipitation of calcium phosphate (mainly carbapatite), nephrocalcinosis and/or lithiasis. Carbapatite calculi formed in RDTA patients have a peculiar morphology (type IVa2 of our classification) – smooth surface, with a brownish yellow glazed appearance – very suggestive of this etiology [17].

Hereditary RDTA is transmitted as an autosomal recessive disease. In the complete form it affects young children, who exhibit hyperchloremic acidosis, bone resorption, growth retardation, polyuria, hypercalciuria, marked hypocitraturia and often hypokalemia [31]. Treatment must be prophylactic, based on alkali supplementation (in the form of sodium potassium bicarbonate, or better, potassium citrate) in sufficient amount to correct acidosis and normalize the excretion of calcium and citrate. When initiated early, such palliative therapy may preserve normal bone mineralization and growth, and limit nephrocalcinosis. In the case of delayed or inadequate treatment, massive nephrocalcinosis with progressive loss of kidney function may ensue.

In adults, RDTA is more often an acquired condition, secondary to a number of systemic disorders, mainly autoimmune diseases, such as Sjögren's syndrome, hypergammaglobulinemia or hepatic diseases, that may be revealed by calcium phosphate stones with or without nephrocalcinosis [1].

Taken together, secondary forms account for no more than 10–15% of cases of calcium stone disease which, in the vast majority of patients, must be considered idiopathic or primary. Of course, any secondary cause must be excluded before accepting the diagnosis of idiopathic calcium urolithiasis.

## 7.5 IDIOPATHIC CALCIUM STONE DISEASE

Primary, or idiopathic, calcium stone disease is about twice as common in males as in females and usually first manifests after the age of 30, although these features are less striking in industrialized countries. Lithogenic factors are the same as in secondary forms, but often the disease is multifactorial, involving a combination of increased urine calcium and/or oxalate concentration, with decreased citrate content and urine volume in variable proportions (Table 7.5).

### 7.5.1 Idiopathic hypercalciuria

The upper limit of 24 hour urinary calcium excretion in healthy adults on a free diet is 0.1 mmol (4 mg) per kilogram of body weight in either sex. Based on such a definition, more than 50% of patients with urinary calcium oxalate stones exhibit idiopathic hypercalciuria (IH). In our patients, the incidence of calcium oxalate crystalluria was found to rise sharply when urinary calcium concentration exceeded 3.8 mmol/l.

Pathophysiology of IH is still largely debated. Obviously, IH is not a homogeneous disorder, but rather involves multiple mechanisms. The classification proposed by Pak distinguishes resorptive, absorptive and renal IH on the basis of the fasting urinary calcium/creatinine ratio (fCa/Cr) and its increment following a standardized oral calcium load [32]. In absorptive hypercalciuria, fCa/Cr is normal ($<0.12$ mg/mg or

**Table 7.5** Lithogenic metabolic urinary abnormalities in idiopathic calcium oxalate stone disease

| Lithogenic factors mmol/24 h (mg) | Male | Female |
|---|---|---|
| Calcium* | $> 7$ (280) | 6 (240) |
| Oxalate | $> 0.5$ (45) | 0.45 (40) |
| Uric acid | $> 5$ (840) | 4.5 (750) |
| Citrate | $< 1.5$ (300) | 1.5 (300) |
| Magnesium | $< 4$ (100) | 3.5 (85) |
| Urea† | $> 350$ (24 g) | 300 (20 g) |
| Sodium | $> 150$ (3.5 g) | 150 (3.5 g) |

* $> 0.1$ mmol/kg BW/day in either sex.
† $> 5$ mmol/kg BW/day in either sex (corresponding to protein intake of 1 g/kg BW/day).

$<0.4$ mmol/mmol), whereas fCa/Cr is supranormal in renal hypercalciuria. In fact, the post-load increment in Ca/Cr is greater than in normal subjects in both groups because all hypercalciuric patients exhibit intestinal hyperabsorption, whether as the primary disorder or as secondary to renal calcium leak [33].

However, a reduction in calcium intake inconsistently results in lowering urinary calcium excretion below 0.7 mmol/kg BW (body weight)/day, even in patients with the 'absorptive' phenotype. Moreover urinary calcium excretion is increased by a high sodium intake [34] or a high animal protein intake [35–37]. This relationship is even more marked in hypercalciuric subjects than in normocalciuric stone formers or in healthy subjects [38]. The mechanism(s) underlying the increased sensitivity of IH patients to the hypercalciuric effects of protein and/or sodium load are not fully understood [39]. However, this finding indicates that environmental factors, such as the current nutritional habits in affluent societies, probably add their effects to underlying endogenous metabolic disorders, thus increasing the predilection to stone formation [1].

The possible mechanisms underlying IH are multiple: (i) primary calcitriol overproduction [40] (nearly one third of IH patients exhibit high normal serum calcitriol values); (ii) increased sensitivity of enterocytes to calcitriol; (iii) vitamin D-independent intestinal calcium hyperabsorption; (iv) primary renal tubular leak of calcium or of phosphate resulting in enhanced PTH secretion and increased calcitriol release [41]; and (v) altered trans-membrane transport of calcium and/or oxalate ions [42]. Some of these defects may be genetically inherited and polymorphism studies will probably improve our knowledge in the near future [43].

### 7.5.2 Other lithogenic factors

Moderate idiopathic hyperoxaluria is often found in calcium stone formers and may be associated with hypercalciuria [24]. An inadequately low calcium intake ($< 600\,\mathrm{mg/day}$) favors enhanced intestinal oxalate absorption and thus hyperoxaluria [44,45] and may explain the increased incidence of calcium stones in adults having a low calcium intake [46]. In our experience, oxalate excretion often exhibits large day-to-day variations, thus resulting in peaks of calcium oxalate supersaturation, all the more deleterious as hypercalciuria is simultaneously present.

Hyperuricosuria has been claimed to favor calcium stone formation through heterogeneous nucleation of calcium oxalate crystals on uric acid crystals [2] or, more likely, because urate in solution induces the precipitation of CaOx crystals by the mechanism of salting out [47].

Moderate hypocitraturia is frequent in calcium stone formers [48] and there is a large day-to-day variation. Hypocitraturia may be induced by high animal protein intake (due to large acid-ash load), high sodium load, potassium depletion and/or low net alkali intake, all conditions favored by current Western dietary habits [15]. Hypocitraturia in IH patients is even more significant when related to urine calcium concentration. Because citrate acts mainly by binding $Ca^{2+}$ ions, a relatively low citrate concentration in the face of a high calcium concentration favors calcium oxalate crystal formation and aggregation [9].

Qualitative, rather than quantitative, defects in macromolecular polyanions such as nephrocalcin and Tamm–Horsfall protein have been reported [49]. In particular, the inhibitory property of the Tamm–Horsfall protein is largely negated when polymerization occurs due to high sodium or calcium concentration, or low urinary pH [50].

Magnesium ions form complexes with oxalate ions, thus reducing urine supersaturation with respect to calcium oxalate, but significant idiopathic hypomagnesuria is very infrequent. A magnesium output lower than 1 mmol/day should alert one to the possibility of some enteric disorder [1].

Last but not least, a persistently low urine volume is a major factor in stone formation, because it increases in the same proportion the concentrations of all prolithogenic solutes, whereas the effects of a higher concentration of inhibitors has much less potent effects. Doubling the concentration of calcium and of oxalate multiplies by a factor of four (approximately) the calcium oxalate product and thus the probability of forming calcium oxalate crystals [1].

### 7.5.3 Prophylactic treatment of idiopathic calcium stone disease

Secondary prevention (or metaphylaxis) of idiopathic calcium urolithiasis is aimed at preventing stone recurrence. Such a goal is now attainable in the great majority of cases. Prophylactic measures mainly consist of readjustment of dietary habits, together with specific pharmacologic measures in the case of persistent hypercalciuria, hyperuricosuria or hypocitraturia. They do not depend on any classification of hypercalciuria. Our decision algorithm for treatment is presented in Figure 7.2.

The first measure in any stone former is to obtain a sufficient urine volume (between 2 and 2.5 l/day) to achieve optimal urine dilution, together with moderation in calcium, animal protein and salt intake,

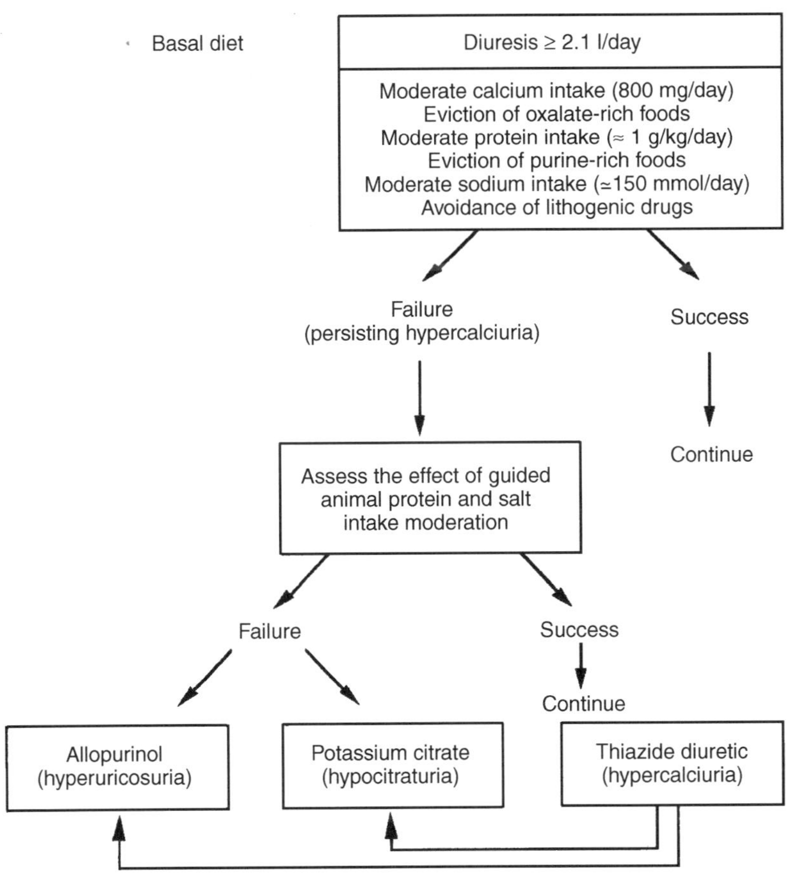


**Figure 7.2** Proposed therapeutic decisional algorithm in calcium stone formers.

increased fiber consumption and exclusion of oxalate-rich foods and of any lithogenic drug. We recently determined that a urine specific gravity (SG) of 1012 in the 24 hour urine collection corresponds to a mean urine volume of 2100 ml, and that a marked reduction in the incidence of CaOx crystallization is observed when urine SG is below 1012.

The optimal calcium intake, whether or not IH is present, is debated. An intake of about 800 mg (20 mmol) per day is now usually recommended. A reduced intake, as recommended by most authorities until the 1980s, results in increased oxalate absorption [44, 45] and negative calcium balance with the risk of decreased bone mineral density [51]. An excessive intake may increase calcium excretion due to intestinal hyperabsorption. About half of the total calcium intake should be provided as dairy products to increase phosphate load. Simultaneously, foods with a high content of absorbable oxalate (mentioned above) should be avoided. Total protein intake, often in excess of 1.3 g/kg BW/day in affluent countries, should be reduced to about 1 g/kg/day, especially with regard to animal proteins such as meat, fish and poultry [52]. Average daily intake of 150 g of such meats is an acceptable restriction in the long term. Salt intake should be reduced in parallel, as well as consumption of refined sugars. Fluid intake should be achieved using drinking water of moderate calcium content such as 100–150 mg/l (2.5–4 mmol/l), avoiding fruit juices (rich in rapidly absorbable sugar and oxalate). There may be a case for limiting beer intake because of its purine content, but there is no strong evidence for this.

The objective of the treatment is, by combining increased urine volume and lowered urinary solute load, to reduce the concentration of both calcium and oxalate. The results of such a policy should be evaluated in terms of urine biochemistry. The proposed goals are indicated in Table 7.6. Twenty-four hour urinary urea excretion closely reflects the daily total protein consumption (urea excretion of 100 mmol roughly corresponding to a 20 g protein intake), and 24 hour sodium excretion similarly reflects sodium intake.

**Table 7.6** Therapeutic goals in idiopathic calcium stone disease: optimal urinary concentrations of solutes in both sexes

| Urinary parameters | mmol/l |
|---|---|
| Calcium | < 3.8 |
| Oxalate | < 0.3 |
| Uric acid | < 2 |
| Citrate | > 1 |
| Magnesium | > 1.5 |

If all the laboratory parameters are stabilized in the optimal zone by these measures, that status should be maintained indefinitely. When hypercalciuria persists unabated, especially with a persistently exaggerated urea and sodium excretion, a greater effort is required from the patient to assess the impact of an effective reduction in animal protein and salt intake [52] over a limited duration of time such as six to eight weeks. If this effort succeeds, the patient should be encouraged to pursue the diet long term. If, despite effective lowering of urea and sodium excretion, hypercalciuria still persists, one should consider prescription of thiazide diuretics, irrespective of the absorptive or renal phenotype of IH [53, 54]. Thiazides should be prescribed at moderate dose (25 mg/day of hydrochlorothiazide or chlorthalidone) in order to avoid impotence and muscle cramps. If symptomatic hypokalemia and/or hypocitraturia occurs, potassium supplementation should be provided in the form of slow-release potassium citrate preparations. The same is true in the case of persistent idiopathic hypocitraturia [55, 56]. If uricosuria persists despite moderation in protein and purine intake, especially if urine pH is $<5.5$, or if hyperuricemia develops while on thiazide therapy, allopurinol should be added (200 to 300 mg/day).

Regular clinical and laboratory monitoring, about every six months during the first three years, is an important part of the 'stone clinic effect' [57]. This encourages the patient to comply with diuresis [58] and diet recommendations, and allows the assessment of tolerance of treatment and monitoring of stone recurrence by X-ray and/or echography. In our experience, assessment of SG in the first morning urine (in addition to the determination of SG in the 24-hour urine sample) is a simple and useful means to assess that fluid intake is well distributed throughout day and night. In 25% of our patients we observed a high SG in early morning urine despite a satisfactory 24 hour urine volume and SG, thus indicating insufficient overnight dilution, often in association with persistent crystalluria and risk of stone recurrence. In such cases, the patient should be advised to ingest a large amount of water at bedtime, and again have a drink of water sometime in the middle of the night.

## 7.6 NON-CALCIUM STONE DISEASE

### 7.6.1 Uric acid stones

Stones mainly or exclusively made of uric acid account for about 10% of renal stones. Uric acid stone disease is twice as frequent in males as in females in all age classes, and its relative incidence is higher in subjects over 60 in both sexes [1]. Pure uric acid calculi are totally radiolucent. They can be differentiated from tumors of the renal pelvis, blood clots or fragments of papillary necrosis by computerized tomography. The $pK_a$ of the first proton of uric acid is about 5.5 at 37°C, and at a lower pH more than half of the total urate urinary content is in the form of undissociated uric acid. The solubility of uric acid in urine at body temperature is only 0.6 mmol/l (100 mg/l) at pH 5, whereas the solubility of sodium urate (the predominant form above pH 5.5), is 11.9 mmol/l (nearly 2 g/l) at pH 7. Other risk factors are a high daily urate excretion and a low urine output, the latter contributing *per se* to a low urine pH [6]. Thus, formation of uric acid crystals is virtually unavoidable whenever urinary pH is consistently lower than 5.5, especially in the presence of hyperuricosuria.

### *Secondary forms of uric acid lithiasis*

The main causes of uric acid urolithiasis are listed in Table 7.7. Uric acid crystalluria and urolithiasis may occur as a consequence of uric acid overproduction resulting from rapid cell turnover in myeloproliferative disorders (such as polycythemia vera) or from massive nucleolysis during cytotoxic chemotherapy in lymphoproliferative diseases, preventable by appropriate hydration and alkalinization, and allopurinol. Inborn errors of purine metabolism are responsible for uric acid overproduction, hyperuricemia, hyperuricosuria and urolithiasis. Hyperuricosuria without hyperuricemia may result from the use of uricosuric drugs, probenecid, tienilic acid or suprofen, especially when they are used in gouty patients.

Hyperuricosuria in the presence of hypouricemia indicates a disorder of tubular reabsorption of uric acid, as observed in the Fanconi syndrome (idiopathic or secondary to cystinosis). Occasionally, light-

**Table 7.7** Main causes of uric acid lithiasis

| |
|---|
| Hyperuricosuria with hyperuricemia |
| Nucleolysis in myelo- or lymphoproliferative disorders |
| Inborn errors in purine metabolism |
| Primary uric diathesis with gout |
| Hyperuricosuria with normo- or hypouricemia |
| Uricosuric drugs |
| Proximal renal tubular disorders (hereditary or acquired Fanconi syndromes) |
| Purine gluttony |
| Persistently acid urine |
| Diarrheal diseases (ileostomy, enteropathy) |
| Laxative abuse |
| Primary idiopathic uric stone disease |

chain multiple myeloma or Sjögren syndrome, due to proximal tubule involvement, may lead to the formation of uric acid stones. By contrast, familial renal hypouricemia is a benign condition.

Chronic diarrhea or ileostomy induces fluid and alkali losses, resulting in excretion of concentrated, highly acidic urine, thus favoring the production of uric acid gravel and stones. The same is observed in the case of occult laxative abuse. Because the kidneys respond to alkali loss by increased ammoniagenesis, stones in the latter case are typically made of acid ammonium urate [59]. Similar composition is also observed in endemic bladder stones in young children in developing countries, who at the end of breast-feeding receive a diet poor in phosphate, thus resulting in enhanced ammoniagenesis and production of urine with low pH and high ammonium content.

### *Idiopathic uric acid stone disease*

The most common uric acid stone disease is idiopathic, occurring in most cases without a personal or familial history of gout. Usually blood and urine concentrations of uric acid are normal (of note, the normal values for both in the general population have increased markedly during the past few decades), but those patients exhibit a permanently low urinary pH, often in the range of 4.8 to 5.2, with lack of diurnal or nocturnal variation [7]. The accepted cause for low urinary pH is impaired enzymatic deamination of glutamine in the kidneys, resulting in the production of urines with both low pH and low ammonium content. However, the molecular basis for such a disorder has not been so far elucidated. Thus, in idiopathic uric acid stone disease, low urinary pH is the dominant lithogenic factor, hyperuricosuria and low urine volume acting only as additional factors. Climatic and ethnic factors certainly contribute, because the incidence of uric acid-containing stones is especially high in tropical countries and in the Middle East.

Treatment is based on urine dilution and alkalinization. Prophylaxis of stone recurrence is usually achieved with a moderate alkali intake, such as 4 to 6 g per day of sodium bicarbonate or potassium citrate or a mixture of sodium and potassium citrate, in divided doses. The goal is to maintain urinary pH constantly in the range of 6 to 6.5, but no more than 7 to avoid calcium phosphate precipitation [60]. Patients with severe, recurrent disease should be instructed to monitor urine pH and dilution by means of dipsticks, in order to adjust the dose and time of alkali supply. The French Vichy mineral water (which contains about 3.5 g/l sodium bicarbonate) conveniently achieves both urine dilution and alkalinization. Dissolution of calculi present in the kidney may be obtained by more intensive alkalinization under close supervision. In addition to alkali, 250 mg of acetazolamide can be given at bedtime to sustain nocturnal alkaline diuresis. Moderation of purine-rich food intake is recommended and, in the case of persistent marked hyperuricosuria (>5 mmol, or 800 mg/day), allopurinol should be added.

Patients with idiopathic uric acid stone disease require close clinical surveillance with frequent echographic examination, because the abnormally low urine pH is permanent and often leads to rapid recurrence whenever urine dilution or alkalinization is neglected. There also exist mixed stones, combining uric acid and calcium oxalate, which often exhibit a particularly severe and recurrent course [61].

### 7.6.2 Cystinuria

Cystinuria is a genetic defect of dibasic amino acid transport in the kidney and intestine. Because cystine is very poorly soluble in aqueous solution, the consequence is the formation of cystine stones in the kidneys. Cystinuria accounts for 1 to 2% of stones in adult patients and for nearly 10% in children. The disorder is inherited as an autosomal recessive trait. There are several variants of cystinuria but their differentiation does not affect the management of patients. The only lithogenic factor is the high cystine concentration in the urine. Homozygotes commonly excrete 800–1200 mg/day (3.2 to 4.8 mmol/day) of cystine, whereas heterozygotes excrete intermediate values between homozygotes and healthy subjects (<50 mg or 0.2 mmol/day) and usually are asymptomatic. Cystine solubility in urine over the pH range from 4.5 to 7 is at best 250 mg/l. Only at a urinary pH of more than 7.5 does cystine solubility rise to 800 mg/l [62]. The disease usually manifests itself in the 2nd or 3rd decade, but may occasionally present before the age of ten or as late as in the seventh decade of life. Cystine stones are weakly radio-opaque due to sulfur content.

Microscopic analysis of urine sediment in untreated patients shows characteristic large hexagonal crystals and provides immediate diagnosis. The classic cyanide–nitroprusside screening test detects cystine concentrations exceeding 75 mg/l. In the absence of effective therapy, repeated stone episodes with ureteric obstruction and/or staghorn-like development are likely to occur, requiring multiple percutaneous nephrolithotomy or classical surgery (because cystine stones are poorly fragmented by ESWL). Ultimately this can lead to nephrectomy, progressive renal failure and the need for supportive therapy. Prophylactic treatment is aimed at increasing the capacity of urine to dissolve cystine and at reducing urinary free cystine excretion [63]. Although there is variation in the therapeutic approach to cystinuric patients amongst experienced groups, there is a consensus with regard to the primary measure, i.e. the need to sustain a diuresis of at least 3 l per day, to achieve the maximum possible solubilization of the total daily output of cystine. Such a regimen implies that the patient should ingest water at bedtime and again during the night, taking advantage of the provoked nocturia [60]. However, even maintaining such a large urine volume is rarely sufficient to avoid stone formation. Alkalinization of urine will assist in solubilizing cystine crystals. Approximately 2 mmol/kg body weight of sodium bicarbonate in divided doses are required to maintain the urine pH at around 7.5, but no more than 8 to avoid calcium phosphate precipitation that would surround pre-existing stones, rendering them insoluble. This is usually achieved by the administration of 3 to 4 g of sodium bicarbonate four times a day. Salt intake should be reduced to compensate for this large sodium load. Potassium citrate (60 to 80 mEq/day) may be preferable to sodium bicarbonate. Patients should be instructed to check both urine SG and pH with dipsticks (with appropriate correction of SG reading for pH) in order to maintain urine pH in the range of 7.5 to 8 and urine density constantly under 1010. Disappearance of cystine crystals in the first morning urine is an indicator of treatment efficacy. Combined urine dilution and alkalinization allows prevention of stone formation in the long term.

If despite such measures stones recur, or a pre-existing stone fails to dissolve, it would be reasonable to use dimethylcysteine (D-penicillamine) or alpha-mercaptopropionylglycine (Tiopronin). Both compounds are sulfhydriles which cleave cystine to form mixed disulfides 50 times more soluble than cystine [64]. Although 1 g D-penicillamine solubilizes at best 0.5 g cystine, the daily dose should be limited to no more than 600 or 900 mg taken at bedtime. Side effects are frequent when using larger doses. They include skin rash, leukopenia, thrombocytopenia, proteinuria or the nephrotic syndrome. Some patients who do not tolerate D-penicillamine may tolerate Tiopronin. Patients have been successfully treated with D-penicillamine for more than 20 years without significant side effects [64]. However, like others we prefer to try, in the first instance, just dilution and alkalinization (preferably with potassium citrate) for as long as possible, and reserve long-term use of sulfhydriles for refractory patients.

### 7.6.3 Infection stones

The incidence of infection stones, characterized by the presence of struvite and carbapatite as major components, has dramatically decreased in all industrialized countries over the past three decades, in parallel with improved detection and treatment of urinary tract infection. At the present time, infection stones account for less than 3% of the stones observed in industrialized countries, with a higher incidence in female patients. Precipitation of MAP and carbonate apatite (CA) is due to the extreme alkalinity of urine ($pH \geqslant 8$). The latter is a consequence of urea splitting by microorganisms producing the enzyme urease, mainly the *Proteus* group or, less commonly, *Ureaplasma urealyticum* [2]. Stones are radio-opaque with a lamellar structure, and if left untreated may develop and enlarge in the pelvis and calyces, leading to the well-known staghorn calculi. The presence of numerous 'coffin-lid' struvite crystals in alkaline urine is pathognomonic. Careful examination of removed stones has led, in several of our patients, to the recognition of a core made of calcium oxalate, surrounded by struvite, thus suggesting that MAP stones may occur as the consequence of the superinfection of a pre-existent calculus during an episode of urinary tract infection (UTI). Therefore, all UTI episodes due to *Proteus*, especially pyelonephritic episodes, should be vigorously treated, until complete eradication of infection is achieved.

Treatment of infection stones is based on three principles. First, obtain total removal of all the stones, usually by means of PCNL supplemented by ESWL [13]. Second, obtain total and stable eradication of infection by means of appropriate and sufficiently prolonged antibiotherapy, using antibacterial agents with a high tissue penetration. Third, search for underlying metabolic disorder(s) that may favor stone production, and treat them accordingly. Such a policy usually allows stable cure in the great majority of cases. The use of urease inhibitor drugs such as acetohydroxamic acid, which exert a minor palliative effect and often result in severe side effects such as leukopenia and thromboembolism, appears to be of limited interest.

### 7.6.4 Infrequent stones

The autosomal recessive defect in adenine phosphoribosyltransferase results in a tissue accumulation of 2,8-DHA (including in the renal parenchyma), increased urinary excretion and formation of stones. 2,8-DHA nephrolithiasis is certainly an underdiagnosed disease. In addition, it is often misdiagnosed as uric acid lithiasis, because 2,8-DHA stones also are radiolucent and may be confused with uric acid on the basis of similar routine chemical reactions [65]. This has deleterious consequences because 2,8-DHA stones are insoluble in alkaline urine, the sole treatment being allopurinol. When undiagnosed and thus improperly treated, 2,8-DHA lithiasis may lead to end stage renal failure [66].

Xanthinuria is a very rare autosomal recessive defect of the enzyme xanthine oxidase, resulting characteristically in hypouricemia and hypouricosuria together with increased excretion of xanthine. Both 2,8-DHA and xanthine are easily identified by infrared spectroscopy [1, 17].

Drug-induced nephrolithiasis accounts for about 1% of stones. The most frequently involved drugs are triamterene, glafenine (previously used as antalgic in France, now withdrawn from the market) and silica-containing gastrointestinal preparations. Acetazolamide induces mild acidosis with alkaline urine and hypocitraturia, thus resulting in calcium phosphate precipitation, similar to phosphate stones induced by cadmium intoxication. Sulfadiazine is now often used at high dose for treating cerebral toxoplasmosis in HIV-positive patients and may result in massive crystalluria and tubular obstruction [1, 17]. Protease inhibitors such as indinavir sulfate, recently introduced as combination therapy in HIV-positive patients, induce frequent formation of radiolucent stones [67].

In conclusion, major advances have been made in both the non-invasive treatment of urinary stones and in the pathophysiology of stone formation. Etiological evaluation is therefore essential in all stone formers. Based on the identification of lithogenic risk factors, individualized therapeutic measures will now be able to prevent, or at least substantially decrease, stone recurrence, and may largely prevent the development of progressive renal failure in virtually all patients.

## REFERENCES


1. Jungers, P., Daudon, M. and Le Duc, A. (1989) *Lithiase Urinaire*. Flammarion Médecine-Sciences, Paris.
2. Robertson, W.G. (1993) Aetiological factors in stone formation, in *Oxford Textbook of Nephrology*, Oxford University Press, Oxford, pp. 1822–46.
3. Whitfield, H.N. (1993) The surgical management of renal stones, in *Oxford Textbook of Clinical Nephrology*, Oxford University Press, Oxford, pp. 1869–82.
4. Consensus Conference: Prevention and Treatment of Kidney Stones (1988) *J. Am. Med. Assoc.*, **260**, 977–81.
5. Rose, G.A. (1993) The medical management of renal stone disease, in *Oxford Textbook of Nephrology*, Oxford University Press, Oxford, pp. 1847–69.
6. Coe, F.L., Favus, M.J., Pak, C.Y.C. *et al.* (1996) *Kidney Stones, Medical and Surgical Management*, Lippincott-Raven, *Philadelphia, New York*.
7. Coe, F.L., Parks, J.H. and Asplin, J.R. (1992) The pathogenesis and treatment of kidney stones. *N. Engl. J. Med.*, **32**, 1141–52.
8. Daudon, M., Hennequin, C., Bader, C. *et al.* (1995) Inhibitors of crystallization., *Adv. Nephrol.*, **24**, 169–218.
9. Kok, D.J., Papapoulos, S.E. and Bijvoet, O.L.M. (1986) Excessive crystal agglomeration with low citrtate excretion in recurrent stone formers. *Lancet*, **i**, 1056–9.
10. Robertson, W.G. and Peacock, M. (1980) The cause of idiopathic calcium stone disease: hypercalciuria or hyperoxaluria? *Nephron*, **26**, 105–10.
11. Daudon, M., Réveillaud, R.J., Levasseur, H. and Jungers, P. (1989) Combined influence of urinary calcium and oxalate concentration on crystal formation in stone formers, in *Urolithiasis* (eds V.R. Walker, R.A.L. Sutton, G.C.B. Cameron *et al.*), New York, London, pp. 155–7.

12. Ehreth, J.J., Drach, G.W., Arnett, M.L. *et al.* (1994) Extracorporeal shock wave lithotripsy: Multicenter study of kidney and upper ureter versus middle and lower ureter treatments. *J. Urol.*, **152**, 1379–85.
13. Segura, J.W., Preminger, G.M., Assimos, D.G. *et al.* (1994) Nephrolithiasis clinical guidelines panel summary report on the management of staghorn calculi. *J. Urol.*, **151**, 1648–51.
14. Lingeman, J.E., Woods, J., Toth, P.D. *et al.* (1989) The role of lithotripsy and its side effects. *J. Urol.*, **141**, 793–7.
15. Robertson, W.G. (1987) Diet and calcium stones. *Miner. Electrolyte Metab.*, **13**, 228–34.
16. Wrong, O. (1993) Nephrocalcinosis, in *Oxford Textbook of Clinical Nephrology*, Oxford University Press, Oxford, pp. 1882–904.
17. Daudon, M., Bader, C.A. and Jungers, P. (1993) Urinary calculi: review of classification methods and correlations with etiology. *Scann. Microsc.*, **7**, 1081–106.
18. Broadus, A.E., Horst, R.L., Lang, R. *et al.* (1980) The importance of circulating 1,25-dihydroxyvitamin D in the pathogenesis of hypercalciuria and renal stone formation in primary hyperparathyroidism. *N. Engl. J. Med.*, **302**, 421–6.
19. Patron, P., Gardin, J.P. and Paillard, M. (1987) Renal mass and reserve of vitamin D: determinants in primary hyperparathyroidism. *Kidney Int.*, **31**, 1174–80.
20. Marx, S.J., Spiegel, A.M., Levine, M.A. *et al.* (1982) Familial hypocalciuric hypercalcemia: the relation to primary parathyroid hyperplasia. *N. Engl. J. Med.*, **307**, 416–26.
21. Lemann, J. Jr. and Gray, R.W. (1989) Idiopathic hypercalciuria. *J. Urol.*, **141**, 715–8.
22. Ahlstrand, C. and Tiselius, H.G. (1987) Urine composition and stone formation during treatment with acetazolamide. *Scand. J. Urol. Nephrol.* **21**, 225–8.
23. Hildebrandt, F., Jungers, P. and Grünfeld, J.P. (1997) Medullary cystic and medullary sponge kidney, in *Diseases of the Kidney*, 6th edn (eds R.W. Schrier and C.W. Gottschalk), Little, Brown and Co, Boston, pp. 499–520.
24. Rose, G.A. (ed.) (1988) *Oxalate Metabolism in Relation to Urinary Stone*, Springer-Verlag, London.
25. McLeod, R.S. and Churchill, D.N. (1992) Urolithiasis complicating inflammatory bowel disease. *J. Urol.*, **148**, 974–8.
26. Watts, R.W.E. (1994) Primary hyperoxaluria type I. *Q. J. Med.*, **87**, 593–600.
27. Marangella, M., Petrarulo, M. and Vitale, C. *et al.* (1992) Plasma and urine glycolate assays for differentiating hyperoxaluria syndromes. *J. Urol.*, **148**, 986–9.
28. Watts, R.W.E. (1994) Treatment of primary hyperoxaluria type I. *J. Nephrol.*, **7**, 208–14.
29. Cochat, P., Deloraine, A., Olive, F. *et al.* (1995) Primary hyperoxaluria type 1: the therapeutic dilemma. *Adv. Nephrol.*, **24**, 229–44.
30. Chlebeck, P.T., Milliner, D.S. and Smith, L.H. (1994) Long-term prognosis in primary hyperoxaluria type II (L-glyceric aciduria). *Am. J. Kidney Dis.*, **23**, 255–9.
31. Caruana, R.J. and Buckalew, V.M. (1988) The syndrome of distal (type 1) renal tubular acidosis: clinical and laboratory findings in 58 cases. *Medicine* (Baltimore), **67**, 84–99.
32. Pak, C.Y.C., Britton, F., Peterson, R. *et al.* (1980) Ambulatory evaluation of nephrolithiasis: classification, clinical presentation and diagnostic criteria. *Am. J. Med.*, **69**, 19–30.

33. Broadus, A.E., Dominguez, M. and Bartter, F.C. (1978) Pathophysiological studies in idiopathic hypercalciuria. Use of an oral calcium tolerance test to characterize distinctive hypercalciuric subgroups. *J. Clin. Endocrinol. Metab.*, **47**, 751–60.
34. Muldowney, F.P., Freaney, R. and Moloney, M.F. (1982) Importance of dietary sodium in the hypercalciuria syndrome. *Kidney Int.*, **22**, 292–6.
35. Fellström, B., Danielson, B.G., Karlström, B. *et al.* (1984) Effects of high intake of dietary animal protein on mineral metabolism and urinary supersaturation of calcium oxalate in renal stone formers. *Br. J. Urol.*, **56**, 263–9.
36. Breslau, N.A., Brinkley, L., Hill, K.D. and Pak, C.Y.C. (1988) Relationship of animal protein-rich diet to kidney stone formation and calcium metabolism. *J. Clin. Endocrinol. Metab.*, **66**, 140–4.
37. Jaeger, Ph., Hess, B., Takkinen, R. and Zipperle, L. (1995) Nutritional determinants of nephrolithiasis. *Adv. Nephrol.*, **24**, 219–27.
38. Jungers, P., Daudon, M., Hennequin, C. and Lacour, B. (1993) Correlation between protein and sodium intake and urinary calcium excretion in calcium stone formers. *Néphrologie*, **14**, 287–90.
39. Wasserstein, A.G., Stolley, P.D., Soper, K.A. *et al.* (1987) Case-control study of risk factors for idiopathic calcium nephrolithiasis. *Miner. Electrolyte Metab.*, **13**, 85–95.
40. Broadus, A.E., Insogna, K.L., Lang, R. *et al.* (1984) Evidence for disordered control of 1,25 dihydroxyvitamin D production in absorptive hypercalciuria. *N. Engl. J. Med.*, **311**, 73–80.
41. Bordier, P., Ryckewaert, A. and Guéris, J. (1977) On the pathogenesis of so-called hypercalciuria. *Am. J. Med.*, **63**, 398–409.
42. Bianchi, G., Vezzoli, G., Cusi, D. *et al.* (1988) Abnormal red-cell calcium pump in patients with idiopathic hypercalciuria. *N. Engl. J. Med.*, **319**, 897–901.
43. Favus, M.J. (1989) Familial forms of hypercalciuria. *J. Urol.*, **141**, 719–22.
44. Marshall, R.W., Cochran, M. and Hodgkinson, A. (1972) Relationships between calcium and oxalic acid intake in the diet and their excretion in the urine of normal and stone-forming subjects. *Clin. Sci.*, **43**, 91–9.
45. Bataille, P., Charransol, G., Grkgoire, I. and Fournier, A. (1983) Effect of calcium restriction on renal excretion of oxalate and the probability of being a stone former. *J. Urol.*, **130**, 218–21.
46. Curhan, G.C., Willett, W.C., Rimm, E.B. and Stampfer, M.J. (1993) A prospective study of dietary calcium and other nutrients and the risk of symptomatic kidney stones. *N. Engl. J. Med.*, **328**, 833–8.
47. Grover, P.K., Ryall, R.L. and Marshall, V.R. (1993) Dissolved urate promotes calcium oxalate crystallization: epitaxy is not the cause. *Clin. Sci.*, **85**, 303–7.
48. Nicar, M.J., Skurla, C., Sakhaee, K. and Pak, C.Y.C. (1983) Low urinary citrate excretion in nephrolithiasis. *Urology*, **21**, 8–14.
49. Hess, B., Nakagawa, Y. and Coe, F.L. (1989) Inhibition of calcium oxalate monohydrate crystal aggregation by urine proteins. *Am. J. Phisiol.*, **257**, F99–F106.
50. Hess, B., Zipperle, L. and Jaeger, P. (1993) Citrate and calcium effects on Tamm–Horsfall glycoprotein as a modifier of calcium oxalate crystal aggegration. *Am. J. Physiol.*, **265**, F1–F8.
51. Bataille, P., Achard, J.M., Fournier, A. *et al.* (1991) Diet, vitamin D and vertebral mineral density in hypercalciuric stone formers., *Kidney Int.*, **39**, 1193–205.

52. Goldfarb, S. (1988) Dietary factors in the pathogenesis and prophylaxis of calcium nephrolithiasis. *Kidney Int.*, **34**, 544–55.
53. Ettinger, B., Citron, J.T., Livermore, B. and Dolman, L.I. (1988) Chlorthalidone reduces calcium oxalate calculous recurrence but magnesium hydroxide does not. *J. Urol.*, **139**, 679–84.
54. Coe, F.L., Parks, J.H., Bushinsky, D.A. *et al.* (1988) Chlortalidone promotes mineral retention in patients with idiopathic hypercalciuria. *Kidney Int.*, **33**, 1140–6.
55. Pak, C.Y.C. (1987) Citrate and renal calculi. *Miner. Electrolyte Metab.*, **13**, 257–66.
56. Pak, C.Y.C. (1991) Citrate and renal calculi: New insights and future directives. *Am. J. Kidney Dis.*, **17**, 420–5.
57. Hosking, D.H., Erickson, S.B. and Van den Berg, C.J. *et al.* (1983) The stone clinic effect in patients with idiopathic calcium urolithiasis. *J. Urol.*, **130**, 1115–8.
58. McCormack, M., Dessureault, J. and Guitard, M. (1991) The urine specific gravity dipstick: a useful tool to increase fluid intake in stone forming patients. *J. Urol.*, **146**, 1475–7.
59. Dick, W.H., Lingeman, J.E. and Preminger, G.M. *et al.* (1990) Laxative abuse as a cause for ammonium urate renal calculi. *J. Urol.*, **143**, 244–7.
60. Lemann, J. Jr. (1983) Nephrolithiasis, in *Textbook of Nephrology* (eds S.G. Massry and R.J. Glassock), Williams and Wilkins, Baltimore, pp. 6.266–6.282.
61. Millman, S., Strauss, A.L., Parks, J.H. and Coe, F.L. (1982) Pathogenesis and clinical course of mixed calcium oxalate and uric acid nephrolithiasis. *Kidney Int.*, **22**, 360–70.
62. Singer, A. and Das, S. (1989) Cystinuria: a review of the pathophysiology and management. *J. Urol.*, **142**, 669–73.
63. Scriver, C.R. (1986) Cystinuria. *N. Engl. J. Med.*, **315**, 1155–7.
64. Crawhall, J.C. (1987) Cystinuria. An experience in management over 18 years. *Miner. Electrolyte Metab.*, **13**, 286–93.
65. Céballos-Picot, I., Pérignon, J.L., Hamet, M. *et al.* (1992) 2,8-Dihydroxyadenine urolithiasis, an underdiagnosed disease. *Lancet*, **339**, 1050–1.
66. Gagné, E.R., Deland, E., Daudon, M. *et al.* (1994) Chronic renal failure secondary to 2,8-dihydroxyadenine deposition: the first report of recurrence in a kidney transplant. *Am. J. Kidney Dis.*, **24**, 104–7.
67. Daudon, M., Estépa, L., Viard, J.P., Joly, D. and Jungers, P. (1997) Urinary stones in HIV-1-positive patients treated with indinavir. *Lancet*, **349**, 1294–5.

# 8

# Interstitial, toxic and metabolic nephropathies

*M. Jadoul*

In this chapter, we review the clinical characteristics, diagnosis, specific management and prevention of interstitial, toxic and metabolic chronic interstitial kidney diseases induced by analgesics, cisplatin and other cytostatic agents, cyclosporin A, amphotericin B, heavy metals (lead, cadmium) and lithium. We further discuss the controversial role of uric acid as a cause of kidney disease and review Balkan endemic nephropathy and Chinese herbs nephropathy.

General measures for renal protection useful in most, if not all, renal diseases, such as optimal blood pressure control, nutritional management and treatment of dyslipidemia will not be alluded to, as these are discussed in other chapters of this book.

## 8.1 ANALGESIC NEPHROPATHY

Analgesic nephropathy (AN) is a tubulo-interstitial kidney disease characterized by the frequent development of papillary necrosis and caused by continuous analgesic abuse.

### 8.1.1 Etiology

Phenacetin was initially implicated as the causal agent ('phenacetin kidney'). However all of the ingredients of analgesic mixtures including aspirin, paracetamol, pyrazolones and caffeine have been implicated at some time so that the cause(s) of analgesic nephropathy remain(s)

*Renal Disease.* Edited by G. Venkat Raman. Published in 1998 by Chapman & Hall, London. ISBN 0 412 45700 8.

controversial. Earliest reports were from Switzerland: a change in the pattern of interstitial kidney disease was observed and ascribed to analgesic abuse. Many case reports and series have subsequently confirmed this association.

Case control studies further confirmed an association between heavy analgesic consumption and the risk of end stage renal disease (ESRD). Sandler *et al.* [1] performed a multicentre case control study of 544 adults with newly diagnosed kidney disease (serum creatinine $\geqslant 1.5\,mg/dl$) and 560 matched control subjects from North Carolina, USA. Histories of use of analgesics were obtained by telephone interviews with the patients or proxies. Daily users of analgesics had a higher risk of renal disease than infrequent users, especially for phenacetin (odds ratio 5.11) but also for acetaminophen (odds ratio 3.21). There was no increased risk in daily aspirin users.

More recently, Perneger *et al.* [2] made a similar case control study in 716 patients treated for ESRD and 361 control subjects of similar age from Maryland, Virginia, West Virginia and Washington DC, USA using telephone interviews. Heavier acetaminophen use was associated with an increased risk of ESRD in a dose-dependent fashion. When persons who had taken fewer than 1000 pills containing acetaminophen in their lifetime were used for reference, the odds ratio was 2 for those who had taken between 1000 and 4999 pills and 2.4 for those who had taken 5000 or more pills. Interestingly, the pattern of risk associated with analgesic abuse differed little according to the labeled causes of ESRD (diabetes mellitus, hypertension, any other specified cause or no known cause). This was interpreted by the authors as evidence for a deleterious influence of heavy acetaminophen use on kidney function in patients with other nephropathies. Alternatively, this may reflect the low degree of accuracy of the diagnoses registered as cause of ESRD, especially in the USA where many patients do not undergo a kidney biopsy. Finally, the criticism has been raised that the case patients took more acetaminophen because physicians recommend it as the analgesic of choice in renal failure. This controversy is unlikely to be resolved before a longitudinal cohort study is performed in heavy consumers of acetaminophen.

Not all case control studies have demonstrated a significant risk of ESRD due to analgesic use: Murray *et al.* [3] studied in a similar manner 527 patients and 1047 matched control subjects from the north-eastern USA. They failed to demonstrate a statistically significant risk of ESRD for analgesics used alone or in combination. This may simply reflect the fact that long-term high-dose use of such drugs was less usual in this study population.

In 1968, the only prospective controlled cohort study of the consequences of analgesic abuse was initiated in Switzerland by Dubach and colleagues [4]. They identified 623 Swiss women, 30 to 49 years of age, who were thought to be regular users of phenacetin, as suggested by the presence of acetaminophen in the urine. A group of 621 controls was selected. Both groups had normal renal function at baseline. By 1975, 260 women in a high-analgesic use group (defined by a urinary *n*-acetylparaaminophenol concentration $\geqslant 0.77$ mmol/l), 231 in a low-use group and 506 in the control group were available for analysis. Urinary-concentrating ability and serum creatinine were measured, and acetaminophen detected in the urine. In the high-use group, 4.6% of the women had reduced urinary-concentrating ability compared to 1.3% in the low-use group and 1% of the controls. Increases in serum creatinine were detected in 5.3% of the high-use group compared to 0.4% and 0% in the low-use and control groups respectively. After 11 years' follow-up, urinary-concentrating ability was reduced in 23% of the high-use group compared to 6.7% of controls. Serum creatinine was increased in 6.7% of the high-use group and 0.9% of the controls. Thirty-nine patients (6.7%) had died in the study group, primarily due to renal and cardiovascular causes compared to 13 patients (2.2%) in the control group. Twenty year mortality (in 89% of the original cohort members) showed a significantly increased risk of overall mortality (relative risk 2.2) and of death due to urologic or renal disease (relative risk 16.1), death due to cancer (relative risk 1.9) and death due to cardiovascular disease (relative risk 2.9). The relative risk of cardiovascular disease (fatal or non-fatal myocardial infarction, heart failure or stroke) was also significantly increased. Whereas phenacetin abuse was associated with higher mortality, salicylate use had no effect on either mortality or morbidity.

Experimental studies in animals suffer from the fact that studies in rats are difficult to extrapolate to humans, as the rat kidney has a single papilla and longer nephrons than the human kidney. Yet papillary necrosis has been demonstrated in rats only following administration of very large doses of phenacetin. In contrast, papillary necrosis readily occurs in animals given aspirin or acetaminophen, both alone and in combination.

Finally, some ecologic studies, but not all, have demonstrated a reduction in the prevalence of analgesic nephropathy following the removal or regulation of phenacetin distribution: after early restriction of access to phenacetin in Sweden, the prevalence of analgesic nephropathy as a cause of ESRD dropped markedly from 20% to below 2% over the last 20 years. Similarly, in Australia, following the introduction of legislative measures restricting access to analgesics, the prevalence of analgesic nephropathy in patients starting dialysis declined significantly [5]. By contrast, access to phenacetin was restricted and subsequently prohibited in Belgium, but the prevalence of analgesic nephropathy declined only moderately [6].

These discrepancies may partly reflect the long delay between analgesic abuse and the resulting chronic renal disease: no change should be expected in ESRD incidence before several years or decades after legislative measures are taken. Alternatively, Elseviers and De Broe have suggested that, despite the fact that phenacetin was banished from the market in Belgium, analgesic abuse still persisted, as abuse of analgesic mixtures containing acetaminophen, caffeine, codeine and/or salicylates. They suggested banning such preparations from the pharmaceutical market [6]. It remains surprising that such mixtures have been available throughout these years in other countries like France, in which the prevalence of analgesic nephropathy has remained consistently low.

Overall, case series, case control studies and the prospective study from Dubach have convincingly demonstrated that heavy analgesic abuse, mainly phenacetin, usually in analgesic mixtures, causes renal disease. The causal role of acetaminophen alone has more recently been suggested by US investigators [2] but remains controversial. Salicylate use does not appear to carry a significant risk.

### 8.1.2 Clinical features

Typically, analgesic nephropathy develops slowly in middle-aged women and is frequently asymptomatic until the late stage of renal insufficiency. Sterile leukocyturia is common. Hematuria is less common and suggests either recent renal papillary necrosis or urothelial carcinoma. Arterial hypertension is present in about 50% of patients, not infrequently in association with renal arterial stenosis [5]. Papillary necrosis may be clinically silent or give rise to ureteric obstruction.

Extra-renal complications of chronic analgesic consumption are also observed in such patients. They include peptic ulcers, related to the salicylate component. Anemia inappropriate for the severity of renal insufficiency is also rather common and may reflect either chronic gastrointestinal hemorrhage or mild hemolysis with methemoglobinemia due to phenacetin [5]. The prevalence of such extra-renal complications of analgesic consumption appears lower in patients with a diagnosis of analgesic nephropathy in recent years than in the 1970s [5].

Increased cardiovascular mortality has been clearly demonstrated in analgesic abusers by Dubach *et al.* [4]. However, it remains unclear whether this increased mortality is due to analgesic abuse itself or to the associated renal insufficiency, arterial hypertension and/or other risk factors, such as smoking. Indeed many studies pointed to an 'accelerated atherosclerosis' in patients with analgesic nephropathy, but most studies were retrospective and not controlled with regard to other cardiovascular risk factors. More recently the European Dialysis and Transplant Association (EDTA) registry re-evaluated this issue [7]. The mortality in general and the death rates due to cardiovascular causes were found not to differ in renal replacement therapy patients with analgesic nephropathy from those in patients with standard primary renal disease.

### 8.1.3 Diagnosis

Diagnosis will rest on careful questioning for analgesic use and/or urinary screening for analgesic metabolites. Sterile pyuria and mild (lower than 1 g/24 h) proteinuria are common but not specific. Renal papillary necrosis may be detected in the early stages by intravenous urography and by plain or computerized tomography. Renal biopsy is of little use unless there are signs of glomerular disease: Nanra *et al.* found, in nine out of 62 patients with analgesic nephropathy and proteinuria higher than 0.5 g/day who underwent kidney biopsy, additional renal diseases such as allopurinol-induced hypersensitivity and various forms of glomerulonephritis [5].

In patients with ESRD, the diagnostic criteria for analgesic nephropathy were recently refined [8]. A comparison of 60 Belgian analgesic abusers with 188 controls, all of whom underwent renal ultrasonography plus plain kidney tomography, showed that a decrease in kidney length combined with bumpy contours of both kidneys had a sensitivity of 90% and a specificity of 95% for AN, analgesic abuse, defined as the daily use of analgesic mixtures for $\geqslant 5$ years, being taken as gold standard for the diagnosis of AN. The additional finding of signs of renal papillary necrosis resulted in an overall sensitivity of 72% and a specificity of 97% for a positive predictive value of 92%. Other signs such as hypertension, anemia and sterile pyuria had insufficient sensitivity and/or specificity to be of diagnostic value in patients starting renal replacement therapy. The validity of these criteria has subsequently been tested in a multicentre European study (ANNE study), in 598 patients starting renal replacement therapy (RRT) for ESRD of unclear etiology. The sensitivity and specificity for AN of decreased kidney length with bumpy contours were 85 and 93% respectively, thus somewhat lower than in Belgium. These criteria may help in the future to obtain a more reliable insight into the magnitude of AN as a problem in different countries [9].

Differential diagnosis should include other causes of renal papillary necrosis, such as diabetic, obstructive, reflux and sickle-cell nephropathies.

### 8.1.4 Management

The reduced urinary-concentrating capacity increases the risk of dehydration in patients with analgesic nephropathy. This dehydration may favor papillary necrosis and should be prevented by meticulous control of the hydration state. Ureteric obstruction due to shed papillae should be relieved by appropriate urological intervention. Patients should regularly be screened for urothelial carcinoma by urine cytology and more extensive investigations whenever hematuria develops. This also applies to patients already on renal replacement therapy, even after renal transplantation.

Other therapeutic measures are similar to those in patients with other chronic renal diseases: antihypertensive therapy, treatment of urinary tract infection, therapy of acid–base and electrolyte disturbances. Obviously, analgesic abuse should be stopped as soon as possible in patients with analgesic nephropathy: this may result in stabilization of renal function, as recently highlighted by Hauser *et al.* [10]. They evaluated 23 patients with analgesic nephropathy and apparent cessation of drug abuse. Blood samples for the determination of acetaminophen and salicylate were drawn on the occasion of routine examination. These proved positive in only two out of 12 patients whose renal function remained stable over one year, but in nine out of 11 patients whose renal function deteriorated over the same time. These data emphasize the importance of a continuing analgesic abuse, unknown to the medical staff, with regard to the progression of renal insufficiency.

## 8.2 CISPLATIN AND OTHER CYTOSTATIC AGENTS

Cisplatin is a very potent chemotherapeutic agent whose nephrotoxicity limits the dosage administered. It is used in the treatment of testicular, bladder, ovarian and various squamous cell carcinomas (lung, head and neck, uterine cervix).

### 8.2.1 Pathophysiology

Within two hours of cisplatin administration, 90% of the platinum is tightly bound to plasma proteins. It is presumed that only the freely filtered unbound platinum has cytotoxic activity. In rats the kidneys have the highest somatic cisplatin concentration and this is presumed to be the mechanism of the nephrotoxicity. Chronic cisplatin nephrotoxicity is characterized by focal acute tubular necrosis, with cystic dilated tubules lined by flattened epithelium showing atypical nuclei and atypical mitotic figures. A permanent and often progressive decrease in the glomerular filtration rate (GFR) is observed. Both the proximal and distal tubules are affected.

At the ultrastructural level, an increased number and size of apical pinocytotic vesicles and lysosomal bodies are observed, together with loss of brush borders and rounded mitochondria. The distal tubule and collecting duct epithelium show hydropic degeneration. Increased DNA synthesis with a sharp increase in cell proliferation rate is observed and affects both tubular epithelium and interstitial tissue. Interstitial fibroblastic proliferation leads to interstitial fibrosis.

### 8.2.2 Risk factors

Dehydration is the major risk factor and should be avoided at all costs. Elderly patients have no greater risk of cisplatin nephrotoxicity than their younger counterparts, and should not be excluded from therapy on the basis of age. Renal irradiation and cisplatin may result in combined toxicity, irrespective of time sequence or interval. For instance, low-dose cisplatin given immediately before or as long as nine months after irradiation causes a decrease in the latent period for radiation nephritis, whose severity is increased. When given more than three months prior to radiation, the effect is less severe [11, 12].

### 8.2.3 Prevention

Aggressive hydration and the avoidance of other nephrotoxic agents such as aminoglycosides have been the time-tested means to reduce cisplatin nephrotoxicity. Even though days, weeks or months are required for the severe changes in renal function to fully develop, the critical events seem to occur almost immediately. Therefore, protective measures should be applied before, during and very soon after cisplatin infusion.

Preventing cisplatin-bound exchange and subsequent damage is perhaps a mechanism by which co-administration of NaCl reduces toxicity. Hydration may function also by reducing the time during which cisplatin and renal tubule are in contact. In rats, prevention of nephrotoxicity by hydration correlates directly with increased urine chloride concentration.

Efforts to further reduce toxicity have led to the use of hypertonic saline drug vehicle, mannitol and furosemide diuresis. Hypertonic saline vehicle is recommended for patients with a cisplatin dosage of $100\,mg/m^2$ or more. Hypertonic saline still requires intense hydration to prevent cisplatin nephrotoxicity. It does not reduce the cisplatin antitumor effect and does not provide protection from other toxic effects like neuropathy, ototoxicity and vomiting. There are no convincing data regarding the specific protective effect of mannitol apart from during the first cisplatin course, perhaps by reducing cisplatin urine concentration. Furosemide has no advantage compared to hydration alone in preventing nephrotoxicity but does prevent fluid overload during aggressive hydration in patients at risk of cardiac failure. Several pharmacological agents are currently under evaluation for the prevention of toxicity: these include probenecid, DDTC (dithiocarbamate), methionine, sodium thiosulfate, intravenous glutathione, etc. Some of these agents appear promising in experimental studies and are currently being evaluated in phase I human trials [11, 12]. Finally, newer platinum analogs with a lower nephrotoxic potential are being developed (carboplatin, ormaplatin).

### 8.2.4 Other cytostatic agents

The nephrotoxicity of many other anticancer chemotherapeutic agents has been occasionally reported or suspected. Some of them, like cisplatin, cause a progressive chronic tubulo-interstitial fibrosis resulting in chronic renal failure. These include nitrosoureas, streptozotocin and ifosfamide, among others. One point of major importance for all these agents is that renal failure may not develop for months after stopping the cytostatic treatment. Nephrotoxicity is cumulative, resulting in a higher risk of renal failure in patients treated for longer periods, with higher dosages.

Adequate hydration is recommended to ensure the lowest possible concentration of the drug passing through the renal tubule. For nitrosoureas, the first indication of renal abnormalities develops a median of 24 months after starting treatment, even if therapy was discontinued. The mechanism of the nephrotoxicity remains as yet unknown and histology shows tubulo-interstitial lesions [13].

More recently, the potential nephrotoxicity of ifosfamide both in adults and children has been emphasized. Chloral acetaldehyde, a major metabolite of ifosfamide, may be at least partly responsible for the renal toxicity of the drug. Again, overt toxicity may only develop months after withdrawal of the drug [14].

The urothelial toxicity associated with cyclophosphamide may be ameliorated by administration of uromitexan (Mesna).

## 8.3 CYCLOSPORIN A NEPHROTOXICITY (see also Chapter 15)

Nephrotoxicity is a major side effect of cyclosporin A (CsA). Data obtained in organ transplant recipients are reviewed first. The prevalence, risk factors and histological pattern of chronic cyclosporin A nephrotoxicity in patients treated for indications other than organ transplantation are described later.

### 8.3.1 Organ transplant recipients

Many reports have documented the potential of cyclosporin A to produce chronic nephropathy. The most striking was from Stanford [15]. Thirty-seven cardiac transplant recipients receiving cyclosporin A for 12 to 24 months were compared with 24 recipients receiving azathioprine for more than 24 months. Despite equivalent cardiac performance, GFR in those treated with CsA was much lower ($47 \pm 3\,\text{ml/min/1.73}\,\text{m}^2$) than in azathioprine-treated patients ($94 \pm 4$) ($P < 0.001$). Longitudinal examination over 48 months in 15 CsA-treated patients showed persistently reduced GFR, with three members of the CsA-treated group developing ESRD. Admittedly these patients were treated in the early 1980s with high cyclosporin A dosages: 17 mg/kg initially, 10 mg/kg one month after transplantation, 7.5 mg/kg six months after transplantation.

Other groups have reported less worrying findings: for example, Gonwa *et al.* [16] followed up 45 heart transplant recipients for one year, 27 of whom were followed for two years. GFR declined from 71 ml/min before operation to 59 ml/min eight weeks later, but did not change significantly over the subsequent two years. Cyclosporin A dosage averaged 6 mg/kg two months after transplantation and 3.5 mg/kg one year after transplantation, a much lower dosage than in the previous study.

Still more recently, the clinical relevance of CsA nephrotoxicity in renal transplant recipients has been challenged by a controversial report [17]. Burke *et al.* retrospectively reviewed the effect of cyclosporin A on renal function and graft rejection in 1663 renal transplant recipients followed at six US centers. The rate of graft survival was 78% after a median of 36 months. Grafts were lost in 179 patients mostly because of acute rejection (25%) or chronic renal dysfunction unresponsive to a reduction in cyclosporin A dosage (40%). The median change in the serum creatinine concentration in all patients after transplantation was less than 0.001 mg/dl/month. The authors concluded that the majority of renal transplant recipients tolerate long-term CsA therapy without evidence of progressive toxic nephropathy.

Unfortunately, rejection was defined merely by the initiation of anti-rejection therapy and was histologically confirmed in only 39% of the episodes. Thus the elimination of cyclosporin A as a contributing factor in graft failure relies on the lack of decrease of serum creatinine concentration after reduction of cyclosporin A dosage. In the absence of more detailed data, especially pathological, implicating cyclosporin A, the real question remains: why should some patients have progressive chronic nephropathy due to CsA (see below) whereas others (e.g. renal transplant recipients) do not? The denervation of the transplanted kidney might be held responsible, but chronic CsA-induced nephropathy can be produced experimentally, regardless of whether the kidney is innervated.

This does not detract from the fact that cyclosporin A has been a major advance in the field of organ transplantation but emphasizes the fact that the search for ways to minimize chronic nephrotoxicity and for less toxic but equally effective compounds must continue (see below).

### 8.3.2 Other immunological diseases

Several investigators have recently evaluated the impact of cyclosporin A therapy on renal function in psoriasis patients. Young *et al.* followed, by iothalamate clearance, 16 patients receiving CsA (average 3.9 mg/kg/day) for three years [18]. GFR declined at an average rate of 3.1 ml/min/1.73 $m^2$ per year.

Kidney biopsies from 19 cyclosporin A-treated patients, compared to 38 age-matched transplant donors, showed increased interstitial fibrosis and tubular atrophy at one year (scale: 0 = normal, 4 = severe): $1.9 \pm 0.2$ versus $0.3 \pm 0.1$ and $1.6 \pm 0.2$ versus $0.3 \pm 0.1$ ($P < 0.0001$ in both cases). Eleven patients had a second biopsy after two more years of cyclosporin A, showing further progression of fibrosis and tubular atrophy and the onset of cyclosporin A-associated arteriolopathy [18].

Pei *et al.* [19] similarly followed fifteen psoriatic patients treated with low-dose (average 3.9 mg/kg/day) cyclosporin A for thirteen months. Serum creatinine rose during the study period from 0.94 mg/dl to 1.2 mg/dl. GFR was significantly reduced at follow-up in seven out of 15 patients. Four patients had moderate tubulo-interstitial scarring and arteriolopathy while the remaining patients had mild structural abnormalities.

### 8.3.3 Risk factors for cyclosporin A nephrotoxicity

Several investigators have addressed this important question. Feutren *et al.* compared 41 patients with histologically defined CsA nephrotoxicity with patients on CsA but without similar renal lesions [20]. All of them were treated for autoimmune diseases. Risk factors for cyclosporin A nephrotoxicity included a large initial dose, a larger maximal increase in serum creatinine above baseline value and older age [20]. They proposed minimizing the risk of nephrotoxicity by restricting the dose of CsA to no more than 5 mg/kg/day and avoiding increases in serum creatinine of more than 30% above the patients baseline value. Similar findings were made by Pei *et al.* [19]: severe acute nephrotoxicity (defined as a reversible increase of serum creatinine >90% of baseline value) was a marker for moderate chronic nephrotoxicity.

### 8.3.4 Management of chronic nephrotoxicity

Vigorous treatment of cyclosporin A-induced hypertension is warranted and will usually start with a calcium channel blocker. Many other pharmacological attempts have been made to minimize chronic CsA nephrotoxicity. These include calcium channel blockers (even in the absence of hypertension), misoprostol, and other drugs in experimental models, such as endothelin-receptor antagonists, fish oils, etc. Although some data are promising, there is still a long way to go, as illustrated by the report of Hunley *et al.* [21]. These investigators were able to show, in a salt-depleted rat model of cyclosporin A nephrotoxicity, that simultaneous treatment with a specific endothelin A receptor antagonist prevented CsA-induced decrease of GFR but unfortunately completely failed to prevent renal structural damage!

The search for alternative immunosuppressive agents remains imperative. Tacrolimus (FK506), a new potent immunosuppressive drug, does also induce substantial chronic nephrotoxicity. A CsA analog, cyclosporin G (OG 37 3/5), was found, in a small (a total of 40 patients) randomized double-blind trial, to be slightly less nephrotoxic but as effective as cyclosporin A. This will require confirmation. Finally the most effective way to minimize cyclosporin A nephrotoxicity may well be to use as low dosages as possible, to avoid the numerous drug interactions with CsA, to prescribe cyclosporin A only if absolutely indicated, and to consider carefully the possibility of discontinuing the drug, even in renal transplant recipients, in whom this may be safely performed in selected groups. This possibility may become reality with the advent of new drugs such as mycophenolate.

## 8.4 AMPHOTERICIN B AND THE KIDNEY

The nephrotoxicity of amphotericin B has been recognized for some forty years and remains an important cause for concern, especially as the incidence of severe fungal infections is high in patients with human immunodeficiency virus infection, organ transplants or undergoing cancer chemotherapy.

### 8.4.1 Clinical picture

This typically includes impaired concentrating ability, renal sodium, potassium, and magnesium wasting with dehydration, hypokalemia and hypomagnesemia, renal tubular acidosis and azotemia. Serum creatinine begins to rise within a few days to weeks of therapy. Patients are typically non-oliguric. Urinalysis can reveal hematuria and/or pyuria. Decreased renal blood flow, increased renal vessel resistance and direct tubular toxicity with increased membrane permeability have been demonstrated.

### 8.4.2 Management and prevention

In patients with renal failure, renal function usually improves after withdrawal of the drug, although improvement may be very slow. Co-administration of other nephrotoxic agents such as aminoglycosides, etc. should be avoided. Long-term, dialysis may be occasionally required.

It has long been suggested that salt loading protects against amphotericin B-induced nephrotoxicity. Llanos *et al.* [21] tested this hypothesis in two groups of ten patients treated with amphotericin B 50 mg/dose, three times per week for ten weeks, for muco-cutaneous leishmaniasis. Patients were randomized to receive either one litre of saline or 5% dextrose in water administered intravenously over one hour in a double blind manner directly prior to amphotericin B administration. Interestingly, none of the patients sustained an increase in creatinine to values greater than 1.7 mg/dl but the mean serum creatinine increased slightly over time in the dextrose group, and remained unchanged in the saline group (0.6 to 1.0 mg/dl versus 0.8 to 0.8 mg/dl respectively). This nephroprotection was observed at the expense of a higher need for potassium supplementation in the saline than in the dextrose group. The lower overall incidence of nephrotoxicity in this study may be due to the high (around 250 mmol/day) basal salt intake and/or the lack of co-administration of other nephrotoxic drugs and to racial variation in responsiveness (the study was performed in Peru).

### 8.4.3 Perspectives

The nephrotoxicity of amphotericin B should be less frequently observed in the not too distant future, for several reasons. Firstly, new, chemically unrelated drugs are currently under evaluation for the treatment of various mycotic infections; for instance, fluconazole has recently been shown to be as effective and less toxic than amphotericin B in the treatment of candidemia in patients without neutropenia [23]. Secondly, major developments in new modalities of administering amphotericin B are under way, e.g. liposomes or other lipid vehicles. Current preliminary data are very encouraging and several preparations are already commercially available in some countries. An improved therapeutic toxic ratio is strongly suggested in humans but trial evidence is needed to establish the definite role and indications of the various preparations [24]. Thirdly, sensitive and specific tests for the diagnosis of invasive mycosis and fungal febrile episodes may well be available soon and this should reduce the need for empirical amphotericin B treatment [25].

## 8.5 LEAD NEPHROPATHY

### 8.5.1 Pathophysiology

Lead concentrates in kidney, bone, teeth and hair within an hour after absorption from the gut. Acute administration of lead results in excretion by glomerular filtration and tubular secretion. In patients intoxicated with lead, the fraction of uric acid reabsorption is disproportionately high for the degree of renal failure. Complex toxic interaction of lead occurs with trace elements such as cadmium, zinc, copper, silicium and arsenic. Lead can also induce immunologic abnormalities in mice. This raises the possibility that the kidney also could be injured by immune mechanisms after chronic low-level lead exposure. The sources of lead are numerous and may be both occupational and non-occupational (for instance, battery burning, ceramics making, cooking in leaden pots, ingesting contaminated herbal medicines, etc.) [26].

### 8.5.2 Clinical features

Typically, renal failure is evident only after years of excessive lead absorption and is frequently associated with hypertension. Fifty per cent of the patients suffer from gout. As gout is unusual in renal failure, when both conditions occur together and neither intratubular uric acid deposition nor stone diseases are present, lead nephropathy should be suspected [27]. Urinary protein excretion is usually low ($\leqslant 1\,g/24\,h$).

Histopathology shows a relatively acellular tubulo-interstitial nephritis without intranuclear inclusion bodies if there is no current exposure to lead. The appearance of arterial nephrosclerotic lesions before hypertension develops suggests that the primary injury from lead is in the microvascular endothelium.

### 8.5.3 Diagnosis

Diagnosing lead nephropathy is difficult because symptoms of lead intoxication are variable and non-specific. Occupational or environmental lead exposure should be carefully looked for. An elevated blood lead level correlates best with recent exposure but a normal value does not exclude a remote exposure with an increased body burden.

An ethylene diamino tetra-acetic acid (EDTA) lead mobilization test can establish excessive body stores; since renal failure reduces the rate of lead chelate excretion urine collections should be extended to three or four days after the administration of EDTA. The degree of renal failure that precludes reliance on the lead mobilization test has not been precisely determined but the chelation test is probably inappropriate when serum creatinine exceeds 700 μmol/l. Urinary lead excretion after EDTA in excess of 650 μg per day (or per four days in patients with renal failure) strongly suggests an excessive lead load. This demonstration, together with a history of progressive renal disease and uniformly contracted kidneys, still remain the most satisfactory diagnostic criteria, in the absence of other known causes of nephropathy [27].

### 8.5.4 Management and prevention

Treatment of excessive lead absorption depends on the total amount of lead in the body, the rate of absorption, the age of the patient and the degree of organ dysfunction. The value of chelation therapy in chronic tubulo-interstitial nephritis caused by chronic moderate lead absorption is doubtful; obviously one should not expect much improvement in established interstitial fibrosis. The effectiveness of chelation therapy can be monitored by repeated chelation testing.

Low-level lead absorption should be minimized by environmental control. Leaded gasoline was considered to contribute to 60% of lead emission in the Federal Republic of Germany in 1984 and an inquiry of the European Community came to the conclusion that approximately 25% of blood lead concentration was accounted for by exposure to gasoline lead aerosols. The potential beneficial effect of the increasing use of lead-free gasoline is thus awaited with interest.

This may be of particular interest as Staessen *et al.* [28] recently showed that in a random Belgian population sample of 965 men and 1016 women the creatinine clearance rate was inversely correlated with blood lead and zinc protoporphyrin values both before and after adjustments for body mass index and diuretic treatment. A ten-fold increase in blood lead concentration was associated with a reduction of 10 to 13 ml/min in creatinine clearance. Low-level exposure to lead may thus contribute to impairment of renal function in the general population, although the converse hypothesis that renal impairment may lead to an increase in the blood lead concentration cannot be dismissed.

## 8.6 CADMIUM NEPHROPATHY

The association between kidney disease and cadmium was first noted at the end of the 19th century but the characteristic low-molecular-weight proteinuria and osteomalacia were only recognized in the 1940s. Moreover, uncertainty persisted as to whether the nephropathy was the result of concomitant nephrolithiasis or lead nephropathy, so that it is only recently that cadmium has been identified as a definite, independent cause of nephropathy.

### 8.6.1 Epidemiology

Cadmium is widely used in the manufacture of plastics, pigments, glass and electrical equipment. The heaviest exposure occurs in smelting, electroplating and welding operations. Recent data have again emphasized that cadmium exposure may be both occupational and non-occupational, for example, in residents of areas with zinc smelters in the past in Belgium. Cadmium in the soil of such areas was positively correlated with cadmium in some vegetables, e.g. celery or beans, and in the residents' urine [29].

### 8.6.2 Metabolism

Absorption occurs primarily by inhalation and cadmium is subsequently transported to the liver bound to albumin. A carrier protein, metallothioneine, is synthesized within 24 hours and the cadmium–thioneine complex is released from the liver and filtered in the glomerulus. It is subsequently reabsorbed by proximal tubules and transferred to lysosomes. The catabolism of the complex with the release of unbound cadmium into the cytoplasm probably contributes to the proximal tubule injury. Once concentrated in the kidneys, cadmium has a half-life exceeding 10 to 20 years [29].

### 8.6.3 Clinical features

Proteinuria is usually less than 1 g/day. Low-molecular-weight proteinuria, aminoaciduria, renal glucosuria, hypercalciuria and increased urinary excretion of cadmium are observed in people exposed to cadmium. Low-molecular-weight proteinuria is, of course, not specific for cadmium nephropathy but is a useful index of early cadmium nephrotoxicity when other causes of renal dysfunction have been excluded. Osteomalacia with pseudofractures and severe bone pain was the major clinical manifestation of environmental cadmium intoxication in Japan after the Second World War. This arose from consumption of rice contaminated by cadmium. Mean serum creatinine increased from 1.19 to 1.68 mg/dl in 21 individuals followed for nine to 14 years after tubular proteinuria had been detected.

A longitudinal study of occupational cadmium nephropathy by Roels *et al.* [30] provides further evidence that clinical renal disease may result from excessive occupational cadmium absorption and that low-molecular-weight proteinuria predicts the adverse outcome. Twenty-three male workers exposed to cadmium dust in a non-ferrous smelter up to five years previously were examined annually for five years. They had been selected for study because of low-molecular-weight proteinuria. Serum creatinine increased over five years from 1.2 to 1.5 mg/dl. The estimated reduction in GFR averaged 30 ml/min per 1.73 $m^2$, about five times the anticipated age-adjusted reduction for males over five years.

Urine cadmium concentrations in excess of 10 μg/l or 10 μg/g creatinine are considered indicative of nephrotoxicity. For screening purposes, a urine $\beta_2$-microglobulin concentration >200 μg/l should raise the suspicion of excessive cadmium absorption.

### 8.6.4 Management

Unfortunately, cadmium nephropathy cannot be reversed once tubulo-interstitial disease has progressed sufficiently to produce clinical renal failure. The disease may even progress when exposure has been terminated after the discovery of isolated low-molecular-weight proteinuria. Chelation therapy is ineffective.

## 8.7 URIC ACID NEPHROPATHY

Uric acid is the end product of purine catabolism in man, by oxidation of xanthine and hypo-xanthine, mainly by the liver. Renal handling of uric acid differs widely from species to species: the results of studies performed on experimental animals may thus not be applicable to man. Four different mechanisms have classically been postulated in renal handling of urate: glomerular filtration, reabsorption, tubular secretion and post-secretory reabsorption. A large number of physiological maneuvers, pathophysiological factors, toxins and drugs are known to affect the renal handling of urate.

### 8.7.1 Renal failure as a complication of gout?

In the 1960s Gonick *et al.* described intratubular crystal deposition in the medullary interstitium, frequently surrounded by an inflammatory reaction, in patients with gout and renal failure. This was interpreted as a specific renal lesion in gout. Subsequently, however, urate deposits were found in the interstitium in many patients with renal failure without a history of gout, together with nephro-angiosclerosis, glomerular sclerosis and interstitial fibrosis, non-specific lesions probably linked to the associated hypertension, obesity, diabetes mellitus and arteriosclerosis. Yu and Berger [31] have longitudinally studied a large cohort of patients with gout: in patients without other disorders renal function remains stable or decreases 'normally' (as a function of age, over a period of more than twenty years). Uric acid lowering therapy, did not alter the evolution of kidney function. In gouty patients with other associated disorders, deterioration of renal function was linked to coexistent hypertension, ischaemic heart disease or pre-existing renal insufficiency. Similarly, Rosenfeld followed eighty patients with creatinine clearance between 40 and 18 ml/min and elevated serum uric acid. The patients were stratified according to the presence or absence of hypertension and the patients in each group were randomly allocated to a control group or a group treated with allopurinol to effectively lower serum uric acid. After more than 30 months' follow-up, no difference in the rate of change of renal function was observed, despite effective lowering of serum uric acid by allopurinol in the treated group. Similar results have been reported by other groups. Thus present evidence does not suggest that hyperuricemia is an important factor in the onset or progression of renal failure; the treatment of asymptomatic hyperuricemia is thus not indicated, at least to preserve renal function, and a requiem for gouty nephropathy has been proposed [32].

A small subgroup of patients with hyperuricemia, gout and renal failure deserves special emphasis. Since the first report by Duncan and Dixon [33] in 1960, several kindreds have been identified with the combination of hyperuricemia and gout, usually presenting at an early age in both sexes, a syndrome referred to as 'familial juvenile hyperuricemic nephropathy'. Hyperuricemia and/or gout were associated with progressive renal failure, with an autosomal dominant pattern, although in a few kindreds the disease was manifest only in women. As reports documented prolonged hyperuricemia and/or low-fractional urate excretion before signs of renal disease or renal failure, the hypothesis was raised that hyperuricemia may be the cause of renal failure. However, specimens of kidney tissue in such kindreds have usually failed to demonstrate urate crystals.

Recent reports from Guy's Hospital [34, 35] have suggested that early allopurinol therapy may contribute to the preservation of renal function, but reports from other groups have shown that allopurinol perhaps slowed but did not fully prevent progression of renal failure, though it effectively prevented gout [36].

Of importance, the dosage of allopurinol should be carefully titrated as GFR declines, thereby reducing renal excretion of oxypurinol, the main metabolite of the drug.

Overall, the absence of crystals in the renal tissue coupled with the failure to halt progression with the control of hyperuricemia suggests that in this autosomal dominant renal disease hyperuricemia and/or gout are only sensitive early indicators of renal involvement by an as yet unknown hereditary defect. Further progress in this field awaits the identification by linkage analysis of one or more candidate's loci for this disease.

## 8.8 LITHIUM NEPHROPATHY

In 1859, the British physician Garrod first proposed lithium in the treatment of mood disorders. In the last forty years, the place of lithium in psychiatric practice has been well established, so that nowadays about 0.1% of the populations of western countries is at any one time on lithium prophylaxis (see also Chapter 12).

### 8.8.1 Pathophysiology and clinical features

Lithium is not bound to plasma proteins and freely filtered by glomeruli like other ions, the kidney being its almost exclusive route of excretion. Normally the clearance of lithium is approximately 25% of the GFR. Lithium is reabsorbed in the proximal tubule in a proportion of the GFR comparable to that of sodium and water, but is neither reabsorbed nor secreted in the distal nephron. Hypovolemia increases the proximal reabsorption of sodium, water and lithium, thus decreasing lithium clearance.

Polyuria and polydipsia were recognized in the 1970s as frequent (up to 40% of treated patients) consequences of lithium therapy. The precise site of lithium inhibition of the action of vasopressin remains incompletely defined but is likely to be at the level of vasopressin-sensitive adenyl cyclase activity. Interestingly, Marples *et al.* [37] have recently demonstrated a profound downregulation of Aquaporin-2 (AQP-2) expression in lithium-fed rats, coincident with severe polyuria, both partly reversible after one week on a lithium-free diet. AQP-2 is probably the predominant vasopressin-sensitive water channel of the renal collecting duct [1]. It is, of course, tempting to speculate that this AQP-2 downregulation is causally related to the lithium-induced diabetes insipidus.

Lithium-induced impairment of distal urinary acidification was also described during the 1970s: as fractional excretion of bicarbonate at normal plasma bicarbonate values was very low and excretion of phosphate and ammonia was normal, incomplete distal renal tubular acidosis was diagnosed by exclusion.

Much more worrying was the lack of reversibility of the urinary concentrating ability after lithium discontinuation. Hestbeck *et al.* [38] reported in 1977 a correlation between impaired urinary-concentrating ability and the duration of lithium therapy. Boton *et al.* reviewed in 1987 twenty studies of patients treated with lithium (over 1500 patients in total) of whom up to 87% had impaired urinary-concentrating ability with, in more than half of the studies, a correlation between impaired ability and duration of lithium therapy or total lithium dose [39]. A similar progressive defect in distal renal tubular acidification was identified.

Cross-sectional studies evaluating the influence of lithium administration on GFR have suffered from various limitations, including inappropriate control groups and poor methods of measurement of GFR. Overall, Boton *et al.* estimated that 15% of patients on maintenance lithium had a significantly reduced GFR. Still very few of them have a GFR below 55 ml/min/1.73 $m^2$ [39]. Most studies do not find a relationship between the duration of lithium therapy and impaired GFR. Prospective studies similarly failed to show a declining GFR in patients on stable lithium, in the absence of acute lithium intoxication.

The differential diagnosis of polyuria and polydipsia in patients with psychiatric disorders includes, in addition to lithium therapy, mainly psychogenic polydipsia.

### 8.8.2 Pathology

Hestbeck *et al.* [37] described interstitial fibrosis, tubular atrophy and glomerular sclerosis in 13 of 14 patients on lithium therapy for more than one year. Several other cross-sectional studies subsequently reported similar findings in lithium-treated patients. However, all these studies lacked an appropriate control group and more recently the specificity of the chronic tubulo-interstitial changes attributed to lithium has been questioned: psychiatric patients without previous lithium therapy showed similar changes on renal biopsy; more specific features include distal tubular dilation and microcyst formation, probably due to the proliferation of distal tubular cells [40].

### 8.8.3 Prevention and management

Annual measurement of 24 hour urinary volume and creatinine clearance is indicated in patients on lithium therapy. More importantly, patients on lithium should be provided with information about precautions: a low threshold for contacting a physician, if unusual symptoms or signs develop; the avoidance of acute lithium intoxication is the single most useful way to preserve GFR. In particular extra-renal (diarrhea, vomiting, febrile illness) or renal losses of salt and water may precipitate lithium intoxication. Similarly the potential harmful effects of drug interactions must be emphasized. Many non-steroidal anti-inflammatory drugs, especially indomethacin, ibuprofen and naproxen, increase serum lithium levels and may precipitate toxicity. Sulindac and aspirin appear relatively safer [41]. Similarly, several case reports have strongly suggested an interaction between angiotensin-converting enzyme (ACE) inhibitors and lithium, resulting in lithium toxicity [42]. Thus careful monitoring of renal function and serum lithium levels is mandatory whenever such drugs are introduced in patients on lithium therapy, especially if they have other risk factors like old age, diuretic therapy, chronic renal or cardiac disease.

Although thiazide diuretics are effective in controlling lithium-induced polyuria, they should be avoided as they encompass the risk of increased lithium reabsorption and subsequent intoxication. Amiloride, a potassium-sparing diuretic, appears much safer and may be at least partially effective [43].

Finally, as several studies noted a correlation between trough serum lithium concentration and 24 hour urine volume, a once-daily schedule has been advocated, whenever possible, to achieve the lowest possible trough serum lithium level. The risk of discontinuation of maintenance lithium therapy in patient with severe psychiatric disorders should be considered in relation to the small risk of significant chronic renal damage.

## 8.9 BALKAN ENDEMIC NEPHROPATHY

Balkan endemic nephropathy (BEN) is a familial chronic tubulo-interstitial disease confined to parts of the former Yugoslavia, Bulgaria and Romania, first described in the mid-1950s. The disease occurs along the tributaries of the Danube, in the plains and low hills at an altitude of 150 to 500 m above sea level in a region of high humidity and high rainfall.

### 8.9.1 Epidemiology

Between 30 and 50 years of age the disease becomes clinically overt, requiring replacement therapy in the sixth decade, with a slight female predominance. An occupational history of farming is common. The disease develops only in the inhabitants of affected villages. The familial character of the disease is striking. Within the affected villages, there are many unaffected households living in close relationship to affected families.

### 8.9.2 Etiology and pathology

Etiology remains unknown [44]. Numerous investigations have been conducted into the possible role of trace elements (lead, cadmium and silica), bacteria and viruses, fungal and plant toxins, genetic factors and immune mechanisms.

Of particular interest is the potential role of ochratoxin A and aristolochic acid. Ochratoxin A is a mycotoxin contaminating plant products. A feed-related chronic renal disease in pigs, porcine nephropathy, has been linked to ochratoxin A. This disease resembles Balkan nephropathy, suggesting a common cause. The available evidence incriminating ochratoxin A in BEN remains inconclusive but compatible with an etiological role for this toxin. Similarly aristolochic acid, a known nephrotoxin, has been incriminated but few studies are available as yet on its role. Extensive studies on the role of fungal and plant toxins in the etiology of BEN are needed, especially in view of the likely role of aristolochic acid as the cause of Chinese herbs nephropathy: the two conditions share many characteristics (see Section 8.10).

Marked focal and segmental atrophy is observed with rather severe hyperplastic intimal changes and narrowing of blood vessels. Glomerular lesions are usually mild and focal and probably secondary to the tubulo-interstitial lesions. Fluorescence microscopy is not contributive.

### 8.9.3 Clinical characteristics

The onset is insidious with slowly progressive renal failure. Anemia, usually of the normocytic, normochromic and non-regenerative type, is a constant feature and can be demonstrated in the early stages. Urinary tract infection is uncommon whereas nocturia due to the decreased concentrating capacity of the kidneys is the rule. Hypertension is either absent or mild. Kidneys are small with a smooth outline. Proteinuria is mild and mainly of tubular origin, $\beta_2$-microglobulinuria preceding clinical disease by decades. Other renal functional changes characteristic of tubular disease are observed: impaired urinary acidification, impaired concentrating capacity, etc.

The urinary sediment is usually unremarkable with a few red and/or white blood cells per high power field. Macroscopic hematuria should prompt the search for urothelial tumors, whose prevalence is high in patients with BEN.

As the etiology of BEN remains unknown, effective prevention is currently impossible. Treatment remains supportive. Patients at risk should be carefully screened for the development of urinary tract tumors. Patients with ESRD may be treated by dialysis and kidney transplantation, without recurrence in the graft.

## 8.10 CHINESE HERBS NEPHROPATHY

In 1993, rapidly progressive interstitial renal fibrosis was reported in nine young women who all had attended the same slimming clinic in Brussels. This newly described nephropathy, the so-called Chinese herbs nephropathy (CHN), was quickly ascribed to the Chinese herbs *Stephania tetrandra* and *Magnolia officinalis* taken as part of the slimming regimen, and is now known to affect over eighty women [45].

### 8.10.1 Clinical picture

Virtually all affected patients are women, aged 23–65 years. This probably reflects the predominant female attendance of this slimming clinic. Hypertension usually develops only in the later stages of the disease. Anemia is unusually severe for the degree of renal failure. Proteinuria is mild and of tubular origin. The renal failure is frequently discovered only by routine blood testing. Even after termination of the offending treatment, renal failure frequently progresses relentlessly, leading to ESRD within a few months to years [45–47].

### 8.10.2 Pathology

Cosyns *et al.* [42] examined four nephro-ureterectomy specimens obtained from three patients prior to or at the time of transplantation for CHN. They observed extensive hypocellular interstitial sclerosis, tubular atrophy and global sclerosis of glomeruli, decreasing from the outer to the inner cortex, including the columns of Bertin, together with irregular thickening of interlobular and afferent arterioles. In addition atypical urothelial cells were observed in all three cases. Fibrosis may further extend beyond the kidneys, as demonstrated by intense periureteral fibrosis in one patient, submesothelial fibrosis in two patients and further suggested by the observation of aortic insufficiency in up to a third of patients with CHN [45].

### 8.10.3 Etiology

The unusual, subacute course of the disease in patients who had all followed the same slimming regimen suggested a common, toxic etiology. The possibility of adulteration of the slimming regimen by known toxic compounds was excluded [46]. As the Chinese herbs were prescribed from 1990 onward, whereas the previous slimming regimen from the same clinic appeared innocuous for up to fifteen years, these Chinese herbs were incriminated. Interestingly, the alkaloid derived from *Stephania tetrandra* (Fangji) could not be identified suggesting that this herb might have been replaced by another more toxic herb. Subsequently the presence of *Aristolochia fangchi* was demonstrated in batches of Chinese herbs imported in Belgium [45]. Aristolochic acid thus appears to be the potential offending drug: it is known to be nephrotoxic and mutagenic. Still, as the same Chinese herbs, originating from batches imported at the same time, have been utilized by other slimming clinics in Belgium without apparent untoward effects, an interaction between Chinese herbs and other compounds included in the slimming cure is a distinct possibility.

### 8.10.4 Management

As soon as the toxicity of the slimming regimen was recognized, its prescription was stopped. Unfortunately, even after discontinuation of the toxic agents, CHN usually runs a relentless course. In an attempt to prevent this, Vanherweghem *et al.* [46] tried steroid therapy in 12 cases with biopsy-proven CHN and a serum creatinine ranging from 1.8 to 3.7 (average: 2.8 mg/dl) at the time of steroid therapy. A control group of 12 female patients was selected on the basis of biopsy-proven CHN, similar serum creatinine levels at the onset of follow-up and no steroid therapy. After twelve months' steroids (1 mg/kg for one month tapered by 0.1 mg/kg per fortnight) serum creatinine was significantly lower in treated ($4 \pm 0.7$) than untreated ($7.1 \pm 0.8$) patients. This steroid regimen had however substantial side effects and did not fully prevent the progression of renal failure. This apparent steroid sensitivity of CHN suggests that the renal fibrosis may be at least partly immune-mediated.

All patients with Chinese herbs nephropathy will need, in addition, careful follow-up for the development of urothelial malignancy, already diagnosed in three of them, as in analgesic and Balkan endemic nephropathies, and for valvular disease.

## 8.11 CONCLUSIONS

From the review of this large range of interstitial, toxic and metabolic nephropathies, several guidelines emerge for the prevention of the onset and progression of such diseases. These include avoiding or discontinuing potentially toxic agents whenever possible (e.g. analgesics, lithium, cyclosporin A, etc.), choosing an alternative less toxic treatment (e.g. for amphotericin B), careful monitoring if the nephrotoxic treatment is deemed absolutely necessary (e.g. lithium, cyclosporin A, cisplatin), avoiding dehydration (analgesics, cisplatin, amphotericin B) and drug interactions (lithium, cyclosporin A), avoiding unorthodox medicine (CHN), and finally adequate legislative and environmental measures to prevent avoidable toxicities such as those derived from analgesics, lead, cadmium and Chinese herbs.

## REFERENCES


1. Sandler, D.P., Smith, J.C., Weinberg, C.R. *et al.* (1989) Analgesic use and chronic renal disease. *N. Engl. J. Med.*, **320**, 1241–3.
2. Perneger, T.V., Whelton, P.K. and Klag, M.J. (1994) Risk of kidney failure associated with the use of acetaminophen, aspirin and nonsteroidal antiinflammatory drugs. *N. Engl. J. Med.*, **331**, 1675–9.
3. Murray, T.G., Stolley, P.D., Anthony, J.C. *et al.* (1983) Epidemiologic study of regular analgesic use and end-stage renal disease. *Arch. Intern. Med.*, **143**, 1687–93.
4. Dubach, U.C., Rosner, B. and Sturmer, T. (1991) Effects of phenacetin and salicylate on mortality and cardiovascular morbidity. *N. Engl. J. Med.*, **324**, 155–60.
5. Nanra, R.S. (1993) Analgesic nephropathy in the 1990s – an Australian perspective. *Kidney Int.*, **42**, S86–S92.
6. Elseviers, M.M. and De Broe, M.E. (1994) Analgesic nephropathy in Belgium is related to the sales of particular analgesic mixtures. *Nephrol. Dial. Transplant.*, **9**, 41–6.
7. Brunner, F.P. and Selwood, N.H. (1994) End-stage renal failure due to analgesic nephropathy, its changing pattern and cardiovascular mortality. *Nephrol. Dial. Transplant.*, **9**, 1371–6.
8. Elseviers, M.M., Bosteels, V., Cambier, P. *et al.* (1992) Diagnostic criteria of analgesic nephropathy in patients with end-stage renal failure: results of the Belgian study. *Nephrol. Dial. Transplant.*, **7**, 479–86.
9. Elseviers, M.M., Waller, I., Nenov, D. *et al.* (1995) Evaluation of diagnostic criteria for analgesic nephropathy in patients with end-stage renal failure: results of the ANNE study. *Nephrol. Dial. Transplant.*, **10**, 808–14.
10. Hauser, A.C., Derfler, K. and Balcke, P. (1991) Progression of renal insufficiency in analgesic nephropathy: impact of continuous drug abuse. *J. Clin. Epidemiol.*, **44**, 53–6.
11. Anand, A.J. and Bashey B. (1993) Newer insights into cisplatin nephrotoxicity. *Ann. Pharmacotherapy*, **27**, 1519–25.
12. Cornelison, T.L. and Reed, E. (1993) Nephrotoxicity and hydration management for cisplatin, carboplatin and ormaplatin. *Gynecol. Oncol.*, **50**, 147–58.
13. Narins, R.G., Carley, M., Bloom, E.J. and Harrison, D.S. (1990) The nephrotoxicity of chemotherapeutic agents. *Semin. Nephrol.*, **10**, 556–64.
14. Berns, J.S., Haghighat, A., Staddon, A. *et al.* (1995) Severe, irreversible renal failure after ifosfamide treatment. *Cancer*, **76**, 497–500.
15. Myers, B.D., Sibley, R., Newton, L. *et al.* (1988) The long-term course of cyclosporine-associated chronic nephropathy. *Kidney Int.*, **33**, 590–600.
16. Gonwa, T.A., Mai, M.L., Pilcher, J. *et al.* (1992) Stability of long-term renal function in heart transplant patients treated with induction therapy and low-dose cyclosporine. *J. Heart Lung Transplant*, **11**, 926–8.
17. Burke, J.F., Pirsch, J.D., Ramos, E.L. *et al.* (1994) Long-term efficacy and safety of cyclosporine in renal-transplant recipients. *N. Engl. J. Med.*, **331**, 358–63.
18. Young, E.W., Ellis, C.N., Messana, J.M. *et al.* (1994) A prospective study of renal structure and function in psoriasis patients treated with cyclosporin. *Kidney Int.*, **46**, 1216–22.
19. Pei, Y., Scholey, J.W., Katz, A. *et al.* (1994) Chronic nephrotoxicity in psoriatic patients treated with low-dose cyclosporine. *Am. J. Kidney Dis.*, **23**, 528–36.

20. Feutren, G. and Mihatasch, M.J. (1992) Risk factors for cyclosporine-induced nephropathy in patients with autoimmune diseases. *N. Engl. J. Med.*, **326**, 1654–60.
21. Hunley, T.E., Fogo, A., Iwasaki, S. and Kon, V. (1995) Endothelin A receptor mediated functional but not structural damage in chronic cyclosporine nephrotoxicity. *J. Am. Soc. Newphrol.*, **5**, 1718–23.
22. LLanos, A., Cieza, J., Bernando, J. *et al.* (1991) Effect of salt supplementation on amphotericin B nephrotoxicity. *Kidney Int.*, **40**, 302–8.
23. Rex, J.H., Bennett, J.E., Sugar, A.M. *et al.* (1994) A randomized trial comparing fluconazole with amphotericin B for the treatment of candidemia in patients without neutropenia. *N. Engl. J. Med.*, **331**, 1325–30.
24. Meunier, F. (1994) Alternative modalities of administering amphotericin B: current issues. *J. Infect.*, **28**, 51–6.
25. Obayashi, T., Yoshida, M., Mori, T. *et al.* (1995) Plasma (1→3)-$\beta$-D-glucan measurement in diagnosis of invasive deep mycosis and fungal febrile episodes. *Lancet*, **345**, 17–20.
26. Ritz, E., Mann, J. and Stoeppler, M. (1988) Lead and the kidney. *Adv. Nephrol.*, **17**, 241–74.
27. Bennett, W.M. (1985) Lead nephropathy. *Kidney Int.*, **28**, 212–20.
28. Staessen, J.A., Lauwerys, R.R., Buchet, J.P. *et al.* and the cadmibel study group (1992) Impairment of renal function with increasing blood lead concentrations in the general population. *N. Engl. J. Med.*, **327**, 151–6.
29. Staessen, J.A., Lauwerys, R.R., Ide, G. *et al.* (1994) Renal function and historical environmental cadmium pollution from zinc smelters. *Lancet*, **343**, 1523–7.
30. Roels, H., Lauwerys, R.R., Buchet, J.P. *et al.* (1989) Health significance of cadmium induced renal dysfunction. *Br. J. Ind. Med.*, **46**, 755–64.
31. Yu, T. and Berger, L. (1982) Impaired renal function in gout. *Am. J. Med.*, **72**, 95–100.
32. Beck, L.H. (1986) Requiem for gouty nephropathy. *Kidney Int.*, **30**, 280–7.
33. Duncan, H. and Dixon, A.S. (1960) Gout familial hyperuricaemia, and renal disease. *Q. J. Med.*, **29**, 127–35.
34. Simmonds, H.A., Warren, D.J., Cameron, J.S. *et al.* (1980) Familial gout and renal failure in young women. *Clin. Nephrol.*, **14**, 176–82.
35. Moro, F., Ogg, C.S., Simmonds, H.A. *et al.* (1991) Familial juvenile gouty nephropathy with renal urate hypoexcretion preceding renal disease. *Clin. Nephrol.*, **35**, 263–9.
36. Yokota, N., Yamanaka, H., Yamamoto, Y. *et al.* (1991) Autosomial dominant transmission of gouty arthritis with renal disease in a large Japanese family. *Ann. Rheum. Dis.*, **50**, 108–111.
37. Marples, D., Christensen, S., Christensen, E.I. *et al.* (1995) Lithium-induced downregulation of aquaporin-2 water channel expression in rat kidney medulla. *J. Clin. Invest.*, **95**, 1838–45.
38. Hestbech, J., Hansen, H.E., Amdisen, A. and Olsen, S. (1977) Chronic renal lesions following long-term treatment with lithium. *Kidney Int.*, **12**, 205–13.
39. Boton, R., Gaviria, M. and Batlle, D.C. (1987) Prevalence, pathogenesis and treatment of renal dysfunction associated with chronic lithium therapy. *Am. J. Kidney Dis.*, **10**, 329–45.
40. Walker, R.G. (1993) Lithium nephrotoxicity. *Kidney Int.*, **44**, S93–S98.
41. Ragheb, M. (1990) The clinical significance of lithium-nonsteroidal anti-inflammatory drug interactions. *J. Clin. Psychopharmacol.*, **10**, 350–4.

42. Lehmann, K. and Ritz, E. (1995) Angiotensin-converting enzyme inhibitors may cause renal dysfunction in patients on long-term lithium treatment. *Am. J. Kidney Dis.*, **25**, 82–7.
43. Batlle, D.C., Von Riotte, A.B., Gaviria, M. and Grupp, M. (1985) Amelioration of polyuria by amiloride in patients receiving long-term lithium therapy. *N. Engl. J. Med.*, **312**, 408–14.
44. Hall, P.W. (1992) Balkan endemic nephropathy: more questions than answers. *Nephron.*, **62**, 1–5.
45. Van Ypersele De Strihou, C. and Vanherweghem, J.L. (1995) The tragic paradigm of Chinese herbs nephropathy. *Nephrol. Dial. Transplant.*, **10**, 157–60.
46. Vanherweghem, J.L., Depierreux, M., Tielemans, C. *et al.* (1993) Rapidly progressive interstitial renal fibrosis in young women: association with slimming regimen including Chinese herbs. *Lancet*, **341**, 387–391.
47. Cosyns, J.P., Jadoul, M., Squifflet, J.P. *et al.* (1994) Chinese herbs nephropathy: a clue to Balkan endemic nephropathy? *Kidney Int.*, **45**, 1680–8.

# 9

# Lipids and renal disease

*J.F. Moorhead, C. Brunton and Z. Varghese*

## 9.1 INTRODUCTION

Abnormalities of lipid metabolism are nearly always present in renal disease. Characteristic patterns of abnormality occur in the nephrotic syndrome, end stage renal failure (ESRF), dialysis and transplantation, and many patients with progressive renal disease suffer each in turn as they experience each phase. In addition a high proportion of renal patients die from atherosclerotic cardiovascular events. Unsurprisingly, more attention has been accorded to these phenomena in recent times. Most studies of risk factors in renal failure have emphasized cardiovascular and cerebrovascular disease since these have proved to the major causes of death in dialysis and transplant patients. Severe arterial disease, to which atherosclerosis makes an important contribution, is common by the time patients reach dialysis, so it is inevitable that this should have received attention in hyperlipidaemic states such as the nephrotic syndrome. Excluding immunological diseases and vasculitides, the largest patient groups with progressive kidney disease are patients with hypertension and/or diabetes, and the strongest clinical associations with progression are proteinuria [1] and hypercholesterolaemia. Since diabetic patients form an increasing proportion of renal failure populations, management of atherosclerotic major vascular disease is of increasing importance.

The need to devise treatments for the syndrome of progressive renal disease (PRD), conventionally characterized in terms of gradual and inexorable loss of glomerular filtration rate (GFR), has focused some

*Renal Disease.* Edited by G. Venkat Raman. Published in 1998 by Chapman & Hall, London. ISBN 0 412 45700 8.

interest on the possibility that the nephron might be directly damaged by lipoproteins in nephrotic hyperlipidaemic patients. Whatever the cause, PRD leads to end stage renal failure (ESRF) and has therefore become an increasingly important economic and scientific challenge. Quite apart from the role of the lipids in PRD, there is an overwhelming need to address the cardiovascular risk in these patients.

## 9.2 PATHOPHYSIOLOGY AND PATHOGENESIS

The syndrome of PRD includes some or all of the following: hypertension, derangement of calcium and phosphate metabolism, abnormalities of renal endocrine functions giving rise to renal osteodystrophy and erythropoietin deficiency anaemia. Abnormalities of renal tubular function and responses are common. In addition, abnormal lipid metabolism is a systemic complication of renal disease which has not been shown to be due to intrinsic renal physiological dysfunction, but rather a consequence of renal diseases. Hyperlipidaemia is most readily recognized in the hypercholesterolaemia of the nephrotic syndrome and after renal transplantation, and in the hypertriglyceridaemia of haemodialysis patients. In animals substantial experimental evidence supports a concept of lipoprotein-mediated exacerbation of renal disease, and the severity and ubiquity of lipid abnormalities in renal diseases pose important therapeutic and research questions in their own right.

In a substantial proportion of patients the time of onset and cause of the original renal disease are unknown, and many patients present for the first time with significantly impaired renal function or advanced renal failure. At the clinical level, other systemic diseases such as hypertension and diabetes contribute to individual patients' declining renal function, and careful control of these may slow progression. At the cellular and molecular level many contributory factors still remain to be identified and related to different stages of PRD. Thus far no useful therapeutic tools have been fashioned from the research effort devoted to these latter factors. The scope of intervention is limited to the diligent clinical control of known risk factors, rather than the biological events which produce them. Within the spectrum of renal diseases, the cellular and molecular interactions of lipoproteins could vary with their concentration, composition and post-secretory modifications.

A clearer understanding of lipoprotein metabolism followed the work of Brown and Goldstein. Of particular interest to nephrology was the observation that smooth muscle cell proliferated [2] and became foam cells [3]. This led us to surmise that the mesangial cell, which has smooth muscle characteristics, would behave much as arterial smooth muscle, provided lipoproteins could gain access to it, and that (as in atherosclerosis) inflammatory cells would be attracted to the site. Progressive glomerular disease would result, the end result being 'glomerular atherosclerosis'. It has long been known that apoprotein A (apo-A) passes the glomerular filter and that lipids are excreted directly into the urine. This excretion implies direct contact of lipids with renal tubular cells and it was suggested that this could mediate tubulo-interstitial disease. We argued that in nephrotic patients and animals, circulating excess lipoprotein would supersede the original disease as the main cause of persistent glomerular injury [4].

An aid to understanding this process in the context of progressive glomerular disease is that the original disease need not persist: lipid-mediated disease may be self-perpetuating. In support of a concept of initiating injury [5] there is only sparse evidence of lipoproteins causing renal disease. For example, it was recently suggested that a specific pattern of lipid abnormality, characterized by abnormal isoforms of apo-E, caused lipoprotein thrombi in glomeruli with renal failure [6], and Gjone and coworkers reported that congenital lecithin cholesterol acyl transferase (LCAT) deficiency was associated with progressive disease in some Norwegian families [7]. Apart from these examples however it seems most likely that lipoproteins damage previously injured glomerular structures.

The persistent proteinuria of many glomerular diseases acts as a (possibly indirect) stimulus to the synthesis of excess lipoprotein by the liver, so maintaining the vicious cycle. As nephrons are lost and serum albumin rises the few remaining nephrons may be exposed by hyperfiltration to proportionally more lipoprotein than before. Frequently systemic diseases with a renal component, e.g. systemic lupus erythematosus coexist with hyperlipoproteinaemia, thus adding to the complexity of contributory pathophysiological processes. In this review we shall examine some of the possible roles of lipoproteins in the pathogenesis of progressive renal disease, and the means by which their pathological effects may be reduced. Because lipid metabolism is complex it will be useful to briefly describe the major plasma lipids and indicate how they vary in renal diseases.

## 9.3 THE STRUCTURE AND FUNCTIONS OF LIPOPROTEINS

Plasma lipids comprise seven major classes of compounds: fatty acids, prostaglandins, glycerides, phospholipids, sphingolipids and steroids. These water-insoluble plasma lipids are transported in a family of complex particles known as lipoproteins, which are specifically structured for the emulsification of lipids in plasma. The non-polar lipids, cholesterol ester and triglycerides are confined to the lipoprotein core

**Table 9.1** Proteins and lipid concentrations of human lipoproteins (%W/W)

| Lipoproteins | Density | TG | FC | CE | PL | PROT | MW |
|---|---|---|---|---|---|---|---|
| Chylomicrons | < 0.95 | 85–90 | 1–3 | 2–4 | 8–10 | 2–4 | $0.4 \times 10^9$ |
| VLDL | 0.95–1.006 | 50–65 | 5–10 | 10–15 | 16–20 | 8–12 | $5–10 \times 10^6$ |
| IDL | 1.006–1.019 | 25–30 | 7–8 | 18–22 | 18–22 | 15–20 | $4–4.8 \times 10^6$ |
| LDL | 1.019–1.063 | 6–10 | 7–10 | 35–40 | 20–24 | 20–25 | $2.8 \times 10^6$ |
| Lp(a) | 1.070–1.107 | 4–9 | 6–10 | 26–38 | 22–24 | 26–36 | $3–8 \times 10^6$ |
| HDL2 | 1.063–1.125 | 4–6 | 5 | 12–18 | 25–30 | 42–45 | $3.6 \times 10^5$ |
| HDL3 | 1.125–1.210 | 3–5 | 3–4 | 10–12 | 22–25 | 50–55 | $1.8 \times 10^5$ |

TG = triglycerides.
FC = free cholesterol.
CE = cholesterol ester.
PL = phospholipids.
PROT = proteins.
MW = molecular weight.

which is surrounded by a monolayer of proteins (apoproteins) and more polar lipids, free cholesterol and phospholipids.

Lipoprotein classification, conventionally based on their density by ultracentrifugation techniques [8], has provided a useful basis for studying the physiological interactions and pathophysiology of these complex particles (Table 9.1). Centrifugation separates lipoproteins into chylomicrons, very low-density lipoproteins (VLDL), intermediate-density lipoproteins (IDL), low-density lipoproteins (LDL), lipoprotein(a) (Lp(a)), and high-density lipoproteins (HDL). This scheme is, however, an oversimplification because each lipoprotein class is heterogeneous, encompassing a continuum of particles of various sizes and densities. Lipoprotein particles are modified, enter and leave these compartments at many points along the density spectrum [9].

Lipid synthesis and assembly into lipoproteins, and the transport, storage and metabolism of lipoproteins are regulated by apoproteins (Table 9.2), lipid modifying enzymes, cholesterol ester transfer protein (CETP) and membrane receptors (Table 9.3). All regulatory mechanisms are potential sites for generating imbalances between synthesis and catabolism, thereby giving rise to a variety of dyslipidaemias. The genes for most apoproteins and membrane receptors have been isolated, sequenced and mapped in the human genome [10].

**Table 9.2** Apoproteins of plasma lipoproteins

| Apoprotein &I | Distribution | MW | Chromosomal localization | Function |
|---|---|---|---|---|
| AI | CM, HDL, VLDL | 28 000 | 11 | Structural component of HDL<br>LCAT activator |
| AII | HDL, CM, VLDL | 17 000 | 1 | ? |
| AIV | CM, VLDL, HDL | 44 500 | 11 | LCAT activator |
| B48 | CM | 264 000 | 2 | Structural component of CM |
| B100 | VLDL, IDL, LDL | 594 000 | 2 | Structural component of LDL<br>Ligand for LDL receptor |
| CI | VLDL, CM, IDL, HDL | 6600 | 19 | LCAT activator |
| CII | VDL, CM, HDL | 8900 | 19 | Activator of LPL |
| CIII | VLDL, CM, HDL | 8800 | 11 | Inhbitor of LPL |
| E | CM, VLDL, IDL, HDL | 34 000 | 19 | Ligand for LDL receptor |

**Table 9.3** Lipoprotein receptors

| Receptor | Major lipoprotein bound | Specificity | Present in |
|---|---|---|---|
| LDL | LDL, VLDL | Apo-B, Apo-E | Liver<br>Adrenals<br>Kidney<br>Macrophages<br>Fibroblasts<br>Mesangial cells |
| Scavenger | Modified LDL | Modified apo-B | Macrophages |
| Remnant | CM and VLDL remnants | Apo-E | Liver |
| LDL receptor-related protein (LRP) | Remnants | Apo-E, LPL<br>$\alpha_2$-Macroglobulin protease complexes | Liver |

### 9.3.1 Chylomicrons

Chylomicrons are, by virtue of their low-protein and high-fat content, the largest and 'lightest' of lipoproteins and are rich in triglycerides derived from food. Dietary lipids are hydrolysed in the small intestine by pancreatic lipases and the major components of this hydrolysis, fatty acids, monoglycerides and cholesterol, are taken up by the absorptive cells of the small intestine and incorporated into chylomicrons. The latter are secreted into the lymphatics and subsequently enter the circulation through the thoracic duct. They become emulsified through the addition of apo-B48, apo-AI, apo-AII and apo-AIV, then acquire apo-CI, -CII, -CIII and apo-E from HDL. They are available for early metabolism at the endothelial surface where 80% of triglycerides in chylomicrons are removed by the action of lipoprotein lipase (LPL). Apo-CII activates LPL and apo-CIII inhibits this enzyme. Some of their apoproteins, namely apo-AI and apo-AII, are transferred to HDLs during this delipidation process and the partially delipidated chylomicrons are known as chylomicron remnants. This progressive change in particle size seems to provide some benefit for its binding to apo-E receptors on hepatocytes and facilitates the delivery of dietary cholesterol to the liver. Apo-CIII may also have an inhibitory effect on the hepatic uptake of chylomicron remnants [11]. The chylomicron-mediated pathway represents exogenous lipoprotein metabolism. Both normal subjects and hypertriglyceridaemic patients have a post-prandial increase in triglycerides, reflecting transport of dietary fat as chylomicrons.

Increased concentrations of chylomicron remnants are frequently found in patients with renal failure, in particular in dialysis patients where their formation is related to the reduced activities of both LPL and hepatic lipase (HL) [12, 13]. In haemodialysis patients Nestel *et al.* [14] detected increased plasma concentrations of apo-B48 and apo-AIV, apolipoproteins normally associated with chylomicrons.

Hypertriglyceridaemia associated with CRF is usually moderate, but the atherogenic potential of chylomicron remnants is far greater than VLDL. Apo-E appears to be the principal ligand for both chylomicron and VLDL remnants, so chylomicron remnants devoid of apo-E are cleared very slowly from the circulation [14, 15].

A relationship between the apo-B/E receptor and the recently described LDL receptor-related protein (LRP) and its interaction with LPL in the removal of chylomicron remnants is just beginning to emerge. Chylomicron remnant binding to LRP requires apo-E and is inhibited by C apoproteins. LRP molecules have distinct binding sites for LPL and it seems that LPL may substitute for apo-E and mediate the binding of chylomicron remnants to LRP [16].

The degree to which LRP receptor-associated protein (RAP) regulates the binding characteristics of various ligands associated with LRP is not known, but RAP seems to have the ability to block the binding of remnants to LRP. Therefore, a deficiency of apo-E and LPL and an increase in RAP may be able to delay the clearance of chylomicron remnants from the circulation. Whether this phenomenon applies in renal failure is unknown, but severe chylomicronaemia may also occur in nephrotics [17, 18] possibly as a result of slower removal of chylomicron remnants.

### 9.3.2 Very low-density lipoproteins

Synthesis of triglyceride-rich VLDL occurs from endogenous sources. The site of this lipogenesis is the liver, where fatty acids are synthesized from glucose and acetate, a process which is regulated by changes in insulin and glucagon levels that occur with the feeding cycle. Fatty acids in the cytosol of the hepatocytes can either enter mitochondria for beta-oxidation or can remain in the cytosol where they are esterified into triglycerides. Insulin favours the synthesis of triglycerides and glucagon stimulates the mitochondrial oxidation of fatty acids [19,20]. However, whether or not insulin also increases the assembly and secretion of VLDL particles is unresolved.

Cholesterol and triglycerides are synthesized in the liver together with cholesterol ester, apo-B100, phospholipids and free cholesterol, then assembled in the endoplasmic reticulum of hepatocytes and secreted into hepatic venous outflow as VLDL. VLDL also carries apo-E, apo-CI, -CII and -CIII. The delipidation pathway of VLDL is similar to that of chylomicrons in that LPL on the endothelial surface converts VLDL to IDL, also known as VLDL remnants or LDL1. About 50% of IDL is removed directly by the liver and the remaining fraction is further delipidated by hepatic lipase and converted to LDL. During the delipidation process of VLDL, surface phospholipids and apoproteins other than apo-B100 are transferred to HDL as they are from chylomicrons. Cholesteryl ester, which is formed in the plasma as a result of the action of LCAT on the HDL particle, is transferred from HDL to VLDL and IDL through the mediation of CETP.

VLDL is a heterogeneous mixture of particles ranging from 25 to 70 nm in size; comparison of the kinetic disappearance of large and small particles revealed that the size is an important determinant of metabolic clearance. Large VLDL particles behave like chylomicrons and after partial delipidation, they are directly removed by a receptor-mediated mechanism. Thus carbohydrate feeding promotes the synthesis of large triglyceride-enriched VLDL particles which fail to be converted to LDL. In this situation, LDL levels will be low. On the other hand, a high cholesterol diet favours the assembly and secretion of smaller VLDL particles which will undergo delipidation to generate proportionately more LDL [21,22].

Hypertriglyceridaemia occurs in 20–70% of patients with CRF, reflecting increased VLDL triglyceride levels [23]. Infusion of glucose via dialysate fluid in both haemodialysis and peritoneal dialysis patients has the same effect as carbohydrate feeding in promoting the synthesis of large VLDL particles. This would facilitate the direct removal of VLDL via the apo-B/E receptor in the liver or through LRP without first being converted to LDL. In a small group of dialysis patients and normal controls, VLDL apo-B turnover studies have demonstrated normal IDL apoB fluxes in the context of raised VLDL apo-B fluxes in patients with raised VLDL. This again suggests direct hepatic removal of VLDL apo-B without its being converted to LDL [24]. This probably explains why hypercholesterolaemia is not so prevalent in haemodialysis patients.

Most studies support decreased triglyceride and VLDL removal as the cause of hypertriglyceridaemia in patients with renal failure [25, 26]. We have studied the rate of triglyceride clearance by administering intravenous lipid emulsion to dialysis patients and measuring the decrease in light scattering using nephelometry in serial samples as LPL digests the particles. The fractional removal rate of intralipid expressed as *K*2, the slope of the log-transformed light-scattering value over time, is reduced in uraemia in the presence or absence of intravenous heparin administration [27].

The structure and functional properties of LPL have been reviewed by Wang *et al.* [28]. It is an acylglycerol hydrolase, highly conserved in mammals and widely distributed on endothelium, which breaks down the triacylglycerol (TG) of TG-rich lipoproteins, chylomicrons and VLDL. It requires a cofactor, apo-CII, present in VLDL, chylomicrons and HDL. It is non-competitively inhibited at high concentration by apo-CIII; it has a heparin-binding domain which may explain heparin releasability during haemodialysis. In the nephrotic syndrome LPL activity may be deficient [29] possibly due to loss of a cofactor in nephrotic urine [30]. However a role for LPL in the pathogenesis of atherosclerosis was suggested by Zilversmit [31], and recently Saxena *et al.* reported that LPL increases LDL retention by subendothelial matrix [32]. Clearly LDL trapped by affinity to subentholelial matrix could be subject to oxidative modification, macrophage influx and foam cell formation.

### *Lipolytic activity in uraemia*

LPL plays an important role in the metabolism of VLDL. In uraemic patients this enzyme is decreased in adipose tissue [33] and there is evidence to suggest that the basis of defective triglyceride removal is decreased activity of this enzyme [12]. A significant impact was made on understanding lipid metabolism in dialysis patients by the observation that patients who were uraemic or on haemodialysis had fasting hypertriglyceridaemia and a decrease in post-heparin lipolytic activity [34]. Reduction in fat clearance after heparin was found to be related to plasma HDL, part of which activates LPL. Moreover, heparin inhibited LCAT, an important enzyme for cholesterol transport. These abnormalities in dialysis patients were partly explained by a low HDL cholesterol, high HDL triglyceride and lower fractional clearance rates of intravenous fat. These findings suggest that the severe abnormalities of fat metabolism present in both uraemic predialysis and haemodialysis patients may increase the risk of developing atheromatous vascular disease in this population.

Impairment of LPL activity may be due to a number of factors: decreased synthesis due to insulin resistance, decreased releasable pool of LPL due to repeated heparinization (in haemodialysis patients), decreased activator concentration (low apo-CII/apo-CIII ratio), or the presence of other LPL inhibitors [23]. A number of observations lend support to the idea that parathyroid hormone (PTH) is an inhibitor of LPL: type IV hyperlipidaemia is reported relatively frequently in patients with primary hyperparathyroidism [35], plasma triglyceride levels often fall precipitously after total parathyroidectomy in haemodialysis patients (Z. Varghese and J.F. Moorhead, personal observation) and Lacour *et al.* observed hypertriglyceridaemia in rats following PTH administration [36]. Parathyroidectomy in uraemic dogs normalized triglyceride levels, abnormal intravenous fat tolerance test and impaired post-heparin LPL activity [37].

An additional mechanism for the decreased catabolism of VLDL triglyceride is the reduced LCAT activity in uraemic patients. Usually, increased concentrations of VLDL and triglycerides stimulate LCAT activity. LCAT activity is further reduced by heparinization during haemodialysis [38]. A reduced LCAT activity may contribute to reduced VLDL catabolism by altering the cholesterol esterification rate in nascent HDL and HDL3. Thus, impaired catabolism of VLDL and reduced LCAT activity may provide an explanation for reduced HDL concentration in chronic renal failure (CRF) patients with hypertriglyceridaemia. This explanation seems plausible because treatment of chronic ambulatory peritoneal dialysis (CAPD) patients with gemfibrozil resulted in the normalization of LPL, HL, triglycerides and HDL [39].

Some studies also indicate increased synthesis of VLDL in CRF patients. Fasting hyperinsulinaemia, often seen in CRF, is thought to contribute to this overproduction. VLDL and its downstream product LDL are usually raised in nephrotic patients, probably as a result of a combination of overproduction and decreased removal [40, 41].

As indicated previously the degree of hypertriglyceridaemia is mild to moderate in CRF patients. However, the presence of atherogenic remnants derived from the partial degradation of VLDL triglycerides can be an important risk factor in promoting vascular disease. Joven *et al.* [42] have confirmed that the concentration of IDL is increased two to 10-fold in 14 out of the 15 nephrotic patients investigated. The elevation of IDL was independent of the usual association with diabetes or type III dyslipoproteinaemia. They also observed an increase in IDL in normotriglyceridaemic haemodialysis patients. Another feature of hypertriglyceridaemia in renal failure is triglyceride enrichment of VLDL, IDL and LDL. there is also a redistribution of cholesterol from HDL to IDL and VLDL even when the plasma level of cholesterol is within the normal range [43].

### 9.3.3 Low-density lipoproteins

In normal subjects LDL is the major lipoprotein fraction of fasting plasma. A single molecule of apo-B100 is the only apoprotein present in LDL. Normally cholesterol ester forms 80% of core lipids and carries approximately 75% of the total cholesterol in plasma. In normal situations, there is a substrate product relationship between VLDL and LDL, and almost all LDL apo-B can be accounted for as a product of VLDL metabolism. However there is evidence that under some circumstances the liver can secrete LDL directly into the plasma compartment [44]. In patients with familial hypercholesterolaemia (FH) the daily transport of apo-B in the LDL fraction has been found to exceed the transport of apo-B in VLDL. This is an important observation in understanding how LDL can be increased without changes in VLDL levels.

The removal of LDL from the circulation occurs largely by a receptor-mediated process in the liver and extrahepatic tissues. Evidence for the existence of cell surface receptors for apo-B was first provided by Goldstein and Brown in studies of human skin fibroblasts [45]. All body cells, including glomerular mesangial cells but possibly excluding nervous tissue, have LDL receptors. However, only hepatocytes are able to excrete cholesterol either as biliary cholesterol or after conversion to bile salts. The receptor-bound LDL is internalized by the cell in an endocytotic vesicle that fuses with primary lysosome. The protein moiety of LDL is degraded and the cholesterol ester is hydrolysed to free cholesterol by a lysosomal acid cholesterol ester hydrolase. Hydrolysis of triglycerides and cholesterol may also occur in the lysosome. Through a feedback system the cell is able to regulate its own cholesterol content. Intracellular free cholesterol inhibits endogenous cholesterol synthesis by inhibiting the rate-limiting enzyme HMG-CoA reductase. An increase in intracellular free cholesterol also inhibits the synthesis or recycling of the apo-B/E receptor, thereby further reducing LDL uptake. Finally, the increased intracellular free cholesterol stimulates its own re-esterification by activating ACAT activity in the cytosol. The cholesterol content of the cell may be further regulated by a reverse cholesterol transport system orchestrated by HDL.

In normolipidaemic subjects 70–80% of LDL is removed through the apo-B/E receptor pathway, defective in FH patients. Some, probably modified, LDL is removed by the monocyte/macrophage scavenger receptor. The important role of this mechanism is illustrated in patients lacking LDL receptors, where scavenger receptors, abundantly present in macrophages, become a major pathway for cholesterol removal. The uptake of LDL through these receptors is not regulated and this unregulated uptake transforms macrophages to lipid-rich foam cells which accumulate in atherosclerotic lesions, including the glomerulus in some nephrotic patients.

The fact that LDL is heterogeneous, i.e. each particle consists of a mixture of protein, fatty acids, phospholipids and cholesterol, causes some difficulty in relation to the interpretation of lipid levels. The protein moiety provides the ligand for the LDL receptor without which its lipid burden would be unable to gain access to cells. The positively charged protein will bind to glycosaminoglycans (GAGs), including glomerular basement membrane [46]. It is probably the protein moiety which enables the post-secretory modification of its lipids, thought to be mimicked by *in vitro* oxidation.

Plasma cholesterol levels are often within the normal range in CRF patients, but the triglyceride content of LDL is increased. There is a redistribution of cholesterol in IDL and VLDL, the overall cholesterol content often being increased [23]. Single vertical spin ultracentrifugation combined with non-denaturing gradient gel electrophoresis revealed striking heterogeneity in the LDL region with multiple bands between 22 and 28 nm [42]. Recently, it has been demonstrated that in both normal and moderately hypertriglyceridaemic subjects, small dense LDL subfractions were more susceptible to copper-induced oxidative modification. Furthermore, the plasma triglyceride concentration appears to have an influence in generating these small dense LDL particles within the density range of 1.036–1.060 g/ml and diameter of <25 nm. De Graff *et al.* [47] have showed that clofibrate treatment reduced the susceptibility of LDL to oxidation. Oxidatively modified LDL also generates lysophosphatidylcholine which is a powerful chemotactic agent for monocyte recruitment into the arterial wall during the early phase of atherogenesis [48]. Maggi and coworkers demonstrated enhanced LDL oxidation in uraemic patients [49]; they also reported autoantibodies against oxidized LDL in haemodialysis patients [50].

We reported a spontaneous fall in cholesterol concentration in nephrotic patients with progressive renal disease [51]. One explanation for this finding could be the post-translational modification and oxidation of LDL particles and their clearance through scavenger receptors. As renal disease progressed, the characteristic pattern of LPL and LCAT deficiencies, hypertriglyceridaemia and the decreased level of HDL may have altered the phenotypic expression of LDL in favour of small dense

LDL particles. Other modifications of LDL, such as carbamylation of apo-B, may also increase its atherogenicity in CRF [52]. Therefore, functional aberrations in the LDL particle appear to be more significant in increasing the atherogenicity of these particles than an increase in LDL cholesterol concentration in CRF.

### 9.3.4 Lipoprotein(a)

Lp(a) is an LDL-like particle in which apo-B100 is linked to another apoprotein – apo(a). Significantly a high degree of homology is found between apo(a) and plasminogen which contains five typical 'Kringle' domains, characterized by three internal disulphide bridges which create a characteristic pattern, superficially resembling a Danish pastry called a 'kringle'. Apo(a) contains two types of kringles homologous to those in plasminogen: one copy of plasminogen kringle 5 and multiple repeats of plasminogen kringle 4. The number of kringle 4 repeats in apo(a) is highly variable among different individuals, explaining the size polymorphism of apo(a) in the population. One important factor in determining plasma Lp(a) concentration appears to be the variations in apo(a) isoforms. If the apo(a) gene were responsible for Lp(a) levels there should be an inverse correlation between plasma levels and isoform size, but the gene actually accounts for only about 40% of Lp(a) levels, and hence the contribution of genetic or environmental factors to plasma Lp(a) is uncertain [53]. In support of this, one large study of Lp(a) in end stage renal disease (ESRD) found that Lp(a) levels were raised, but no difference in isoform distribution was found in controls [54]. The liver is the major site of Lp(a) synthesis, although the site of assembly and the pathways leading to its catabolism and clearance are unknown. The exact function of Lp(a) and its role in the promotion of atherosclerosis remain unclear, but it is thought to have the potential for both atherogenesis and thrombogenesis. Studies have shown that Lp(a) concentration greater than 30 mg/100 ml is an important risk factor for coronary heart disease particularly in the context of a raised LDL level.

Lp(a) may be raised in a variety of renal patients including nephrotics [55] although this is not always the case. A number of investigators have reported elevated levels of Lp(a) in the context of renal disease. We studied Lp(a) in 76 patients with proteinuria and renal function varying from normal to advanced chronic renal failure. The median Lp(a) levels were elevated more than two-fold but 25% of the patients had values of 30 mg/100 ml or more [56]. Interestingly the levels did not correlate with total cholesterol, other lipoprotein subclasses, or with proteinuria [56]. Shoji *et al.* [57] reported a four-fold increase in median Lp(a) values in CAPD patients, and a two-fold increase in haemodialysis patients. Lp(a) concentration remained high after renal transplantation.

It is possible that the kidney plays a role in Lp(a) metabolism, since its level was found in one study to decrease significantly (though not to normal) in haemodialysis patients after receiving a renal transplant [58]. The decrease was significantly related to increasing creatinine clearance. Another study confirmed that Lp(a) fell initially but remained higher than normal in the first nine months post transplant, and also found higher than normal levels in haemodialysis patients [59]. There seems to be some evidence that loss of renal function in ESRD is associated with raised Lp(a) and restoration after transplantation with a decrease towards the normal. The issue is confused by the fact that it has been suggested that immunosuppressive therapy with cyclosporin may exacerbate the rise in Lp(a) [60].

### 9.3.5 High-density lipoproteins

HDL particles are synthesized and secreted by the liver and the small intestine. Newly secreted particles appear as lamellar discs made up of phospholipids, free cholesterol and apo-E. Upon acquiring apo-AI these discs become the ideal substrate for LCAT which converts free cholesterol, acquired from extrahepatic tissue and other lipoproteins, into cholesteryl esters. During this process HDL becomes a spherical particle having cholesteryl ester as its core lipid. HDL particles undergo a series of remodelling processes in the plasma. In normal human plasma, the major species are the smaller HDL3 and the larger HDL2. The continued LCAT activity in HDL3 converts these particles to cholesteryl ester-rich HDL2. This mature HDL2 is necessary for the transport of the lipoprotein lipase activator apo-CII to nascent chylomicrons and VLDL. Albumin binds the other product of LCAT reaction, lysolecithin, and this prevents product inhibition of this reaction and accelerates the esterification of cholesterol. CETP can exchange cholesteryl ester from HDL for triglycerides in VLDL and IDL. Hepatic lipase can act on this HDL triglyceride and convert HDL2 to HDL3. Thus during the hydrolysis of chylomicrons and VLDL, excess surface components are transferred to HDL2 and this increases the size of these particles. In addition, VLDL triglycerides can exchange with cholesteryl esters in the presence of CETP and the hydrolysis of resulting HDL2 triglycerides by hepatic lipase can cause a decrease in HDL2 size and convert HDL2 to HDL3 [61]. Therefore HDL is a key player in modulating the delipidation cascade of chylomicrons, VLDL and IDL, and also provides a medium for the reverse transport of cholesterol from extrahepatic tissue to the liver.

Apo-AI, the major apoprotein of HDL, is filtered and present in significant amounts in the urine of nephrotic patients. It is not clear whether HDL damages renal tubular cells. In short-term cultures LDL had a much more pronounced effect on proximal renal tubular cells than HDL. However, long-term effects due to filtration of HDL over very long periods may possibly contribute to renal tubular loss in the nephrotic syndrome.

A low HDL cholesterol is a familiar pattern of type IV hyperlipidaemia of CRF [62]. Miller and Miller [63] initially reported an inverse relationship between HDL cholesterol and the risk of developing coronary heart disease (CHD). The mechanism underlying this association is often thought to be due to the reverse cholesterol transport from peripheral sites to the liver. However, there is very little evidence that this transport pathway is increased in subjects with raised HDL concentration. On the other hand it is reasonable to suggest that the increased risk of CHD in subjects with low HDL cholesterol may be in part due to the accumulation of remnant triglyceride-rich chylomicrons and VLDL for the following reasons. Part of the HDL cholesterol pool comes from the delipidation pathways of chylomicrons and VLDL and because of the low levels of LPL in uraemic patients, catabolism of triglyceride-rich lipoproteins is impaired, reducing the amount of HDL cholesterol formed. Reduced HDL cholesterol in CRF may be considered a marker for atherogenic remnant lipoprotein particles.

The recent finding of HDL as an important carrier of lipid hydroperoxides in human plasma provides another explanation for the protective effect of HDL against atherosclerosis [64]. This preferential accumulation of lipid hydroperoxides in HDL reflects the relative lack of antioxidants in HDL particles compared to LDL. It is also reported that oxidized or lipid peroxide carrying HDL is not avidly taken up by macrophages and does not lead to the formation of foam cells.

## 9.4 NEPHROTIC SYNDROME

In both animals and man, the nephrotic syndrome (NS) – proteinuria, hypoalbuminaemia, oedema, hyperlipidaemia and lipiduria – is an easily recognized distinct clinical entity with many primary causes. Dramatic increases in plasma lipids, which often far exceed any other disease, occur in NS and are approximately inversely proportional to hypoalbuminaemia. Nephrotic lipaemic plasma was first recognized more than a century ago, and later lipid deposition was observed in nephrotic kidneys [65]. Many early publications refer to renal lipid deposition at autopsy and later in some renal biopsy specimens but this was not routine, probably because the renal biopsy tissue is routinely treated with lipid solvents.

Hyperlipidaemia nevertheless gave rise to a significant literature starting with Virchow's description of fatty degeneration in the kidneys of patients with Bright's disease [66] and Munk's introduction of the term lipoid nephrosis [67]. Interstitial and arterial lipidosis was found in diabetics by Kimmelstiel and Wilson [68] almost fifty years ago and glomerular lipidosis was noted by Wilens *et al.* in intercapillary lesions in diabetes and other glomerular diseases [69]. Experimental evidence for an influence of lipids on renal disease was obtained by French *et al.* [70] who fed high-cholesterol diets to guinea pigs, animals whose diet would normally contain only plant sterols. These important early observations of the relationship between hyperlipidaemia and renal disease were not conceptualized as contributing independently to the broad range of renal and glomerular disease pathogenesis.

### 9.4.1 Hypoalbuminaemia: lipoproteins versus albumin synthesis

It is not clear why the liver synthesizes excess lipoprotein rather than albumin to correct good nephrotic range urinary protein loss, since albumin is the major urine protein in the earlier stages of NS. However it seems clear that hypoalbuminaemia is implicated in excess hepatic lipoprotein synthesis. Studies have shown that serum cholesterol depends on the renal clearance of albumin [71]. LDL turnover correlates with plasma albumin [72] and LDL catabolic rate correlates with proteinuria [73].

The relationship of plasma albumin to total plasma cholesterol (TC) concentration is approximately inverse but not linear, TC rising precipitously as albumin falls below about 20 g/1. It was suggested that excess hepatic LDL secretion was explained by the fall in plasma oncotic pressure caused by hypoalbuminaemia [74]. Later it was shown that apo-B secretion in HepG2 cells is regulated by albumin, oleic acid and insulin [75], in the case of albumin possibly via viscosity, appearing to support the earlier work of Yedgar *et al.* [76]. Recently Yamauchi *et al.* showed that oncotic pressure regulates gene transcription of both albumin and apo-B in cultured rat hepatoma cells [77].

Therapeutic administration of albumin is probably fruitless in patients with heavy proteinuria, since the rate of administration cannot compensate for urine losses. Since significant proteinuria is associated with most glomerular diseases, it does not on its own offer any important clues as to pathogeneis of glomerular disease, but has great importance as an easily quantifiable marker for loss of glomerular permselectivity. Its value in this respect is however tempered by the fact that the renal tubule contributes to an unknown extent to protein reabsorption and catabolism. Early in disease, renal tubules which are functioning relatively normally reabsorb some filtered protein but that reabsorption falls as renal tubule mass declines. It is possible that fewer hyperfiltering nephrons in advanced disease excrete more protein per nephron than early in the process. Thus the gross plasma protein loss equals tubular reabsorption plus urine protein, the former being unquantifiable; this is presumed highest when the renal tubules are normal in number and function. As renal function declines, gross and net loss become equal. Patients with grossly impaired renal function may lose 10 g of protein per day in the urine, but maintain a normal plasma albumin.

The fact that many investigators have confirmed the value of reduction of proteinuria as a measure of response to treatment in nephrotics could suggest that the improvement is the net effect of reduced filtration and improved tubular reabsorption, the former probably predominating. Reduction of proteinuria therefore remains an important clinical goal, underlined by the fact that progression of disease rarely occurs if proteinuria is reduced or remits [78]. Williams *et al.* noted that progression is proportional to the magnitude of proteinuria [79] as well as renal pathology. As a corollary, analgesic nephropathy and adult polycystic disease in which proteinuria is low usually progress more slowly.

Proteinuria does not reflect glomerular filtration rate. In a retrospective study of 12 nephrotic patients with progressive renal disease, heavy proteinuria continued throughout the time course of renal disease progression, but serum cholesterol gradually fell towards normal as patients approached ESRF. No important dietary or drug changes were made during the course of deterioration in these patients, and the data was analysed when serum creatinine reached 600 μmol/l [51]. At this time serum albumin had returned almost to normal, suggesting that the stimulus to excess lipoprotein synthesis previously provided by hypoalbuminaemia was no longer present. It also seems likely that proteinuria *per se* did not affect liver lipoprotein secretion. The remaining nephrons continued to filter protein and, presumably, lipoprotein.

### 9.4.2 Urine HDL

The kidney is an important organ in the metabolism of HDL and excess HDL excretion could contribute to hyperlipidaemia by a quantitative reduction in cholesterol excretion by the liver. The extent to which HDL metabolism depends on filtration was examined by Saku *et al.* [80] using a filtering and non-filtering isolated perfused rat kidney model. The filtering normal kidney sequestered significantly more rat HDL than controls, and nephrotic kidneys sequestered two to four times as much HDL as non-nephrotic kidneys. Normal kidneys excrete some HDL [81] and the kidney is an important site for HDL catabolism [82]. Although significant excretion of urine HDL, measured in the form of apo-AI [83, 84] or protein of similar molecular weight [85], accompanies proteinuria in humans it is quantitatively insufficient to explain nephrotic hyperlipidaemia. The combination of increased renal metabolism and urine loss of HDL does not result in a significant fall in plasma HDL.

## 9.5 PATHOGENESIS

In recent years improved understanding of atherosclerosis [86] has illuminated the pathology of glomerulosclerosis and supported the concept of lipoproteins as mediators of renal disease [4]. The possible roles of lipoproteins in progressive renal disease may be understood in the more familiar context of atherosclerosis. In major arteries atherosclerosis results from a complex sequence of events in which normal cycling of LDL through vascular endothelium is altered in favour of LDL trapping and oxidation, aided by increased oxidizability of LDL, recruitment of monocytes, proliferation of smooth muscle cells and formation of fibrous tissue. Atherosclerotic heart disease is common in renal failure and it is probable that the high blood cholesterol of nephrotics contributes to this. That this has proved controversial may reflect the shorter exposure time of blood vessels to circulating lipids in nephrotics, in some of whom renal disease may respond to treatment, and the contribution of other, unidentified risk factors.

This concept of atherosclerosis applied to the microvasculature is based on the assumption that the glomerulus possesses cell types which are known to respond to lipoprotein injury in large arteries, namely the endothelium and monocytes, or which resemble smooth muscle, namely the mesangial cell. Moreover the glomerular basement membrane (GBM) is capable of binding human plasma lipoproteins [46]. Clinical examples of focal glomerular sclerosis and diabetic glomerular disease, reinforce the analogy. Placing progressive renal disease within the context of biochemical and molecular cell processes previously associated only with large vessel atherosclerosis stimulated extensive exploration of the mechanisms of lipid-mediated damage to renal cells [87, 88].

In animal models the glomerulus appears to lose protection against lipoproteins, possibly through charge neutralization from combination with apo-B. As a result glomerular cells and basement membrane are subjected to long-term exposure to lipoproteins capable of exerting wide-ranging effects, which include continued glomerular basement membrane binding and the provision of a virtually limitless supply of phospholipid substrate for inflammatory mediators, as well as directly affecting cell metabolism.

In man, diseases are often complex but a connection between vascular disease (retinopathy), hyperlipidaemia and proteinuria has been found in Native Americans [89]. A link has also been found between systolic blood pressure, plasma angiotensin II and serum cholesterol in diabetics, although increased cholesterol concentrations were not associated with more renal damage [90]. A recent analysis of data collected in 1979 for the Diabetic Retinopathy Study emphasized that only hypertension and hypercholesterolaemia were positively linked with rapid progression of renal disease and that hypercholesterolaemia was the major predictor of death [91].

There is considerable evidence for the exacerbation of progressive disease by plasma cholesterol [70] and lipoprotein in animals [92, 93], and possibly in humans. There have been several descriptions of an abnormal accumulation of lipids in glomeruli and tubules since renal biopsy became generally available [94]. Recently Lee *et al.* found that 8.4% of 631 patients had ultrastructurally detectable extracellular lipid in non-sclerotic glomeruli [95], which suggests that there may be an early presclerotic stage of lipoprotein-mediated disease at which lipid-related damage is reversible.

It is assumed that as in large arteries LDL is available in physiological quantities to mesangial and epithelial cells, and although exposure of these cells to LDL in glomerulopathies is probably much greater, there may not be a simple quantitative relationship between the plasma lipoprotein levels and renal cell responses. It is possible for example that hyperlipidaemia may not be a prerequisite for liopoprotein-induced nephron injury: an abnormal degree of access may be sufficient. Presumably LDL is available in physiological quantities to mesangial and epithelial cells, and although exposure of these cells to LDL in glomerulopathies is probably much greater, there is unlikely to be a simple relationship between the plasma lipoprotein levels and renal cell responses. In this regard it is interesting that in a retrospective study of 12 nephrotic patients with progressive renal disease, heavy proteinuria continued throughout the time course of renal disease progression, but serum cholesterol gradually fell to normal levels as patients approached ESRF. No important dietary or drug changes were made during the course of deterioration in these patients [51]. If lipoproteins played a role in mediating progressive renal disease in these patients, it could be assumed either that lipoprotein-mediated injury is most severe when renal function is normal, or that it occurs independently of plasma concentration, only requiring access to glomeruli and tubules.

### 9.5.1 Haemodynamic influences

Examination of the pressure and flow dynamics of glomerular filtration has led some investigators to conclude that increased glomerular pressure plays a leading role in the pathogenesis of glomerular sclerosis

[96]. However, almost all the experimental models from which haemodynamic data were derived are nephrotic, i.e. proteinuria and hyperlipidaemic. In general there have been no controls for hyperlipidaemia, which is even more important in view of the fact that reduction of proteinuria by angiotensin-converting enzyme (ACE) inhibitors may result in a fall in plasma lipoproteins [97–99]. Unfortunately this makes these models difficult to interpret. The topic is discussed in full detail in Chapter 1.

Excluding obvious associations with genetic abnormalities, such as polycystic diseases and persistently active immune diseases, the largest disease groups with declining renal function are patients with hypertension and/or diabetes, and the strongest clinical association with progression is proteinuria [1]. While a major cause of death in these groups is cardiovascular, the presence and influence of renal disease as a causal factor has been inadequately researched in most major studies to date.

### 9.5.2 Oxidized LDL and its cellular interactions

The role of LDL in the pathogenesis of atherosclerosis was emphasized by the demonstration that oxidation of LDL by macrophages caused them to be taken up by the scavenger LDL receptor [100]. The scavenger receptor is equivalent to the acetyl LDL receptor which takes up delipidated OxLDL protein [101]. Monocyte infiltration is a feature of many nephritides. Lipid-stimulated monocyte influx was first shown by French *et al.* [70] in cholesterol-fed rabbits and later characterized more fully in other models [102–104]. In nephrotics, monocytes become foam cells which are a prominent feature of both atherosclerosis and glomerulosclerosis following ingestion of oxidized LDL (OxLDL) via the scavenger receptor.

LDL may undergo oxidative modification *in vitro* by copper ions [105] or spontaneous oxidation *in vivo* [105]. The latter, so-called minimally modified LDL (mOxLDL), may be defined as generating 2–5 mmol of thiobarbituric acid reactive substances (TBARS) per mg of cholesterol. mOxLDL is able to stimulate monocyte endothelial cell interaction [106] and may initiate the enhanced uptake by monocytes of cholesterol-containing particles derived from atherosclerotic lesions [107], a possible cause of foam cell generation. It is also chemotactic for monocytes [106] which secrete transforming growth factor TGF-β, which in turn stimulates fibronectin production by glomerular cells [108]. Since the TGF-β family of polypeptides also stimulates collagen and proteoglycan synthesis this sequence implies a source of glomerular connective tissue. Since LDL also stimulates mesangial cell proliferation [109] and is oxidized by both rat [110] and human mesangial cells the potential for glomerular damage is considerable [111].

The direct interaction of lipids and glomerular structures may be aided by vasomotor influences of LDL on endothelial cells. OxLDL appears especially potent in this regard, its effects being prevented by the antioxidant probucol [112]. Bank [113] showed that the *in vivo* vasodilatory response to acetyl choline in hypercholesterolaemic rats was blunted, possibly because of more rapid inactivation of nitric oxide (NO) in the presence of lipoproteins. It was suggested that elevated levels of LDL may result in excess OxLDL generation by endothelial cells. This in turn stimulates cell membrane phosphatidylinositol turnover, leading to increased generation of prostaglandins $TxA_2$ and $PGH_2$ and accelerated production of reactive oxygen species. This would counterbalance increased NO production by inactivating locally produced NO more rapidly [113]. Post-secretory modification of LDL could confer chemoattractant properties, and, as in atherosclerosis, stimulate glomerular resident monocytes to produce chemoattractants leading to further influx of monocytes [102, 104].

Minimally oxidized LDL stimulates monocyte endothelium interaction [106]. Glomerular macrophages are capable of oxidizing LDL [114], adding to the potential for inflammation. The mesangial cell may also participate directly in this process since rat mesangial cells were shown to promote lipoprotein oxidation in response to LDL [110] and similar data exists for human mesangial cells [111]. Inflammatory mediators, including tumour necrosis factor and interleukin-1, may induce oxygen radical production by mesangial cells [115]. Oxidized LDL binds preferentially to the glomerulus when injected intra-arterially in the rat and binds to mesangial cells *in vitro* [116]. Immune-mediated mesangial injury causes increased oxygen radical and eicosanoid synthesis [117] the inflammatory potential of which can be diminished or eliminated in the mouse model of systemic lupus erythematosus (SLE) by prior administration of eicosapentaenoic acids [118]. Aside from the inflammatory potential of oxidized LDL, lysophosphatidyl choline, an LDL phospholipid, is chemotactic for human monocytes [48].

The glomerular cell response to lipoprotein is therefore affected by a large number of variables, including the physical state of LDL (e.g. whether oxidized or not), the efficiency with which it is metabolized by glomerular cells, glomerular pressures and dynamics, and the type and extent of the original glomerular disease. As in atherosclerosis early inflammatory processes may be replaced by fibrosis; the collagen synthesis which follows lipid-induced damage could continue independently of the initial insult. Short-duration experiments, however, may not reflect *in vivo* processes in man, in whom progressive renal disease may take some years to develop. The duration of exposure may therefore be important if local trapping results in oxidative modification of LDL.

### 9.5.3 Normolipidaemic renal disease

Although the hyperlipidaemia of the nephrotic syndrome still provides the main stimulus to work in this area, it is important to recognize that there may be no level at which the damaged kidney is 'safe' from circulating LDL. Thus even if plasma LDL is normal or adequately controlled by treatment, plasma lipids might still be able to cause or perpetuate glomerular atherosclerosis. For example in experiments with *in vitro* mesangial cell cultures, a low concentration of oxidized LDL (200 $\mu$g/ml) arrested mesangial cell growth as measured by $^3$H incorporation [119].

Lipoproteins seldom cause damage to normal kidneys. Thus, the Watanabe heritable hyperlipidaemic rabbit does not manifest proteinuria (J.F. Moorhead, Z. Varghese and M. Jarmulowicz, unpublished results), and in man familial hypercholesterolaemia is not associated with renal failure. Exceptions are massive obesity in man [120] (although rare) and inherited LCAT deficiency with abnormal LDL which causes renal failure in some families [7]. Extensive renal lipid deposition may occur in patients with arteriohepatic dysplasia (Alagille's syndrome). In this condition, small kidneys, a raised serum creatinine and proteinuria are associated with hypercholesterolaemia and extensive lipid deposition in the mesangium and glomerular and tubular basement membranes [121].

### 9.5.4 Transplantation

One of the most striking features of post-transplant biochemistry is the remarkable rise in plasma cholesterol which takes place within a few days of surgery, contrasting sharply with the hypertriglyceridaemia and (usually) normocholesterolaemia of dialysis patients. This phenomenon has received increased attention in the study of chronic graft failure (CGF) which has many of the hallmarks of chronic atherosclerosis. Accumulating evidence suggests that the vascular component of chronic graft failure has similarities to atherosclerosis.

In a study of chronic rejection in two groups of patients, with stable versus deteriorating renal function [122], it was found that after the histological differences between two groups, the next most significant factor was the total serum cholesterol. It was significantly higher in transplants with deteriorating function, compared to those with stable function ($P$ = $<0.008$). When we divided (Z. Varghese and J.F. Moorhead, unpublished data) 158 transplant patients into two groups with total cholesterol of above or below 5.2 mmol/l, the mean serum creatinine was significantly higher in patients in the higher-cholesterol group (158 $\pm$ 70 versus 172 $\pm$ 158, $P$ $<0.04$). We also found that higher triglyceride levels were associated with the high-cholesterol group (TG = 2.43 $\pm$ 1.17 and 1.38 $\pm$ 0.68, $P < 0.001$). In addition there was no significant difference between 24 hour urine protein excretion rates in the two groups.

It is extremely difficult in this complex area to separate the effects of immune from metabolic processes, and indeed it may be unnecessary so to do. Any immune reaction associated with inflammation requires inflammatory mediators, amongst which are prostaglandin derivatives. Numerous experiments have shown that inflammatory reactions are either prevented or ameliorated by diminishing the supply of arachidonic acid. In transplantation the possibility that the immune arm of the rejection process is facilitated by inflammatory mediators derived from fatty acids is supported by experiments in which kidneys from rats given an essential fatty acid-deficient diet were depleted of glomerular macrophages and were not rejected when transplanted into rats of a different strain [123].

### 9.5.5 Tubulo-interstitial lesions

It was first observed by Risdon *et al.* [124], and subsequently confirmed by others, that tubulo-interstitial disease was a better predictor of progression than glomerular disease [125, 126]. The concept of lipoprotein-related tubulo-interstitial disease derived from histopathological findings of tubular lipidosis and the clinical examination of nephrotic urine for oval fat bodies [127] which are presumably formed in the renal tubules. The original observations of Munk [65] were in fact on fat bodies in the urine and fatty changes in the tubules. In nephrotics, fatty acids are presented in substantial amounts via albumin, their major carrier, and are then probably metabolized into neutral lipids in the tubules [128]. The accumulation of lipids in renal tubular cells was suggested as being potentially toxic, perhaps contributing to tubulo-interstitial disease [4].

In a study of the hyperphagic fa/fa fatty rat, Zucker [129] observed proteinuria and progressive 'glomerulonephrosis' for the first time and described severe interstitial renal disease especially in males. These early descriptions provide clinical and experimental support for a causative link between hyperlipidaemia and progressive tubulo-interstitial disease. Despite the fact that the mass of LDL is probably too great to enable significant filtration of intact particles in measurable quantities in nephrotic urine, both apo-A and apo-B, major apoproteins of LDL, have been found in the tubules and interstitium of nephrotic patients [130, 131]. HDL is excreted in measurable amounts in normal subjects [81] and in larger amounts in nephrotics [83, 132]. Studies in rabbit proximal straight tubule segments microperfused *in vitro* have shown progressive uptake and cellular accumulation of radiolabelled HDL [82].

In order to clarify tubule/lipoprotein interactions we examined human proximal tubular cells in culture [133], finding that native LDL was not toxic to human proximal tubular cells, but both OxLDL and mOxLDL caused cell detachment and death, possibly because of the presence of cytotoxic oxidation products in LDL particles. This study also suggested that LDL may be oxidized by proximal tubular cells, suggesting that any filtered lipid may become toxic in its passage through the tubule. Since mesangial cells which are upstream of the tubules also have this capacity [110], the possibility exists that some oxidatively modified LDL will pass into the tubular lumen. This stimulated us to examine renal tubular cell cytokine response, in the form of endothelin-l (ET-l) synthesis, to *in vitro* challenge to HDL. We found that HDL was mitogenic for these cells and caused a four-fold increase in ET-l secretion. Since ET-l is secreted basolaterally, the high quantities of HDL filtered in nephrotic syndrome could have adverse effects on the renal microcirculation, interstitial fibroblasts and interstitial macrophages [134].

## 9.6 TREATMENT

The rationale for active reduction of plasma cholesterol is based on the similarity between atherosclerosis pathology and the glomerular lesions associated with progressive renal disease in nephrotic patients and animals [4, 135]. Moreover, human atherosclerosis has been reported to regress with reduction of serum cholesterol [136–139]. In renal disease treatment of hyperlipidaemia has at least two objectives – preventing atherosclerotic arterial disease and renal disease progression. The knowledge gained from animal experiments is tantalizingly difficult to translate effectively into immediate benefit for patients. This is partly due to difficulty in designing and interpreting suitable clinical trials on the small number of patients available to any single unit. Further, although there are fundamental similarities between inflammatory processes in man and rat, it may be important to evaluate the relevance of species differences in those aspects of lipid metabolism which contribute to inflammation, since lipid metabolism in the rat has important differences from man.

Progressive renal disease in animal models is exacerbated by high-fat diets [140] and ameliorated by lipid-lowering regimes [141, 142], possibly because of a reduction in arachidonic acid-derived inflammatory mediators. Others [143] noted that lipids and immune complexes acted synergistically in lupus nephritis in mice and that a fish oil rich in eicosapentaenoic acid (EPA) prolonged the life of animals [118]. Total deprivation of eicosanoid precursors through essential fatty acid deficient diets have also been shown to prevent progression in glomerulonephritis [144] in rats. The link between lipoproteins and glomerular inflammation in animal models is therefore quite strong.

The careful management of the lipid abnormalities described in this chapter may reduce risk factors associated with CHD, possibly ameliorate the rate of progression of glomerular and tubulo-interstitial pathology, and reduce the risk of chronic renal graft failure. Four major classes of lipid-lowering agents are available for clinical use: resins, fibrates, vastatins and probucol. However, none of these compounds has been sufficiently evaluated in CRF to recommend their routine use.

Agents which inhibit the synthesis of VLDL, such as fish oil and niacin, and those which increase the catabolism of VLDL may be of use in dialysis patients. Drugs with the ability to induce LDL receptors may be beneficial in nephrotic patients; resins may also be useful in this situation. However, the reduction of total cholesterol produced by vastatins is usually of the order of 30% and they are generally unable to normalize levels when total cholesterol exceeds 8.0 mmol/l. In patients with compromised renal function, side effects may be associated with most types of lipid-lowering agents.

### 9.6.1 Dialysis patients

In spite of the possibility of an increased incidence of CHD in CRF patients on various dialysis modalities, effective and safe modes of treatment for hypertriglyceridaemia and atherogenic remnants have not been systematically evaluated in long-term controlled clinical trials. Dietary regulation is the first step in any lipid-lowering strategy, but long-term compliance with restricted diet is difficult in dialysis patients. Reduction in carbohydrate intake together with an increased ratio of polyunsaturated to saturated fatty acids may be beneficial in reducing the overproduction of VLDL triglycerides by the liver [145]. However, studies involving dietary manipulation must take into account the contribution of glucose from dialysate fluids.

Fibrates have been tested for VLDL-lowering effect in dialysis patients. Their main effect on VLDL triglycerides is to enhance their catabolism through increased LPL activity but they also reduce VLDL synthesis and secretion by the liver. Fibrates also reduce LDL heterogeneity and reduce the level of small dense LDL particles [146]. Many studies suggest a modest increase in HDL cholesterol. Because fibrates are not dialysable, their half life is prolonged in dialysis patients. Early studies by Pierides demonstrated that clofibrate caused myopathy in haemodialysis patients, concluding that the risk is too high to use this drug routinely in renal failure [147]. Others have used bezafibrate and gemfibrozil [39, 148].

HMG-CoA reductase inhibitors or vastatins provide a very useful opportunity to induce apo-B/E receptors, and this increases the removal of circulating atherogeneic remnant particles. This may be a worthwhile strategy for patients on dialysis. Although conventional approaches to treating hyperlipidaemia in CRF may be somewhat limited by toxicity and side effects, the use of vastatins, calcium channel blockers and antioxidants may provide some hope for the future management of patients on dialysis.

### 9.6.2 Transplant recipients

Very limited information is available on treating the hyperlipidaemia of stable renal transplant patients. There is increased awareness that a component of chronic vascular rejection is an extension of the atherosclerotic process in the transplanted kidney. An early study of the treatment of renal transplant patients with fish oil demonstrated a beneficial effect in reducing plasma triglycerides and changing the slope of the reciprocal of plasma creatinine in a favourable direction [149]. We also showed for the first time that low-dose simvastatin, 5 mg/day, is effective and safe in lowering LDL cholesterol and improved the lipid profile in stable renal transplant patients, 14 of whom were receiving cyclosporin A [150]. Apanay and colleagues demonstrated that cyclosporin increases the oxidizability of LDL in renal transplant patients [151], raising the possibility that antioxidant supplements might be useful in protecting these patients from oxidized LDL-induced damage to the transplanted kidneys. Multivitamins are effective antioxidants, at least in the short term. Rabl and colleagues demonstrated that antioxidant treatment by multivitamin infusion reduces the reperfusion-induced damage of transplanted kidneys [152].

### 9.6.3 Nephrotic patients

Although it has long been recognized that hypoalbuminaemia and hyperlipidaemia coexist in NS, the main aim of therapy for many years was to improve the former. If remission or reduction of proteinuria was induced an improvement in the serum albumin would ensue and hyperlipidaemia would correct spontaneously.

Many immunosuppressive regimens are used in the nephrotic syndrome, their effectiveness being highly variable. Spontaneous remissions sometimes occur but many patients relapse and some remain persistently hypoalbuminaemic and hyperlipidaemic. The association of the latter with cardiovascular disease and atherosclerosis has prompted physicians to be more aggressive in managing hyperlipidaemia, but of more direct interest is the possibility that treatment of hyperlipidaemia may actually reduce proteinuria [153, 154] or retard the process of glomerulosclerosis and subsequently renal failure [155, 156].

*Diet*

Low-cholesterol diets, high polyunsaturated to saturated fat ratios, and increased monounsaturated and polyunsaturated fats have produced varying results in hyperlipidaemia. The reduction in total cholesterol has ranged from as little as 6% to almost 30%. Where there has been a more rigorous dietary regimen, as with the vegetarian soya diet [154], the effect has been more consistent, with a 33% reduction in LDL cholesterol over a short time period, and a significant improvement in proteinuria. Extension of these regimens over longer periods may be difficult to achieve because of dietary compliance.

*Fish oil supplements*

Eicosapentanoic and dicosahexanoic fatty acids, both of which are present in fish oil, have the ability to reduce the synthesis and secretion of VLDL [157]. They have not been adequately evaluated in dialysis patients but have been used many times in the nephrotic syndrome. They reduce the synthesis of the more inflammatory eicosanoids and have the added benefit of reducing blood viscosity and platelet aggregation, a potential asset in the prothrombotic state of NS. Recently in a study of patients with immunoglobulin A (IgA) nephropathy and persistent proteinuria 33% of patients in the placebo group had an increase of 50% or more in serum creatinine, compared with 6% of patients taking fish oil supplements [155], but there was no change in the level of proteinuria. A separate study of patients with focal segmental glomerulosclerosis (FSGS) and membranous nephropathy (MN) using *n*-3 fatty acids in differing concentrations [153] showed a significant reduction in proteinuria in the group taking 7.7 g/day of *n*-3 PUFA (polyunsaturated fatty acid) supplementation with no other effects on renal function. Changes in the lipid profile also occur, with reduction in hepatic VLDL synthesis but inconsistent changes in LDL and HDL. A possible drawback of fish oils is their reported tendency to increase the formation of lipid peroxides [158], which are pro-atherosclerotic.

*Resins and fibrates*

These compounds lower total cholesterol by between 10 and 30%, and LDL cholesterol by around 20%. Although effective, gastric side effects and myopathy in the case of fibrates limit their use. Side effects may be reduced when they are used at lower doses in combination with newer agents. Bile acid sequestrants have the added disadvantage of raising triglyceride levels, although overall improvement in the LDL–HDL ratio

[159] has been reported. No reduction of proteinuria or slowing of progression of renal failure has been reported.

### *HMG-CoA reductase inhibitors*

This class of drug increases LDL catabolism by increasing receptor-mediated LDL uptake. HDL cholesterol levels are increased, substantially improving LDL–HDL ratios, and reductions of 25–45% in total cholesterol and triglycerides been reported [156, 159]. It has been suggested [160] that HMG-CoA reductase inhibitors also block the synthesis of isoprenoids that are necessary for mesangial cell proliferation *in vitro*, albeit in far higher concentrations than would be encountered *in vivo*. Myositis, reflected by elevation of plasma creatine kinase (CK), is an established side effect of co-administration of simvastatin and cyclosporin A; however many patients have a rise in CK of two to four times normal which remains stable in spite of increasing dosage, and experience no adverse effects or symptoms of myopathy. Newer formulations of this class of drug are available which claim to reduce Lp(a) levels.

In our report of simvastatin in 23 adult nephrotic patients [161], total and LDL cholesterol fell by 33 and 31% respectively in the simvastatin treatment group, but no significant differences were found between protein excretion in the treatment and placebo groups; others have reported similar results in short-term studies in a smaller number of patients [162]. Another study [156] compared the effects of simvastatin and cholestyramine and demonstrated a 39% reduction of LDL cholesterol in four weeks using simvastatin (cholestyramine was less effective), but no improvement in proteinuria.

### *Vitamin E and probucol*

There is increasing evidence that antioxidants are important when managing hyperlipidaemia [163]. One of these, probucol, is a powerful antioxidant which when used with fish oils has the advantage of lowering LDL cholesterol which accompanies administration of polyunsaturated fatty acids. Probucol alone has a cholesterol-lowering ability of between 12 and 25% although results vary significantly between reports. The role of vitamin E as an antioxidant remains under debate; its potential in NS has not been explored although its dose-dependent inhibition of platelet aggregation could be of benefit. From *in vitro* studies it would seem that administration of vitamin E has less antioxidant effect than probucol [164]. These drugs remain to be evaluated fully in nephrotic syndrome.

Although several drugs reduce lipid levels in nephrotic patients and are well tolerated, the 40% reduction achievable with drugs and diet cannot usually reduce cholesterol levels to normal. This has made long-term studies on lipid lowering and progression of renal failure difficult to achieve. Nonetheless, many of these studies show potentially beneficial effects for nephrotic syndrome in the short term.

### *Management of hyperlipidaemia by LDL apheresis*

Against this background a number of investigators have examined the effect in nephrotic patients of plasma LDL apheresis (LDL-A), which has the advantage of rapidly reducing circulating LDL concentration to normal. In apheresis, selective elimination of LDL, VLDL and Lp(a) is achieved by passing hyperlipidaemic plasma over negatively charged dextran sulphate bound to porous cellulose beads. The method is widely used in the management of familial hypercholesterolaemia when fortnightly treatments are effective [165]. Side effects are rare, except for significant falls in post-apheresis fibrinogen and thromboplastin time possibly due to non-specific binding by dextran sulphate. Clinically, a few patients with pre-existing coronary artery disease may complain of angina; hypotension and migraine have also been reported.

Recently Sakai *et al.* [166] reported a multicentre trial of LDL apheresis in 16 drug-resistant nephrotics, three of whom had MN and the remainder FSGS. Treatment was given twice weekly for three weeks, 2.5–4.0 litres of plasma being treated per session. Total cholesterol and triglycerides were reduced by 60–70% after each treatment, with HDL cholesterol remaining unchanged. One month after treatment, mean TC levels remained at 30–40% of the initial levels, albumin increased significantly by 10–30% and urine protein fell strikingly to less than 1 g/day. Interestingly, although no improvement was shown in MN patients, nine of the FSGS patients showed varying degrees of improvement ranging from 'very useful' to 'slight'. While this technique offers a new approach, possibly in combination with drugs, judgement as to its efficacy must await controlled trials.

## 9.7 CONCLUSION

The evidence cited above provides adequate grounds for concluding that lipoproteins may have a significant adverse effect on human renal disease progression. It is difficult to demonstrate a beneficial effect of lipid lowering in conditions such as the nephrotic syndrome, when the origin of the disease is unknown and the level of cholesterol is so high as to be impossible to normalize. At the other end of the scale hypercholesterolaemia may not be a prerequisite, provided lipoproteins can gain access to the nephron and the interstitium through a damaged glomerular filter. More information is required on the pathophysiology of lipoprotein-mediated disease before a rational range of therapies can be devised for clinical renal disease.

## REFERENCES


1. Cameron, J.S. (1990) Proteinuria and progression in human glomerular diseases. *Am. J. Nephrol.*, **10**, suppl 1, 81–7.
2. Fischer-Dzoga, K. and Wissler, R.W. (1976) Stimulation of proliferation in stationary primary cultures of monkey aortic smooth muscle cells. Effect of varying concentrations of hyperlipemic serum and low density lipoproteins of varying dietary fat origins. *Atherosclerosis*, **24**, 515–25.
3. Buja, L.M., Kovanen, P.T. and Bilheimer, D.W. (1979) Cellular pathology of homozygous familial hypercholesterolemia. *Am. J. Pathol.*, **97**, 327–57.
4. Moorhead, J.F., Chan, M.K., El Nahas, A.M. and Varghese, Z. (1982) Lipid nephrotoxicity in chronic progressive glomerular and tubulo-interstitial disease. *Lancet*, **2**, 1309–12.
5. Ross, R., Glomset, J. and Harker, L. (1977) Response to injury and atherogenesis. *Am. J. Pathol.*, **86**, 675–84.
6. Saito, T., Sato, H., Kudo, K. *et al.* (1989) Lipoprotein glomerulopathy: glomerular lipoprotein thrombi in a patient with hyperlipoproteinemia. *Am. J. Kidney Dis.*, **13**, 148–53.
7. Gjone, E., Blomhoff, J.P. and Skarbovik, A.J. (1974) Possible association between an abnormal low density lipoprotein and nephropathy in lecithin cholesterol acyltransferase deficiency. *Clin. Chim. Act*, **54**, 11–8.
8. De Lalla, O.F. and Gofman, J.W. (1954) Ultracentrifugal analysis of serum lipoproteins, in *Methods of Biochemical Analysis*, (ed. D. Glick), p. 459.
9. Babiak, J. and Rudel, L.L. (1987) Lipoproteins and atherosclerosis. *Clin. Endocrinol. Metab.*, **1**, 515–50.
10. Breslow, J.L. (1987) Genetic regulation of apolipoproteins. *Am. Heart J.*, **113**, 422–7.
11. Windler, E. and Havel, R.J. (1985) Inhibitory effects of C apolipoproteins from rats and humans on the uptake of triglyceride-rich lipoproteins and their remnants by the perfused rat liver. *J. Lipid Res.*, **26**, 556–65.
12. Chan, M.K., Persaud, J., Varghese, Z. and Moorhead, J.F. (1984) Pathogenic roles of post heparin lipases in lipid abnormalities in hemodialysis patients. *Kidney Int.*, **25**, 812–8.
13. Chan, M.K., Varghese, Z., Persaud, J.W. *et al.* (1982) Hyperlipidemia in patients on maintenance hemo- and peritoneal dialysis: the relative pathogenetic roles of triglyceride production and triglyceride removal. *Clin. Nephrol.*, **17**, 183–90.
14. Nestel, P.J., Fidge, N.H. and Tan, M.H. (1982) Increased lipoprotein-remnant formation in chronic renal failure. *N. Engl. J. Med.*, **307**, 329–33.
15. Arbeeny, C.M. and Rifici, V.A. (1984) The uptake of chylomicron remnants and very low density lipoprotein remnants by the perfused rat liver. *J. Biol. Chem.*, **259**, 9662–6.
16. Herz, J. (1993) The LDL receptor related protein – portrait of a multi functional receptor. *Curr. Opin. Lipidol.*, **4**, 107–13.
17. Kaysen, G.A., Mehendru, L., Pan, X. and Staprans, I. (1992) Both peripheral chylomicron catabolism and hepatic uptake of remnants are defective in nephrosis. *Am. J. Physiol.*, **263**, F335–F341.

18. Mehendru, L., Staprans, I. and Pan, X-M. (1991) Peripheral chylomicron (CM) catabolism and hepatic uptake of remnants (RM) are both defective in nephrosis. *J. Am. Soc. Nephrol.*, **2**, 685.
19. McCosh, E.J., Solangi, K., Rivers, J.M. and Goodman, A. (1975) Hypertriglyceridemia in patients with chronic renal insufficiency. *Am. J. Clin. Nutr.*, **28**, 1036–43.
20. McGarry, J.D. and Foster, D.W. (1976) Ketogenesis and its regulation. *Am. J. Med.*, **61**, 9–13.
21. Ginsberg, H.N., Le, N.A., Melish, J. *et al.* (1981) Effect of a high carbohydrate diet on apoprotein-B catabolism in man. *Metabolism: Clinical and Experimental*, **30**, 347–53.
22. Packard, C.J., McKinney, L., Carr, K. and Shepherd, J. (1983) Cholesterol feeding increases low density lipoprotein synthesis. *J. Clin. Invest.*, **72**, 45–51.
23. Chan, M.K., Varghese, Z. and Moorhead, J.F. (1981) Lipid abnormalities in uremia, dialysis and transplantation. *Kidney Int.*, **19**, 625–37.
24. Chan, P.C., Persaud, J., Varghese, Z. *et al.* (1989) Apolipoprotein B turnover in dialysis patients: its relationship to pathogenesis of hyperlipidemia. *Clin. Nephrol.*, **31**, 88–95.
25. Cattran, D.C., Fenton, S.S.A., Wilson, D.R. and Steiner, G. (1976) Defective triglyceride removal in lipemia associated with peritoneal dialysis and haemodialysis. *Ann. Intern. Med.*, **85**, 29–33.
26. Verschoor, L., Lammers, R. and Birkenhager, J.C. (1978) Triglyceride turnover in severe chronic non-nephrotic renal failure. *Metab.: Clin. Exp.*, **27**, 879–83.
27. Chan, M.K., Varghese, Z., Persaud, J.W. *et al.* (1980) Fat clearance before and after heparin in chronic renal failure – haemodialysis reduces post-heparin fractional clearance rates of intralipid. *Clin. Chim. Acta*, **108**, 95–101.
28. Wang, C.S., Hartsuck, J. and McConathy, W.J. (1992) Structure and functional properties of lipoprotein lipase. *Biochim. Biophys. Acta*, **1123**, 1–17.
29. Kashyap, M.L., Mendoza, S.G., Campbell, M. *et al.* (1978) Lipoprotein lipase activator deficiency in very low density lipoproteins in rat nephrotic syndrome. *Experientia*, **34**, 1044–5.
30. Staprans, I., Anderson, C.D., Lurz, F.W. and Felts, J.M. (1980) Separation of a lipoprotein lipase cofactor from the alpha 1-acid glycoprotein fraction from the urine of nephrotic patients. *Biochim. Biophys. Acta*, **617**, 514–23.
31. Zilversmit, D.B. (1973) A proposal linking atherogenesis to the interaction of endothelial lipoprotein lipase with triglyceride-rich lipoproteins. *Circ. Res.*, **33**, 633–8.
32. Saxena, U., Klein, M.G., Vanni, T.M. and Goldberg, I.J. (1992) Lipoprotein lipase increases low density lipoprotein retention by subendothelial cell matrix. *J. Clin. Invest.*, **89**, 373–80.
33. Persson, B. (1973) Lipoprotein lipase activity of human adipose tissue in health and in some diseases with hyperlipidemia as a common feature. *Acta. Med. Scand.*, **193**, 457–62.
34. Bagdade, J.D., Porte, D. and Bierman, E.L. (1968) Hypertriglyceridemia. A metabolic consequence of chronic renal failure. *N. Engl. J. Med.*, **279**, 181–5.
35. Ljunghall, S., Lithell, H., Vessby, B. and Wide, L. (1978) Glucose and lipoprotein metabolism in primary hyperparathyroidism. Effects of parathyroidectomy. *Acta Endocrinol.*, **89**, 580–9.

36. Lacour, B., Basile, C., Drueke, T. and Funck-Brentano, J.L. (1982) Parathyroid function and lipid metabolism in the rat. *Miner. Electrolyte Metab.*, **7**, 157–65.
37. Akmal, M., Kasim, S.E., Soliman, A.R. and Massry, S.G. (1990) Excess parathyroid hormone adversely affects lipid metabolism in chronic renal failure. *Kidney Int.*, **37**, 854–8.
38. Chan, M.K., Ramdial, L., Varghese, Z. *et al.* (1982) Plasma lecithin-cholesterol acyltransferase activities in uraemic patients. *Clin. Chim. Acta*, **119**, 65–72.
39. Chan, M.K. (1989) Gemfibrozil improves abnormalities of lipid metabolism in patients on continuous ambulatory peritoneal dialysis: the role of postheparin lipases in the metabolism of high-density lipoprotein subfractions. *Metab.: Clin. Exp.*, **38**, 939–45.
40. Wheeler, D.C., Mistry, P., Persaud, J. *et al.* (1987) Very low density lipoprotein (VLDL), apolipoprotein B (APO B) kinetics in human nephrotic syndrome (abstract) 10th Int. Cong. Nephrol., London, UK.
41. Warwick, G.L., Packard, C.J., Demant, T. *et al.* (1991) Metabolism of apolipoprotein B-containing lipoproteins in subjects with nephrotic-range proteinuria. *Kidney Int.*, **40**, 129–38.
42. Joven, J., Vilella, E., Ahmad, S. *et al.* (1993) Lipoprotein heterogeneity in end-stage renal disease. *Kidney Int.*, **43**, 410–8.
43. Attman, P. and Alaupovic, P. (1991) Lipid abnormalities in chronic renal insufficiency. *Kidney Int.*, **39**, suppl 31, S-16–S-23.
44. Soutar, A.K., Myant, N.B. and Thompson, G.R. (1995) Simultaneous measurement of apolipoprotein B turnover in very low density and low density lipoproteins in familial hypercholesterolaemia. *Atherosclerosis*, **28**, 247–56.
45. Goldstein, J.L. and Brown, M.S. (1974) Binding and degradation of low density lipoproteins by cultured human fibroblasts. *J. Biol. Chem.*, **249**, 5153–62.
46. Iverius, P.H. (1972) The interaction between human plasma lipoproteins and connective tissue glycosaminoglycans. *J. Biol. Chem.*, **247**, 2607–13.
47. De Graaf, J., Hendriks, J.C., Demacker, P.N. and Stalenhoef, A.F. (1993) Identification of multiple dense LDL subfractions with enhanced susceptibility to *in vitro* oxidation among hypertriglyceridemic subjects. Normalization after clofibrate treatment. *Arteriosclerosis and Thrombosis*, **13**, 712–9.
48. Quinn, M.T., Parthasarathy, S. and Steinberg, D. (1988) Lysophosphatidylcholine: A chemotactic factor for human monocytes and its potential role in atherogenesis. *Proc. Natl. Acad. Sci. USA*, **85**, 2805–9.
49. Maggi, E., Bellazzi, R., Falaschi, F. *et al.* (1994) Enhanced LDL oxidation in uremic patients: an additional mechanism for accelerated atherosclerosis? *Kidney Int.*, **45**, 876–83.
50. Maggi, E., Bellazzi, R., Gazo, A. *et al.* (1994) Autoantibodies against oxidatively-modified LDL in uraemic patients undergoing dialysis. *Kidney Int.*, **46**, 869–76.
51. Moorhead, J.F., Persaud, J.W., Varghese, Z. and Sweny, P. (1993) Serum cholesterol falls spontaneously in nephrotic patients with progressive renal disease. *Renal Failure*, **15**, 389–93.
52. Horkko, S., Savolainen, M.J., Kervinen, K. and Kesaniemi, Y.A. (1992) Carbamylation-induced alterations in low-density lipoprotein metabolism. *Kidney Int.*, **41**, 1175–81.

53. Scanu, A.M. and Fless, G.M. (1990) Lipoprotein (a) heterogeneity and biological relevance. *J. Clin. Invest.*, **85**, 1709–15.
54. Dieplinger, H., Lackner, C., Kronenberg, F. *et al.* (1993) Elevated plasma concentrations of lipoprotein(a) in patients with end-stage renal disease are not related to the size of polymorphism of apolipoprotein(a). *J. Clin. Invest.*, **91**, 397–401.
55. Karadi, I., Romics, L., Palos, G. *et al.* (1989) Lp(a) lipoprotein concentration in serum of patients with heavy proteinuria of different origin. *Clin. Chem.*, **35**, 2121–3.
56. Thomas, M.E., Freestone, A., Varghese, Z. *et al.* (1992) Lipoprotein(a) in patients with proteinuria. *Nephrol. Dial. Transplant.*, **7**, 597–601.
57. Shoji, T., Nishizawa, Y., Nishitani, H. *et al.* (1992) High serum lipoprotein(a) concentrations in uremic patients treated with continuous ambulatory peritoneal dialysis. *Clin. Nephrol.*, **38**, 271–6.
58. Black, I.W. and Wilcken, D.E.L. (1992) Decreases in apolipoprotein(a) after renal transplantation: implications for lipoprotein(a) metabolism. *Clin. Chem.*, **38**, 353–7.
59. Haffner, S.M., Gruber, K.K., Aldrete, Jr, G. *et al.* (1992) Increased lipoprotein(a) concentrations in chronic renal failure. *J. Am. Soc. Nephrol.*, **3**, 1156–62.
60. Webb, A.T., Reaveley, D.A., O'Donnell, M. *et al.* (1993) Does cyclosporin increase lipoprotein(a) concentrations in renal transplant recipients? *Lancet*, **341**, 268–70.
61. Kaysen, G.A. (1991) Hyperlipidemia of the nephrotic syndrome. *Kidney Int.*, **39**, supp 31, S-8–S-15.
62. Rapoport, J., Aviram, M., Chaimovitz, C. and Brook, J.G. (1978) Defective high-density lipoprotein composition in patients on chronic hemodialysis. A possible mechanism for accelerated atherosclerosis. *N. Engl. J. Med.*, **299**, 1326–9.
63. Miller, G.J. and Miller, N.E. (1975) Plasma-high-density-lipoprotein concentration and development of ischaemic heart-disease. *Lancet*, **1**, 16–9.
64. Bowry, V.W., Stanley, K.K. and Stocker, R. (1992) High density lipoprotein is the major carrier of lipid hydroperoxides in human blood plasma from fasting donors. *Proc. Natl. Acad.* Sci. USA, **89**, 10316–20.
65. Munk, G. (1913) Klinische diagnostik der degenerativen nierenerkrankungen. *Z. Clin. Med.*, **78**, 1–52.
66. Virchow, R. (1860) A more precise account of fatty metamorphosis, in *Cellular Pathology* (ed. F. Chance), Churchill, London, p. 342.
67. Munk, F. (1916) Die nephrosen. *Medizinische Klinik*, **40**, 1047–50.
68. Kimmelstiel, P. and Wilson, C. (1936) Intercapillary lesions in the glomeruli of the kidney. *Am. J. Pathol.*, **12**, 83–98.
69. Wilens, S.L., Elster, S.K. and Baker, J.P. (1951) Glomerular lipidosis in intercapillary glomerulosclerosis. *Ann. Intern. Med.*, **24**, 592–607.
70. French, S.W., Yamanaka, W. and Ostwald, R. (1967) Dietary induced glomerulosclerosis in the guinea pig. *Arch. Pathol.*, **83**, 204–10.
71. Hutchinson, F.N. (1993) Proteinuria, hyperlipidemia, and the kidney. *Miner. Electrolyte Metab.*, **19**, 127–36.
72. Wheeler, D.C., Varghese, Z. and Moorhead, J.F. (1989) Hyperlipidemia in nephrotic syndrome. *Am. J. Nephrol.*, **9**, suppl 1, 78–84.
73. Warwick, G.L., Caslake, M.J., Boulton-Jones, J.M. *et al.* (1990) Low-density lipoprotein metabolism in the nephrotic syndrome. *Metabolism*, **39**, 187–92.

74. Conwill, D.E., Granger, D.N., Cook, B.H. *et al.* (1977) The effect of serum oncotic pressure on serum cholesterol levels: a study in normal and nephrotic subjects. *South Med. J.*, **70**, 456–8.
75. Pullinger, C.R., North, J.D., Teng, B.B. *et al.* (1989) The apolipoprotein B gene is consitutively expressed in HepG2 cells: regulation of secretion by oleic acid, albumin and insulin, and measurement of the mRNA half-life. *J. Lipid Res.*, **30**, 1065–77.
76. Yedgar, S., Weinstein, D.B., Patsch, W. *et al.* (1982) Viscosity of culture medium as a regulator of synthesis and secretion of very low density lipoproteins by cultured hepatocytes. *J. Biol. Chem.*, **257**, 2188–92.
77. Yamauchi, A., Fukuhara, Y., Yamamoto, S. *et al.* (1992) Oncotic pressure regulates gene transcriptions of albumin and apolipoprotein B in cultured rat hepatoma cells. *Am. J. Physiol.*, **263**, C397–C404.
78. Zucchelli, P., Ponticelli, C., Cagnoli L. and Passerini, P. (1987) Long-term outcome of idiopathic membranous nephropathy with nephrotic syndrome. *Nephrol. Dial. Transplant.*, **2**, 73–8.
79. Williams, P.S., Fass, G. and Bone, J.M. (1988) Renal pathology and proteinuria determine progression in untreated mild/moderate chronic renal failure. *Q. J. Med.*, **67**, 343–54.
80. Saku, K., Reddy, G.S., Hynd, B.A. and Kashyap, M.L. (1984) Renal handling of high-density lipoproteins by isolated perfused kidneys. *Metabolism*, **33**, 432–8.
81. Segal, P., Gidez, L.I., Vega, G.L., *et al.* (1979) Apoproteins of high density lipoproteins in the urine of normal subjects. *J. Lipid Res.*, **20**, 784–8.
82. Peterson, D.R., Hjelle, J.T., Carone, F.A. and Moore, P.A. (1984) Renal handling of plasma high density lipoprotein. *Kidney Int.*, **26**, 411–21.
83. Short, C.D., Durrington, P.N., Mallick, N.P. *et al.* (1986) Serum and urinary high density lipoproteins in glomerular disease with proteinuria. *Kidney Int.*, **29**, 1224–8.
84. Jungst, D., Caselmann, W.H., Kutschera, P. and Weisweiler, P. (1987) Relation of hyperlipidemia in serum and loss of high density lipoproteins in urine in the nephrotic syndrome. *Clin. Chim. Acta*, **168**, 159–67.
85. Joven, J., Villabona, C., Vilella, E. *et al.* (1990) Abnormalities of lipoprotein metabolism in patients with the nephrotic syndrome. *N. Engl. J. Med.*, **323**, 579–84.
86. Ross, P. (1993) The pathogenesis of atherosclerosis: a perspective for the 1990s. *Nature*, **362**, 801–9.
87. Diamond, J.R. and Karnovsky, M.J. (1988) Focal and segmental glomerulosclerosis: analogies to atherosclerosis. *Kidney Int.*, **33**, 917–24.
88. Kasiske, B.L., O'Donnell, M.P., Cowardin, W. and Keane, W.F. (1990) Lipids and the kidney. *Hypertension*, **15**, 443–50.
89. West, K.M., Erdreich, L.J. and Stober, J.A. (1980) A detailed study of risk factors for retinopathy and nephropathy in diabetes. *Diabetes*, **29**, 501–8.
90. Walker, W.G. (1993) Relation of lipid abnormalities to progression of renal damage in essential hypertension, insulin-dependent and non insulin-dependent diabetes mellitus. *Miner. Electrolyte Metab.*, **19**, 137–43.
91. Krolewski, A.S., Warram, J.H. and Christlieb, A.R. (1994) Hypercholesterolemia – a determinant of renal function loss and death in IDDM patients with nephropathy. *Kidney Int.*, **45**, S-125–S-131.
92. Yoshida, Y., Fogo, A. and Ichikawa, I. (1989) Glomerular hemodynamic changes vs. hypertrophy in experimental glomerular sclerosis. *Kidney Int.*, **35**, 654–60.

93. O'Donnell, M., Kasiske, B.L., Katz, S.A. *et al.* (1992) Lovastatin but not enalapril reduces glomerular injury in Dahl salt-sensitive rats. *Hypertension*, **20**, 651–8.
94. Lim, V.S., Sibley, R. and Spargo, B. (1974) Adult lipoid nephrosis: clinicopathological correlations. *Ann. Intern. Med.*, **81**, 314–20.
95. Lee, H.S., Lee, J.S. and Ko, K.W. (1991) Intraglomerular lipid deposition in routine biopsies. *Clin. Nephrol.*, **36**, 67–75.
96. Anderson, S. and Brenner, B.M. (1988) Intraglomerular hypertension: implications and drug treatment. *Ann. Rev. Med.*, **39**, 243–53.
97. Kaysen, G.A. and Davies, W.R. (1990) Reduction in proteinuria attenuates hyperlipidemia in the nephrotic syndrome. *J. Am. Soc. Nephrol*, **1**, suppl 2, S-75–S-79.
98. Manzato, E., Capurso, A. and Crepaldi, G. (1993) Modification of cardiovascular risk factors during antihypertensive treatment: a multicentre trial with quinapril. *J. Int. Med. Res.*, *21*, 15–25.
99. Pollare, T., Lithell, H. and Berne, C. (1989) A comparison of the effects of hydrochlorothiazide and captopril on glucose and lipid metabolism in patients with hypertension. *N. Engl. J. Med.*, **321**, 868–73.
100. Parthasarathy, S., Printz, D.J., Boyd, D. *et al.* (1986) Macrophage oxidation of low density lipoprotein generates a modified form recognized by the scavenger receptor. *Arteriosclerosis*, **6**, 505–10.
101. Parthasarathy, S., Fong, L.G., Otero, D. and Steinberg, D. (1987) Recognition of solubilized apoproteins from delipidated, oxidized low density lipoprotein (LDL) by the acetyl-LDL receptor. *Proc. Natl. Acad. Sci. USA*, **84**, 537–40.
102. Schreiner, G.F. (1991) The role of the macrophage in glomerular injury. *Semin. Nephrol.*, **11**, 268–75.
103. Magil, A.B. and Frohlich, J.J. (1991) Monocytes and macrophages in focal glomerulosclerosis in Zucker rats. *Nephron*, **59**, 131–8.
104. Pesek-Diamond, I., Ding, G., Frye, J. and Diamond, J.R. (1992) Macrophages mediate adverse effects of cholesterol feeding in experimental nephrosis. *Am. J. Physiol.*, **263**, F776–F783.
105. Palinski, W., Rosenfeld, M.E., Yla-Hertuala, S. *et al.* (1989) Low density lipoprotein undergoes oxidative modification *in vivo*. *Procl. Natl. Acad. Sci. USA*, **86**, 1372–6.
106. Berliner, J.A., Territo, M.C., Sevanian, A. *et al.* (1990) Minimally modified low density lipoprotein stimulates monocyte endothelial interactions. *J. Clin. Invest.*, **85**, 1260–6.
107. Hoff, H.F., O'Neil, J., Pepin, J.M. and Cole, T.B. (1990) Macrophage uptake of cholesterol-containing particles derived from LDL and isolated from atherosclerotic lesions. *Eur. Heart J.*, **11**, suppl E, 105–15.
108. Ding, G., Pesek-Diamond, I. and Diamond, J.R. (1993) Cholesterol, macrophages, and gene expression of TGF-beta 1 and fibronectin during nephrosis. *Am. J. Physiol.*, **264**, F577–F584.
109. Moorhead, J.F., Wheeler, D.C. and Varghese, Z. (1989) Glomerular structures and lipids in progressive renal disease. *Am. J. Med.*, **87**(5N), 12N–20N.
110. Fernando, R.L., Varghese, Z. and Moorhead, J.F. (1993) Oxidation of low-density lipoproteins by rat mesangial cells and the interaction of oxidized low-density lipoproteins with rat mesangial cells *in vitro*. *Nephrol. Dial. Transplant.*, **8**, 512–8.
111. Wheeler, D.C., Chana, R.S., Tolpey, N. *et al.* (1994) Oxidation of low

density lipoprotein by mesangial cells may promote glomerular injury. *Kidney Int.*, **45**, 1628–36.

112. Kaplan, R., Aynedjian, H.S., Schlondorff, D. and Bank, N. (1990) Renal vasocontriction caused by short-term cholesterol feeding is corrected by thromboxane antagonist or probucol. *J. Clin. Invest*, **86**, 1707–14.
113. Bank, N. (1993) Renal hemodynamic consequences of hyperlipidemia. *Miner. Electrolyte Metab.*, **19**, 165–72.
114. Boyce, N.W., Tipping, P.G. and Holdsworth, S.R. (1989) Glomerular macrophages produce reactive oxygen species in experimental glomerulonephritis. *Kidney Int.*, **35**, 778–82.
115. Radeke, H.H., Meier, B., Topley, N. *et al.* (1990) Interleukin 1-alpha and tumor necrosis factor-alpha induced oxygen radical production in mesangial cells. *Kidney Int.*, **37**, 767–75.
116. Coritsidis, G., Rifici, V., Gupta, S. *et al.* (1991) Preferential binding of oxidized LDL to rat glomeruli *in vivo* and cultured mesangial cells *in vitro*. *Kidney Int.*, **39**, 858–66.
117. Oberle, G.P., Niemeyer, J., Thaiss, F. *et al.* (1992) Increased oxygen radical and eicosanoid formation in immune-mediated mesangial cell injury. *Kidney Int.*, **42**, 69–74.
118. Kelley, V.E., Ferretti, A., Izui, S. and Strom, T.B. (1985) A fish oil diet rich in eicosapentaenoic acid reduces cyclooxygenase metabolites, and suppresses lupus in MRL-1pr mice. *J. Immunol.*, **134**, 1914–9.
119. Wheeler, D.C., Persaud, J.W., Fernando, R. *et al.* (1990) Effects of low-density lipoproteins on mesangial cell growth and viability *in vitro*. *Nephrol. Dial. Transplant.*, **5**, 185–91.
120. Kasiske, B.L. and Napier, J. (1985) Glomerular sclerosis in patients with massive obesity. *Am. J. Nephrol.*, **5**, 45–50.
121. Chung-Park, M., Petrelli, M., Tavill, A.S. *et al.* (1982) Renal lipidosis associated with arteriohepatic dysplasia (Alagille's Syndrome). *Clin. Nephrol.*, **18**, 314–20.
122. Isoniemi, H., Nurminen, M., Tikkanen, M.J. *et al.* (1994) Risk factors predicting chronic rejection of renal allografts. *Transplantation*, **57**, 68–72.
123. Schreiner, G.F., Flye, W., Brunt, E. *et al.* (1988) Essential fatty acid depletion of renal allografts and prevention of rejection. *Science*, **240**, 1032–3.
124. Risdon, R.A., Sloper, J.C. and De Wardener, H.E. (1968) Relationship between renal function and histological changes found in renal biopsy specimens from patients with persistent glomerular nephritis. *Lancet*, **2**, 363–6.
125. Wehrmann, M., Bohle, A., Bogenschutz, O. *et al.* (1990) Long-term prognosis of chronic idiopathy membranous glomerulonephritis. *Clin. Nephrol.*, **31**, 67–76.
126. Bohle, A., Mackensen-Haen, S., Von Gise, H. *et al.* (1990) The consequences of tubulo-interstitial changes for renal function in glomerulopathies: a morphometric and cytological analysis. *Pathol. Res. Pract.*, **186**, 135–44.
127. Neuman, M., West, M. and Zimmerman, H.J. (1961) The relationship between proteinuria and fatty elements in the urine sediment. *Am. J. Med. Sci.*, **241**, 617–24.
128. Thomas, M.E. and Schreiner, G.F. (1992) Proximal tubule (PT) cells show differential metabolism of endocytosed fatty acids (FA) into neutral lipids. *J. Am. Soc. Nephrol.* **3**, 752.
129. Zucker, L.M. (1965) Hereditary obesity in the rat associated with hyperlipemia. *Ann. NY Acad. Sci.*, **131**, 447–58.

130. Kashyap, M.L., Ooi, B.S., Hynd, B.A. *et al.* (1979) Sequestration and excretion of high density and low density lipoproteins by the kidney in human nephrotic syndrome. *Artery*, **6**, 108–21.
131. Streather, C.P., Varghese, Z., Moorhead, J.F. and Scoble, J.E. (1993) Lipiduria in renal disease. *Am. J. Hypertens.*, **6**, 353S–357S.
132. Moorhead, J.F., El Nahas, A.M., Harry, D. *et al.* (1983) Focal glomerular sclerosis and nephrotic syndrome with partial lecithin: cholesterol acyltransferase deficiency and discoidal high density lipoprotein in plasma and urine. *Lancet*, **1**, 936–7.
133. Ong, A.C.M. and Moorhead, J.F. (1994) Tubular lipidosis: epiphenomenon or pathogenetic lesion in human renal disease? *Kidney Int.*, **45**, 753–62.
134. Ong, A.C.M., Jowett, T.P., Moorhead, J.F. and Owen, J.S. (1994) Human high density lipoproteins stimulate endothelin-1 release by cultured human proximal tubular cells. *Kidney Int.*, **46**, 1315–21.
135. Moorhead, J.F. (1991) Lipids and progressive kidney disease. *Kidney Int.*, **39**, suppl 31, S-35–S-40.
136. Wissler, R.W. (1978) Progression and regression of atherosclerotic lesions. *Adv. Exp. Med. Biol.*, **104**, 77–101.
137. Superko, H.R. (1991) Prevention and regression of atherosclerosis with drug therapy. *Clin. Cardiol.*, **14**, 1–47.
138. Koga, N. and Iwata, Y. (1991) Pathological and angiographic regression of coronary atherosclerosis by LDL-apheresis in a patient with familial hypercholesterolemia. *Atherosclerosis*, **90**, 9–21.
139. Yamamoto, A. (1991) Regression of atherosclerosis in humans by lowering serum cholesterol. *Atherosclerosis*, **89**, 1–10.
140. Pavlovic, N.M., Malik, S., Chan, M.K. *et al.* (1984) The influence of high fat diet on the proteinuria in puromycin induced nephrotic syndrome in rats. *Clin. Sci.*, **66**, 26P.
141. Kasiske, B.L., O'Donnell, M.P., Garvis, W.J. and Keane, W.F. (1988) Pharmacologic treatment of hyperlipidemia reduces glomerular injury in rat 5/6 nephrectomy model of chronic renal failure. *Circ. Res.*, **62**, 367–74.
142. Wheeler, D.C., Nair, D.R., Persaud, J.W. *et al.* (1991) Effects of dietary fatty acids in an animal model of focal glomerulosclerosis. *Kidney Int.*, **39**, 930–7.
143. Kelley, V.E. and Izui, S. (1983) Synergistic action of immune complexes and lipid in glomerular injury. *Am. J. Pathol.*, **111**, 288–97.
144. Lefkowith, J.B., Rovin, B. and Schreiner, G.F. (1989) Depletion of resident glomerular macrophages by essential fatty acid deficiency protects against glomerulonephritis. *Adv. Prostaglandin Thromboxane Leukotriene Res.*, **19**, 560–3.
145. Sanfelippo, M.L., Swenson, R.S. and Reaven, G.M. (1978) Response of plasma triglycerides to dietary change in patients on hemodialysis., *Kidney Int.*, **14**, 180–6.
146. Grundy, S.M. and Vega, G.L. (1987) Fibric acids: effects on lipids and lipoprotein metabolism. *Am. J. Med.*, **83**, 9–20.
147. Pierides, A.M., Alvarez-Ude, F. and Kerr, D.N. (1975) Clofibrate-induced muscle damage in patients with chronic renal failure. *Lancet*, **2**, 1279–82.
148. Grundy, S.M. (1990) Management of hyperlipidemia of kidney disease. *Kidney Int.*, **37**, 847–53.
149. Sweny, P., Wheeler, D.C. *et al.* (1987) Dietary fish oil supplements preserve renal function in renal transplant recipients with cronic vascular rejection. *Nephrol. Dial. Transplant*, **4**, 1070–5.

150. Martinez Hernandez, B.E., Persaud, J.W., Varghese, Z. and Moorhead, J.F. (1993) Low dose-simvastatin is safe in hyperlipidaemic renal transplant patients. *Nephrol. Dial. Transplant.*, **8**, 637–41.
151. Apanay, D.C., Neylan, J.F., Ragab, M.S. and Sgoutas, D.S. (1994) Cyclosporine increases the oxidizability of low-density lipoproteins in renal transplant recipients. *Transplantation*, **58**, 663–9.
152. Rabl, H., Khoschsorur, G., Colombo, T. *et al.* (1993) A multivitamin infusion prevents lipid peroxidation and improves transplantation performance. *Kidney Int.*, **43**, 912–7.
153. De Caterina, R., Caprioli, R., Giannessi, D. *et al.* (1993) n-3 fatty acids reduce proteinuria in patients with chronic glomerular disease. *Kidney Int.*, **44**, 843–50.
154. D'Amico, G., Gentile, M.G., Manna, G. *et al.* (1992) Effect of vegetarian soy diet on hyperlipidaemia in nephrotic syndrome. *Lancet*, **339**, 1131–4.
155. Donadio, J.V., Bergstralh, E.J., Offord, K.P. *et al.* (1994) Controlled trial of fish oil in IgA nephropathy. *N. Engl. J. Med.*, **331**, 1194–9.
156. Rabelink, A.J., Hene, R.J., Erkelens, D.W. *et al.* (1992) Partial remission of nephrotic syndrome in patient on long-term simvastatin. *Lancet*, **335**, 1045–6.
157. Nestel, P.J., Connor, W.E., Reardon, M.F. *et al.* (1984) Suppression by diets rich in fish oil of very low density lipoprotein production in man. *J. Clin. Invest.*, **74**, 82–9.
158. Dujovne, C.A., Harris, W.S., Colle Gerrond, L.L. *et al.* (1994) Comparison of effects of probucol versus vitamin E on *ex vivo* oxidation susceptibility of lipoproteins in hyperlipoproteinaemia. *Am. J. Cardiol.*, **74**, 38–42.
159. Valeri, A., Gelfand, J., Blum, C. and Appel, G.B. (1986) Treatment of the hyperlipidaemia of the nephrotic syndrome: a controlled trial. *Am. J. Kidney Dis.*, **VIII**, 388–96.
160. Kasiske, B.L., Velosa, J.A., Halstenson, C.E. *et al.* (1990) The effects of lovastatin in hyperlipidemic patients with the nephrotic syndrome. *Am. J. Kidney Dis.*, **XV**, 8–15.
161. Thomas, M.E., Harris, K.P.G., Ramaswamy, C. *et al.* (1993) Simvastatin therapy for hypercholesterolemic patients with nephrotic syndrome or significant proteinuria. *Kidney Int.*, **44**, 1124–9.
162. Vega, G.L. and Grundy, S.M. (1988) Lovastatin therapy in nephrotic hyperlipidemia: effects on lipoprotein metabolism. *Kidney Int.*, **33**, 1160–8.
163. Crook, M.A., Haq, S., Chusney, G. *et al.* (1994) Acute phase proteins and lipoprotein(a) in patients with severe hypercholesterolaemia and normal subjects. *Clin. Chim. Acta.*, **224**, 199–201.
164. Lussier-Cacan, S., Dubreuil-Quidoz, S., Roederer, G. *et al.* (1993) Influence of probucol on enhanced LDL oxidation after fish oil treatment of hypertriglyceridaemic patients. *Arteriosclerosis and Thrombosis*, **13**, 1790–7.
165. Thompson, G.R., Maher, V.M., Matthews, S. *et al.* (1995) Familial hypercholesterolaemic regression study: a randomized trial of low-density-lipoprotein apheresis. *Lancet*, **345**, 811–6.
166. Sakia, S., Muen, M., Iino, Y. *et al.* (1992) Effect of LDL apheresis in patients with drug-resistant nephrotic syndrome. Multi-center cooperative study. *Kidney Dial.*, **33**, 321–8.

# 10

# Complications of chronic renal failure

*K. Erbeck, T.A. Golper and S. Goldfarb*

## 10.1 INTRODUCTION AND PATHOPHYSIOLOGY

The complications of chronic renal failure (CRF) include those of the uremic syndrome as well as those of renal replacement therapies. This chapter will address the complications of uremia, chronic ambulatory peritoneal dialysis (CAPD) and hemodialysis, noting problems that are common as well as those that are unique to each of the three. Guidelines for diagnosis, management and prevention will also be discussed where appropriate. CRF consists essentially of progressive retention of nitrogenous waste products, leading to a state of systemic toxicity that affects (adversely) the function of multiple organ systems. The exact nature of the putative 'toxin(s)' remains a mystery. Fortunately, many of the complications are either treatable or preventable. The success of long-term dialysis has allowed the evolution of novel complications which have been identified recently. Thus, the physician needs to monitor critically a variety of biochemical and clinical functions in the patient suffering from CRF.

## 10.2 LIPID ABNORMALITIES AND ACCELERATED ATHEROSCLEROSIS

There is a 50% incidence of hyperlipidemia in the total dialysis population and the most prevalent pattern is type IV – increased total trigly-

*Renal Disease.* Edited by G. Venkat Raman. Published in 1998 by Chapman & Hall, London. ISBN 0 412 45700 8.

ceride (TG), increased very low-density lipoprotein (VLDL), decreased high-density lipoprotein cholesterol (HDL-C), and normal total cholesterol [1]. The longer a patient is treated by hemodialysis (HD), the lower the cholesterol and the better the ratio of HDL-C/LDL-C.

In CAPD patients the lipid profile is similar to non-dialyzed uremic patients, with both apolipoproteins A and B elevated. Significant losses into peritoneal dialysate of antiatherogenic Apo-A-1 with negligible losses of atherogenic Apo-B is a problem which leads to adverse plasma atherogenic profiles. The selective loss of HDL compared to LDL may increase the risk of coronary disease in CAPD patients more than in HD patients.

In patients with and without uremia these patterns are associated with an increased incidence of ischemic coronary heart disease. Atherosclerotic vascular lesions have been shown to regress in patients whose hyperlipidemia has been successfully treated. Thus, this rationale may be reasonably extrapolated to patients in dialysis. There is a potential role for lipid abnormalities as a cause of progression of renal disease, but this is discussed in detail elsewhere (Chapter 9).

### 10.2.1 Pathogenesis

The mechanisms of hypertriglyceridemia in uremia include increased hepatic production and impaired clearance from the circulation. In uremia there is a low concentration of cell-membrane insulin receptors, poor receptor–insulin affinity, and a post-receptor defect in the glycolytic cycle. This leads to the paradoxical condition of peripheral insulin resistance and relative hyperinsulinemia, which then stimulates hepatic TG synthesis [2].

Hypercalcemia accompanying hyperparathyroidism is associated with reduced tissue sensitivity to insulin. Parathyroid hormone (PTH) contributes to this reduced tissue sensitivity to insulin, impairs insulin secretion and may inhibit lipoprotein lipase, the enzyme responsible for clearing TG from the plasma. Other as yet unidentified inhibitors of this enzyme are also present in uremia. Independent of lipids, PTH may have an effect on the acceleration of atherosclerosis through its effects on cellular calcium movement, particularly in vascular smooth muscle [1].

### 10.2.2 Patient-controlled therapies (*Table 10.1*)

*Ideal weight*

The achievement of ideal body weight is the first step in the management of elevated VLDL. Weight and elevated TG levels are correlated in dialysis patients. Simple hypocaloric diets administered to obese

**Table 10.1** Patient-controlled therapies to lower lipids

| |
|---|
| Achievement of ideal body weight |
| Aerobic exercise |
| Special diet manipulations |
| Control of hyperparathyroidism and phosphate |
| High-carbohydrate, high-fiber, low-fat, low-cholesterol diet high in mono- and polyunsaturates |
| Avoidance of ethanol and simple carbohydrates |
| Fluid and salt restriction in CAPD (to preclude the frequent use of hypertonic peritoneal dialysate, i.e. to avoid the intraperitoneal absorption of glucose) |

hyperlipidemic subjects result in concomitant weight reduction and improvement in serum lipid abnormalities. Since one pound of adipose tissue is equivalent to 3500 calories, weight reduction is often combined with an exercise program. Furthermore, weight loss is associated with improved blood pressure control.

### *Exercise*

A graded exercise program, alone or with weight reduction, provides additional beneficial effects on serum lipid levels. Aerobic exercise training in hemodialysis patients has been shown to result in improvement in type IV hyperlipidemia, glucose uptake, oxygen uptake, anemia, hypertension and mental well-being. For this program to be effective, the patient and physician must have mutually agreed goals, which are realistic and achievable. Lowering lipids is only one aspect and, in certain patients, emphasizing improvement in well-being or lowering blood pressure (and subsequently lowering doses of antihypertensive drugs) should be stressed. Walking, jogging, cycling and swimming are the major exercise modalities for dialysis patients. A cardiologic and orthopedic history and examination and an understanding of the goals are all that are needed to prescribe an individualised exercise program. The key is to know the individual patients, to communicate and to encourage them. Improved hematocrits with erythropoietin (EPO) therapy should assist in improving exercise tolerance.

### *Diet*

Phosphate and calcium control and the subsequent avoidance of hyperparathyroidism may lower the risk of end stage renal disease (ESRD)-related atherosclerosis (see above).

Nitrogen breakdown products may modify lipoprotein composition (carbamylation) in an adverse manner. The low-protein, high-carbohydrate diet of chronic dialysis patients is necessary to avoid symptoms of uremic toxicity. However, in some patients the high carbohydrate intake contributes to hyperlipidemia. Low-carbohydrate and relatively high-fat diets have been shown to lower TG levels in hemodialysis patients without pre-existing hyperlipidemia. A high-carbohydrate, low-fat, low-cholesterol, low-saturated-fat diet also improves the hyperlipidemia in some dialysis patients. A reasonable diet prescription for severe hyperlipidemia in dialysis patients would be 20% of total calories as fats, total cholesterol intake of 100 mg/day, and complex carbohydrates used to maintain a eucaloric state. Unnecessary simple carbohydrates (sucrose and other disaccharides) and alcohol intake should be moderated.

### 10.2.3 Physician-controlled therapies (*Table 10.2*)

*Dialytic adjustments*

*Buffer*

Although uremic hyperlipidemia develops prior to the initiation of dialytic therapy, dialysis or dialysate composition may exacerbate the pre-existing condition. Acetate is a source of calories as well as a

**Table 10.2** Physician-controlled therapies to lower lipids

| |
|---|
| Dialytic manipulation |
| Bicarbonate versus acetate in hemodialysis |
| Lactate versus acetate in peritoneal dialysis |
| Glucose-free hemodialysis |
| Avoidance of 2.5% and 4.25% dextrose peritoneal dialysates |
| Assurance of adequate dialysis |
| Hemofiltration, hemodiafiltration or high-flux dialysis |
| Drugs to avoid (relative contraindication) |
| Beta-adrenergic blocking agents |
| Hormones (androgens, estrogens, glucocorticoids) |
| Diuretics |
| Specific therapeutic agents |
| Activated charcoal, binding resins (e.g. cholestyramine) |
| Nicotinic acid, nicofuranose, acipimox |
| L-carnitine |
| Fish oils rich in PUFAs and EPA |
| Pantethine |
| Fibric acid derivatives (gemfibrozil, bezafibrate, beclobrate, fenofibrate, ciprofibrate) |
| HMG-CoA reductase inhibitors (simvastatin, lovastatin, pravastin) |

precursor of fatty acids and cholesterol. Over time even a small contribution by acetate to lipid production and deposition may contribute to hyperlipidemia and atherosclerosis. A large body of evidence suggests that acetate may play a role in hyperlipidemia. Since lactate is available as an alternative in peritoneal dialysis (PD) and bicarbonate is an alternative for HD, it seems reasonable to offer hyperlipidemic patients on dialysis a trial on non-acetate dialysate as an adjunct to other lipid-lowering maneuvers. Bicarbonate HD is associated with improved patient well-being and lactase PD is associated with a lower incidence of ultrafiltration failure, further supporting the move to avoiding acetate.

*Glucose*

In marginally nourished HD patients, modest glucose dialysate (100 to 200 mg/dl) seems reasonable. In hyperlipidemic or obese HD patients, there appears to be no advantage to the presence of glucose in the dialysate. Several studies have demonstrated a lowering of TG levels in patients switched from glucose-containing dialysate to glucose-free HD. The progressive rise in blood lipids in CAPD patients has been prevented by restricting the use of hypertonic dialysate. Since most CAPD patients are on an unrestricted diet, simple sodium and water restriction will usually suffice to decrease the frequency of hypertonic exchanges.

*Miscellaneous*

Although there is insufficient evidence that heparin is lipogenic, it appears that the use of 4–6 κDa heparin subfractions in hemodialysis patients is associated with a reduction in both TG and cholesterol. Improving dialysis efficiency (delivering more dialysis) by conventional means, as well as hemofiltration and high-flux HD, has been shown to improve lipid profiles. Heparin extracorporeal LDL precipitation in HD patients has been shown to reduce total cholesterol and LDL.

### 10.2.4 Drug therapy

Indications for treatment, levels of intervention and other details are discussed in Chapter 9.

*Drugs to avoid*

Most beta-adrenergic blocking agents, androgens, estrogens, glucocorticoids, diuretics and ethanol have tendencies to exacerbate hyperlipidemia. A few selective beta-blockers (such as pindolol, labetalol and celiprolol), calcium channel blockers, $\alpha_1$-blockers, angiotensin-converting enzyme inhibitors, α-methyldopa and clonidine are not associated with inducing hyperlipidemia. Lower doses or alternate day administration of glucocorticoids and estrogens may be advantageous.

### *Specific drug therapy*

Activated charcoal, ingested as a slurry four times a day, has been employed for the treatment of uremic hyperlipidemia and pruritus. Both situations are improved but patient acceptance has limited this approach. Charcoal capsules are less effective but better tolerated. There are no dose limitations other than patient tolerance.

Nicotinic acid is effective in uremic hypertriglyceridemia but its side effects limit its usefulness. Very low doses of aspirin may attenuate the flushing that follows nicotinic acid ingestion. Dosage of 1.5 g three times per day must be gradually achieved in some cases. Alternative drugs with similar effects are nicofuranose and acipimox.

L-Carnitine is an essential cofactor for fatty acid transport into mitochondria for oxidation. HD (but not necessarily CAPD) results in carnitine depletion. This may be exacerbated by the usual ESRD diet, which is low in carnitine. Carnitine depletion results in depressed mitochondrial oxidation of fatty acids (which leads to muscle weakness) and the cytoplasmic accumulation of lipids. Low-dose (5–10 mg/kg) L-carnitine supplementation (orally, intravenously post-dialysis or in the dialysate) has been shown to improve the type IV picture of both adult and pediatric HD patients. There are few adverse side effects from long-term oral supplements of L-carnitine. Additional benefits include a rise in HDL-C and hematocrit and greater muscle strength. A small proportion of L-carnitine recipients demonstrate a paradoxical rise in the TG level, especially if doses exceed 5 mg/kg/day.

Fish oils rich in polyunsaturated fatty acids (PUFA), especially eicosapentaenoic acid (EPA), are now available in capsule form. They are particularly effective for lowering TG in dialysis patients in doses of 1–4 g/day. Side effects are minimal except for a decrease in platelet count and aggregation. Pantethine, a coenzyme A precursor in the Krebs' cycle, has been shown by one group to reduce both cholesterol and TG in dialysis patients. Side effects include gastric discomfort and pruritus, but the agent is generally well tolerated. While this side-effect profile is attractive, corroborative studies are indicated. Effective doses range from 600 to 1200 mg/day.

Bile acid sequestrants such as cholestyramine and colestipol are generally effective in lowering cholesterol, but tend to cause constipation and drug malabsorption, problems which often already trouble dialysis patients. Probucol is generally used to lower cholesterol levels but is not a first-line drug. Doses of 500 m,g/day should be sufficient as this agent has an exceptionally long half-life even in normal subjects.

Newer fibric acid derivatives are less toxic to both liver and skeletal muscle than the previously used agent clofibrate. Nonetheless, hepatic damage, myositis, hyperkalemia and cholelithiasis are still major side effects. Gemfibrozil is effective in lowering TG in dialysis patients through the enhancement of the activities of the enzymes lipoprotein lipase and hepatic tryglyceride lipase. Fibric acid derivatives may also decrease hepatic uptake of fatty acids and decrease the synthesis of VLDL. Despite pharmacologic data that suggests a gemfibrozil dose reduction is unnecessary in dialysis patients, it is prudent to limit the dose to 600 mg/day, if possible.

HMG (3-hydroxy-3-methylglutaryl) CoA reductase inhibitors upregulate hepatic LDL receptors by inhibiting the rate-limiting step in the cholesterol synthetic pathway. Thus, they are used mainly to lower cholesterol levels, but in the process TGs also are decreased. Simvastatin and lovastatin in doses of 10–40 mg/day will effectively lower cholesterol levels but may cause rhabdomyolysis and liver dysfunction, particularly the latter agent, which is now going out of use. Pravastatin, which is more water-soluble, at the same dosage may have less effect on muscle cells [2].

## 10.3 CARDIAC PROBLEMS

Cardiac failure is common in ESRF and is due to a number of factors, the most important of which is simple fluid overload. Ischemic heart disease frequently coexists, hypertension is extremely common, and anemia is almost invariable. Rarely valvular abnormalities may aggravate the situation. Other potential contributing factors include endocarditis, pericardial effusion, uremic toxins such as phenols, catecholamines, PTH, viral myocarditis and excessive flow through an arteriovenous fistula. The result is often the development of the uremic 'cardiomyopathy'. Both dilated (or congestive) and hypertrophic varieties of cardiomyopathy (CMP) are seen. These classifications overlap and patients may actually change category during the course of the illness.

Dilated CMP is characterized by weak contraction and increased left ventricular end diastolic and left atrial pressures. Hypertrophic CMP is subclassified into obstructive and non-obstructive. Left ventricular hypertrophy (LVH) is defined in adults by maximal left ventricular wall thickness of $\geqslant$15 mm on echocardiogram. In non-obstructive CMP the stimulus for LVH is often unknown, but thought to be chronic hypertension. The LVH of obstructive CMP is secondary to obstruction of left ventricular outflow.

In uremic patients heart disease may be secondary to a number of systemic diseases. Amyloid may be deposited in the myocardium resulting in pump failure. Connective tissue diseases such as lupus erythematosus and polyarteritis nodosa may cause myocarditis. CMP may appear as a complication of diabetes mellitus.

CMP may be a consequence of renal disease and its therapy. It could be secondary to the increased cardiac output through the arteriovenous fistula which may have blood flow rates of over a liter per minute. Prior to the use of erythropoietin blood transfusions were frequently required, with subsequent iron deposition in the myocardium. Long-term steroid therapy of underlying renal disease can predispose to CMP, presumably by the same mechanism that affects skeletal muscle.

Prevention of left ventricular dysfunction is linked to the control of blood pressure and fluid balance. Aggressive treatment of hypertension in the earliest phases of renal disease should be attempted. Target dry weight should be constantly reviewed. In patients who are unable to restrict sodium and fluid intake between hemodialysis sessions, a switch to CAPD may be necessary. The risk of CMP from an arteriovenous (AV) fistula is low if the flow rate through the fistula is less than 20% of the cardiac output. A change to CAPD may be warranted, and the fistula may need to be closed. The hematocrit should be at least 30% for optimal cardiac function.

The management of patients with left ventricular dysfunction is based on distinguishing true myocardial failure from fluid overload or a combination of the two. Acute pulmonary edema may be a result of fluid overload or left ventricular failure secondary to hypertension or myocardial ischemia. Treatment is usually with ultrafiltration, unless hypotension precludes this or dialysis for electrolyte balance is needed. Vasodilatation with transdermal, oral, or intravenous nitrates is often useful, prior to ultrafiltration. The use of angiotensin-converting enzyme (ACE) inhibitors or other vasodilators may also be of benefit [3,4].

## 10.4 HYPERTENSION (see also Chapter 3)

Hypertension is more prevalent in ESRD patients with glomerular and primary vascular diseases (90–100%) than in patients with tubulo-interstitial diseases. Uremic patients tend to have high cardiac output, secondary to anemia, volume expansion, the presence of AV shunts, and the other factors discussed above. Patients on HD tend to have higher and more labile blood pressures (due to the intermittency of treatment) than patients on CAPD. The main reason for high blood pressure in uremic patients is impairment of excretion of salt and water by the diseased kidney. Inappropriate stimulation of the renin–angiotensin system, increased sympathetic activity and changes in vessel wall structure are important additional factors in the pathogenesis.

When high blood pressure is secondary to salt and water retention it is termed 'volume dependent'. Renal dysfunction leads to retention and maldistribution of fluid and electrolytes. Although sodium concentration and extracellular fluid and blood volume are linked, high sodium concentration may directly cause hypertension by increasing vascular wall resistance. Furthermore, hypercalcemia may increase peripheral resistance, and stimulate antidiuretic hormone, angiotensin II and norepinephrine activity.

Patients whose high blood pressure depends on disorders of renal neuroendocrine function demonstrate significant elevation of both plasma renin activity and angiotensin II. These patients may have hypertension refractory to treatment. The renin–angiotensin–aldosterone system may be mechanistically involved in the hypertension even though plasma renin level is normal. Other neuroendocrine factors involved in the pathogenesis of uremic hypertension are norepinephrine, dopamine, vasopressin, atrial natriuretic peptide and neuropeptide Y. The autonomic nervous system impairment reported in uremic patients involves a defect in high-pressure baroreceptors and the afferent limb of the autonomic reflex arc.

Hypertension is probably one of the most important factors in the development of accelerated atherosclerosis in uremic subjects. Left ventricular hypertrophy and eventual heart failure may be secondary to high blood pressure, compounded by problems in myocardial metabolism and coronary blood circulation [4]. In diabetics hypertension accelerates the progression of retinopathy as well as the deterioration of residual renal function. Cerebrovascular accidents occur more frequently in hypertensive uremics than in controls. In diabetics and smokers, peripheral vascular disease is particularly more severe in hypertensives.

For volume-dependent patients, rigid regulation of fluid intake to avoid water and salt overload is of crucial importance, combined with aggressive ultrafiltration at dialysis or hypertonic exchanges at CAPD. Ultrafiltration and intensive HD may exacerbate non-volume-dependent hypertension. Further volume depletion may result in decreased renal perfusion pressure and enhanced renin secretion. For example, angiotensin II activity is increased after HD. CAPD may control refractory hypertension better than HD for several reasons. First, volume removal may be more physiologic, avoiding renin stimulation. PD may clear hypertension-provoking molecules better than HD. Overall volume control may be better with PD. Lastly, the increased intra-abdominal pressure invoked by the presence of the dialysate may retard blood return to the heart, decreasing cardiac output and blood pressure.

Antihypertensive medications must be tailored to the patient. Because of accumulation, a drug with a renal route of excretion may be particularly helpful in non-compliant patients, but these drugs may precipitate hypotension during dialysis. Side effects must be considered. For example, a patient prone to hyperkalemia should not receive ACE inhibitors, and a man with prostatism may benefit from an alpha-adrenoceptor blocker. Treatment is discussed in detail in Chapter 3.

## 10.5 HYPOTENSION

Hypotension may occur in chronic renal failure patients as a consequence of volume depletion or decrease in cardiac output or peripheral vascular resistance. These may be due to coincidental events such as gastroenteritis, cardiac failure or sepsis. Occasionally, this may be secondary to salt-losing nephropathy (Chapter 8).

Hypotension is most frequently a consequence of salt and water loss through over-aggressive dialysis. In patients who are doing well and are eating adequately, 'dry weight' may rise but not be appreciated. To dialyse this patient down to his/her previous dry weight will provoke volume depletion. The distribution of volume may change unfavorably during dialysis. The rapid removal of extracellular solute by diffusion dialysis renders intracellular water hypertonic to extracellular water, causing plasma water to shift inside cells. This might occur in very uremic patients or during rapid high-efficiency dialysis. Dialyzing against a higher dialysate sodium concentration may help to prevent this transcellular water shift.

The rate of ultrafiltration influences blood volume. Cellular water must replace the plasma water lost to the dialyzer. High ultrafiltration rates may be caused by high resistance in the venous limb of the circuit or in the patient's vasculature. Ultrafiltration control machines and careful monitoring of venous pressure and intradialytic weight loss are methods to control this.

Hemorrhage occurs during HD because of anticoagulation during rapid changes in the shape of organs during dehydration, stretching blood vessels. Blood leakage into the dialysate compartment is usually quickly detected, although a large amount of blood may be lost rapidly. Internal hemorrhage into the urinary or gastrointestinal tracts is often silent until overt shock occurs.

Frequent assessment of the dry weight is the most important method to prevent hypotension. Treatment in most cases consists of water volume replacement by high osmolarity solutions and physiologic saline. Sequential treatment with isolated ultrafiltration followed by diffusion HD without any trans-membrane pressure gradient is effective in lowering the incidence of hypotension. The technique of high and low sodium dialysis (HLSD) is another method to avoid hypotension by preserving blood volume. In HLSD $[Na^+]$ alternates every 45 min between 160 and 130 mEq/l. During HLSD the volume of red blood cells fluctuates but not the total volume of blood. Lastly, constant high dialysate osmolarity conserves the blood volume during HD and prevents hypotension. Unlike HLSD, this technique may render the patient thirsty, resulting in larger interdialytic fluid gains.

Risk factors for hypotension during dialysis are advanced age, female sex, administration of antihypertensive drugs, and autonomic dysfunction. Hypotension may not be limited just to the intradialytic period. Factors that can diminish blood pressure without depletion in volume include impaired cardiac contractility or refilling, arrhythmias and pulmonary embolism (air or clot). Hypoxemia can be associated with primary pulmonary disease or the complement activation-mediated event early in dialysis (see below). Abnormalities in electrolyte metabolism impair contractility including hypocalcemia, hypercalcemia, hyperkalemia and severe acidosis (Section 10.3). Magnesium toxicity can cause hypotension and hypoventilation. Treatment includes ventilatory support, intravenous calcium and fluids. Hypercalcemia impairs ventricular compliance causing left ventricular underfilling [5].

Specific disorders of uremia may cause cardiomyopathy and hypotension. Experimental uremia is associated with activation of pericytes and myocardial fibrosis. Myocytes in general are dependent on free fatty acids as a major source of cell energy and carnitine deficiency impairs utilization of this substrate in muscle, possibly contributing to myocardial weakness.

Autonomic dysfunction is most often observed in diabetics, but does occur in other dialysis patients. It may manifest as arterial baroreceptor dysfunction, a primary failure of peripheral vasoconstriction of both arterioles and veins, an impaired cardiovascular response to naturally occurring volume stimuli, or a combination of these. Dialysis with cold dialysate decreases symptomatic hypotension. Bacterial infections may cause hypotension mediated by endotoxins and macrophage-derived inflammatory factors such as the tumour necrosis factor and interleukin-1.

Withholding antihypertensive medication until after hemodialysis treatment, cautious titration, and dose adjustment according to the pharmacokinetics of renal insufficiency will decrease the frequency of intradialytic hypotension secondary to medications.

Many cellulose dialysis membranes activate complement and thus initiate a cascade of immunologic events, including anaphylatoxin formation and sequestration of leukocytes in pulmonary capillaries with subsequent hypoxemia. This can impair myocardial function enough to provoke hypotension. If ethylene oxide sterilant is not completely removed in the rinsing of dialyzers, it can invoke an anaphylactic reaction with shock. This is treated by disconnecting the patient from the extracorporeal circuit and the standard medical care for anaphylaxis. ACE inhibitors also inhibit the metabolism of bradykinin, a vasodilator. There is an increased incidence of severe hypotension shortly after the onset of HD in patients receiving ACE inhibitors, particularly when utilizing polyacrylonitrile membranes (AN 69), but this has also been noted with other membranes. Lower dialysate calcium concentrations may enhance this risk. Should this occur, immediate supportive care and disconnection from the circuit is indicated. Avoidance of this combination of events would then be necessary. Fortunately, this is a rare occurrence. The reverse transport from dialysate to blood of bacterial endotoxin or other small toxic molecules can cause pyrexia and hypotension during the course of a dialysis treatment. While this theoretically would occur more frequently during high-flux dialysis, the frequency of occurrence during conventional dialysis is the same. Control of water quality is the way to avoid this problem. Epidemic hypotension in a dialysis center has been attributed to dialysate contamination with cleansing/disinfectant agents such as azide or formaldehyde. Acetate is a vasodilator and a negative inotrope. Its use as a buffer may contribute to the complement activation mentioned above. This can be eliminated either by avoiding acetate dialysate altogether or limiting its rate of backtransport by using a small surface area dialyzer. Intradialytic electrolyte changes can cause hypotension and are discussed in Section 10.7.

## 10.6 PERICARDITIS

Pericarditis may occur in up to 17% of uremic patients and is responsible for up to 2.5% of deaths. The exact etiology is still unknown but may be related to an increased production and/or ineffective removal of uremic toxins. The frequency of pericarditis is correlated with excessive concentration of urea, creatinine, uric acid and phosphorus, and severe secondary hyperparathyroidism. Immune complexes may be 'uremic toxins', responsible for uremic serositis. Their enhanced removal during PD compared to HD may explain the lower incidence of pericarditis in CAPD patients. Heparin administration in HD may induce hemorrhage into the pericardial cavity and may be one of the reasons why pericarditis complicates HD more often than PD. The impaired immune system in uremic patients may predispose these patients to pericarditis as a complication of a variety of bacterial and viral infections. Underlying systemic diseases (systemic lupus erythematosus, polyarteritis) may also cause direct injury to the pericardium.

The clinical manifestations of pericarditis include fever, jugular venous distension, pulsus paradoxus, chest pain, pleural–pericardial friction rub, hypotension, low cardiac output, and arrhythmias. Large effusions may cause cardiac tamponade. A long-term sequel is the development of constrictive pericarditis. There is a curious association with unexpected clotting of arteriovenous fistulae.

Early diagnosis, aggressive dialysis, non-steroidal anti-inflammatory drugs, close follow-up and prompt surgical intervention may help to improve the prognosis of pericarditis. Medical treatment consists of increased intensity of low-dose heparin hemodialysis and good nutrition with adequate calories and protein to counter tissue catabolism. In some refractory cases peritoneal or high-flux dialysis may be useful. Short courses of high doses of prednisone systemically have been tried, with doubtful results. Intrapericardial non-absorbable steroids may be used, as well as a trial of oral non-steroidal anti-inflammatory agents. Instillation into the pericardial sac of triamcinolone with intermittent drainage has been shown to improve pain, hemodynamics and effusion size. With large effusions or if the effusion progressively increases, surgical decompression by partial or complete pericardiectomy is necessary.

## 10.7 ARRHYTHMIAS

Transcellular $Na^+$, $K^+$, $Ca^{2+}$, and $Mg^{2+}$ transport is crucial to myocardial cell function. Tachycardia, increased excitability and rapid conduction are consequences of cell hyperactivity, where there is increased polarization potential from low extracellular potassium, high extracellular sodium and calcium, or increased activity of membrane ATPases. Junctional arrhythmias and blocks are consequences of hypoactivity, where there is a diminished polarization potential from high extracellular potassium, low intracellular potassium, low extracellular sodium and calcium, and toxicity of digitalis and some antiarrhythmic drugs. Electrolyte-induced alterations in conductivity and contractility are not always so easily classified.

Hyperkalemia decreases myocardial conduction and is exacerbated by hyponatremia, hypocalcemia, acidosis, high extracellular/intracellular potassium ratio and rapid rate of increasing extracellular potassium concentration. Hyperkalemia leads to AV nodal block or sinus arrest (initially manifested by prolonged P–R interval, culminating in a dropping of the P wave) and impairment of intra-atrial and intraventricular conduction (manifested by a widened QRS complex). Death may occur from ventricular tachycardia, fibrillation or asystole.

Hypokalemia may occur during dialysis with low potassium dialysate or during rapid correction of metabolic acidosis. The absolute potassium concentration may not be as important as its rate of decline. Hypokalemia usually manifests as atrial and ventricular extrasystoles, couplets, tachycardias and as mild conduction defects. Severe hypokalemia may cause ventricular fibrillation.

Hypercalcemia diminishes conduction velocity and shortens the refractory period, thereby facilitating re-entry and development of coupled beats, ventricular tachycardia and fibrillation. Hypocalcemia induced by citrate anticoagulation has been associated with potentially fatal cardiac arrhythmias.

Uremic patients are particularly vulnerable to these disorders. Uremic acidosis and vomiting-induced alkalosis are not infrequently seen in this patient population. Other factors may contribute to arrhythmias including anemia, ischemia, autonomic nervous system impairment, structural disease such as accessory pathways or abnormal valve function, cardiomyopathy, pericarditis and impairment in oxygen delivery to the myocardium secondary to dialysis-associated hypoxia. Patients with echocardiographic evidence of left ventricular hypertrophy are particularly at risk for ventricular arrhythmias.

Diagnosis of these disorders by cardiac monitoring during HD in high-risk patients is valuable. Home Holter monitoring is another diagnostic tool. Correction of the arrhythmia may involve changes in the dialysis prescription. For example, the dialysate potassium should be individualized. Increasing the concentration may prevent some arrhythmias but is not without risk of hyperkalemia. Chronic $K^+$ binding resins may be indicated if one is prone to hyperkalemia, but cannot tolerate aggressive intradialytic $K^+$ removal. When hyperkalemia is severe, the gradual lowering of $K^+$ is associated with fewer arrhythmias, compared to rapid changes in $K^+$. Lowering the dialysate calcium concentration from 1.75 to 1.25 mmol/l decreases the number of ventricular and supraventricular beats in selected patients. Cardiovascular instability is less common with bicarbonate rather than acetate buffer. A smaller extracorporeal blood commitment during dialysis may be helpful, utilizing shorter blood lines with hollow fiber and smaller surface-area devices. In patients with proven severe heart disease peritoneal dialysis may be preferable as it does not provoke or aggravate arrhythmias to the same extent as HD [6]. The use of antiarrhythmic medications should be reserved for situations in which treatment of the underlying condition fails. Doses must be adjusted for the degree of renal function and for the type of dialysis. Serum levels should be monitored periodically.

## 10.8 PULMONARY

A pulmonary complication of renal disease, specifically hemodialysis, is hypoxemia during dialysis. The hypoxemia is multifactorial, involving activation of the complement system with subsequent neutrophil sequestration in the pulmonary vasculature. The characteristics of the dialysis procedure also contribute. The combination of cuprophan membrane and acetate dialysate seems to result in the greatest degree of hypoxemia. An additional factor in the hypoxemia of dialysis is hypoventilation provoked by the dialytic removal of $CO_2$ [7].

Uremic pleuritis occurs in predialysis patients or those patients who are inadequately dialyzed. The fluid may have leukocytes, red blood cells, an elevated protein and low glucose. As in the treatment of pericarditis, tight heparinization should be used, especially if the fluid is hemorrhage. The presence of hydrothorax in the setting of CAPD may be due to communication of the peritoneal space with the pleural space. Thoracentesis reveals fluid with the characteristics of dialysate. Instillation of methylene dye in the dialysate with subsequent thoracentesis may be used to diagnose this phenomenon. The use of 99m technetium-labeled albumin is an accurate, non-invasive alternative test. Management of the problem may be difficult. Discontinuing CAPD in an effort to allow the defect to close is usually unsuccessful; surgical closure of the defect is the definitive form of treatment. On occasion, the patient may require transfer to hemodialysis, particularly if there is respiratory compromise.

## 10.9 ANEMIA

Under normal circumstances in healthy kidneys, the production of EPO (erythropoietin) is determined by oxygen supply and demand, with influence from epinephrine and sex hormones. It stimulates late committed erythroid precursors to grow into mature erythrocytes. Both impaired production and abnormal regulation are factors affecting plasma levels in uremic patients. Regulatory dysfunction includes changes in oxygen delivery and demands, impairment of the marrow precursors to respond to low levels of the hormone (receptor dysfunction), and uremic plasma factors that may inhibit normoblast maturation (post-receptor dysfunction).

Therapy with androgens may improve the biological effect of EPO. Initiation of dialysis improves hematocrit. The most effective treatment for impaired erythropoiesis is the addition of exogenous EPO or transplantation. Clinical effects of EPO include increased hematocrit, improved cognition, improved libido and sexual function, restoration of menses, lactation, decrease in iron overload, and overall a significant improvement in quality of life.

EPO therapy is not without side effects. The most common of these are changes in hemodynamics such as increased arterial pressure and systemic vascular resistance, and decreased cardiac index and heart rate. Microcirculatory changes occurring after several months include impaired skin capillary flow.

Anastassiades *et al.* studied peritoneal dialysis patients and uremic, predialysis patients treated with EPO [10]. They found that plasma volume decreased in the peritoneal dialysis patients as red cell volume increased, with no net increase in blood volume. However, in the predialysis patients plasma volume failed to contract, causing a net increase in blood volume as hematocrit increased. Mean arterial pressure increased from 95 to 103 mm Hg in the predialysis group, leading the authors to conclude that changes in blood volume contribute to hypertension with EPO therapy. This may explain why the hypertension is generally controlled with volume removal on dialysis. Other potential mechanisms of erythropoetin-induced hypertension include inhibition of nitric oxide production (a vasodilator) or increase in endothelial cell production of endothelin-1, a vasoconstrictor. Other side effects of EPO include flu-like symptoms and headache. Initial concerns about the potential for increased vascular access thrombosis related to increased hematocrits have not been validated so far. The drug may be given to predialysis patients as well as those on dialysis if hematocrit is $<30\%$. The starting dose is 50–100 units/kg once to thrice weekly and titrated.

Resistance to EPO should be suspected if the hematocrit rate of increase is less than 1% per week in a patient receiving at least 50 U/kg three times weekly intravenously. Iron deficiency is a common cause of EPO resistance. Other underlying disorders such as aluminium toxicity, chronic infection, hyperparathyroidism and bone marrow disease can also contribute to resistance [9, 11].

## 10.10 OTHER HAEMATOLOGICAL ABNORMALITIES

Hemolysis may occur either as part of chronic uremia and/or as a complication of treatment (drug-induced or hemodialysis-induced hemolysis). In CRF there is a slowly dialyzable substance which causes hemolysis by decreasing red blood cell (RBC) pentose phosphate shunt activity, impairing cell membrane integrity and contributing to the formation of unstable oxidized hemoglobin compounds. There may be other substances in uremic plasma that contribute to hemolysis by impairing RBC NaK ATPase. Hypersplenism occurs in some HD patients, perhaps in part as a reaction to spallation products from the dialysis circuit entering the circulation and lodging in the spleen. Underlying systemic diseases (such as systemic lupus erythematosus, polyarteritis, malignant hypertension) can cause microangiopathy and hemolysis. Treatment of the primary disorder is indicated. If serum phosphorus is lowered abruptly or severely with phosphate binders or renal replacement therapy, RBCs become more fragile and hemolysis can ensue. Hemodialysis may cause hemolysis due to membrane contact with cells, other mechanical trauma, or chemical RBC damage from the dialysate solution (high concentrations of copper, aluminium, chloramines or zinc; or hypotonic, hyponatremic or hyperthermic dialysate).

Common sites of blood loss in uremic subjects include the gastrointestinal tract and vascular access, oozing at needle puncture sites and clotted dialyzers. Rarely one sees recurrent hemoperitoneum in women on CAPD. Operations on vascular access for infection, thrombosis, repair or creation are all associated with significant blood loss. Many patients demonstrate one or more defects of coagulation, including defective platelet aggregation, decreased platelet adhesiveness and bleeding time prolongation. The latter may be caused by urea, phenols and guanidinosuccinic acid inhibition of platelet function, increased vessel wall prostacyclin, impaired platelet arachidonic acid metabolism, increased level of PTH, severe anemia and by defects in relationships between platelets and vessel wall, factor VIII and fibrinogen. Repeated heparinization during hemodialysis may also be contributory.

To reduce the bleeding risk in these patients, it is necessary to exclude drugs that impair platelet function, e.g. non-steroidal anti-inflammatory drugs. Underlying diseases that contribute to coagulation defects should be treated. In susceptible individuals, intradialytic bleeding risks may be minimized by heparin-free hemodialysis, low-dose heparin dialysis, regional anticoagulation (reversal of heparin effect with protamine) and anticoagulation with citrate. If heparin-free dialysis is not possible, in the presence of systemic bleeding epoprostenol (prostacyclin) may be useful.

Adequate dialysis is partially defined as that dose necessary to improve platelet function. Substitutional therapy such as blood transfusion, cryoprecipitate and factor VIII may be helpful. Parenteral and oral estrogens as well as *d*,D-arginine vasopressin (DDAVP) have been shown to decrease bleeding time in uremic patients. Episodes of intraperitoneal hemorrhage during CAPD can be treated by room temperature 1.5% dextrose exchanges.

Iron deficiency may occur due to chronic gastrointestinal blood loss (from peptic ulceration or AV malformations), malabsorption of iron, low dietary iron, loss of blood during the dialysis procedure or during access surgery and frequent phlebotomies. To avoid further deficiency, replacement therapy with oral iron is indicated as early as possible and certainly when serum ferritin falls below 100 ng/ml. Parenteral therapy with iron dextran should be considered if enteral therapy is ineffective or poorly tolerated. Folic acid, which is readily dialyzable, should be replaced if deficient, or even routinely in patients on dialysis. Aluminium bone marrow toxicity may manifest as microcytic, hypochromic anemia. Secondary hyperparathyroidism causes bone marrow fibrosis. Chronic or recurrent infection in the partially immunosuppressed dialysis patient often exacerbates anemia. This may be due to down-regulation of the erythron response to EPO.

## 10.11 ENDOCRINE

The metabolism of thyroid hormone is altered in the patient with renal disease, probably related to changes in thyroid binding globulin (TBG) levels and the affinity of thyroxine for TBG. Consistent findings include a reduced total T4, low total T3, low free T4 index and a normal TSH. The response to TRH stimulation is blunted. However, the patient is clinically euthyroid.

Gonadal hormone levels are abnormal in patients of both sexes with renal disease. Testicular dysfunction is common, with elevated follicle-stimulating hormone (FSH) and luteinizing hormone (LH) levels, low sperm counts and low testosterone levels. In the female, the low estradiol and progesterone levels (with concomitant lack of response of LH and FSH) are associated with infertility. Menses are irregular or cease. Another common finding is an elevation of the prolactin level. No treatment is recommended for improving fertility or hyperprolactinemia. Testosterone preparations may be worth trying in impotent males, but the effect is variable.

## 10.12 MUSCULOSKELETAL

Although the association of carpal tunnel syndrome and chronic hemodialysis was recognized in the mid-1970s, the etiology was not clarified until the 1980s. A form of amyloid protein known as beta-2 microglobulin (B2M) is deposited in the synovia, bone and blood vessel walls of patients on dialysis for more than five years. The search for a way to eliminate the accumulation of this protein is under way, including the use of different dialysis membrane properties such as sieving and adsorption of the protein. There is evidence that B2M clearance can be significantly enhanced by the newer biocompatible membranes such as polyacrylonitrile and polysulfone; clearance also seems better with CAPD than with HD [12].

The development of a hernia of the abdominal musculature is a problem commonly seen in patients on CAPD. Umbilical, inguinal and diaphragmatic herniation may also occur. These are due to the increased intra-abdominal pressure incurred from the presence of dialysate, particularly in those patients requiring large volume exchanges. The use of IPD, CCPD, avoidance of exercise when full, and lowering the volume of exchange may all reduce the incidence of herniation. Surgical repair is usually necessary once the hernia has developed.

With the advent of recombinant human EPO, many of these problems have been solved. However, the drug is expensive. The most efficient way to administer it is by the subcutaneous route and the beta preparation is less painful than the alpha preparation. In addition, some CAPD patients demonstrate efficacy with large doses administered as infrequently as once a month. The most common cause of apparent EPO 'resistance' is iron deficiency [8, 9].

## 10.13 RENAL

The incidence of acquired cystic disease (defined as four or more cysts per failing kidney) ranges from less than 10% in the predialysis population to approximately 80% in patients on dialysis for more than three years, including hemodialysis and CAPD. The cysts by themselves however are generally of no clinical significance. Complications related to the presence of these cysts include infection, hematuria and tumor formation, all of which are fortunately rare [13].

Nephrolithiasis may occasionally develop in the patient with renal failure. Much more common is the primary occurrence of stone disease (see Chapter 7). The usual stone composition includes calcium oxalate monohydrate, calcium apatite and protein matrix (B2 microglobulin). Accumulation of oxalate occurs in patients with renal failure. Clearance of oxalate by CAPD is less efficient than hemodialysis. Risk factors for the development of calcium oxalate stones are the administration of 1,25-dihydroxycholecalciferol, which increases the ionic calcium concentration in the urine, and ascorbic acid, which increases the absorption of oxalate in the diet. The daily dose of ascorbic acid, if given as routine replacement, should not therefore be much in excess of the recommended daily allowance of 30 mg.

## 10.14 ACID/BASE DISTURBANCE

The metabolic acidosis of renal failure is due to the inability of the kidneys to excrete titratable acid and ammonium ion. Typically the serum bicarbonate is maintained at 15–20 mmol/l. This is because of the presence of non-bicarbonate buffers such as bone. The $PCO_2$ is decreased due to respiratory compensation for the metabolic acidosis. Occasionally, chronic tubulo-interstitial disease produces a distal form of renal tubular acidosis, with hypokalaemia.

The correction of this acidemia in the predialysis patient can be achieved with oral supplementation in the form of sodium bicarbonate, calcium carbonate, potassium citrate or calcium acetate. Metabolic acidemia adversely affects skeletal muscle protein metabolism. One of the goals of dialysis is to provide adequate base to correct acidemia as well as to provide buffer for the interdialytic period. The induction of alkalosis can result in headache and nausea post-dialysis. The use of bicarbonate as the base on hemodialysis causes less hemodynamic instability compared to acetate.

## 10.15 IMMUNOLOGICAL

The increased incidence of infection in the patient with renal disease is a consequence of such contributory factors as malnutrition and defects in granulocyte chemotaxis, adherence and phagocyte function [14]. The additional effect of iron bioavailability due to blood transfusion increases the virulence of unusual organisms such as *Listeria* and *Yersinia*. The side effect of mucormycosis with the use of desferoxamine (DFO) is discussed in Section 10.16. The chronic activation of complement during hemodialysis has been described with maximal activation occurring within 15 min of initiation. The use of cuprophan membranes has been demonstrated to activate the complement system more readily than cellulose acetate or polyacrylonitrile. The consequences of the activation of complement include leukocyte aggregation and sequestration.

First-use hypersensitivity reactions occur when utilizing an unused, unreprocessed dialyzer. They may be classified into types A and B. Type A is an anaphylactic reaction with urticaria, hypotension and angioedema. It occurs within 20 min of initiation of dialysis, and may necessitate discontinuation of dialysis as well as the standard treatment of anaphylaxis with bronchodilators, epinephrine and steroids. The etiological factors include exposure to the sterilant ethylene oxide in the potting of fresh cuprammonium cellulose dialyzers the dialyzer membrane itself, cytokine activation and contaminated dialysate. Type B reactions are more common and less dramatic than type A. The symptoms are non-specific including back and chest pain, usually described within the first hour. These symptoms tend to resolve spontaneously without discontinuation of or alterations in the dialysis. These reactions may be a mild form of type A reactions, but a different pathogenesis is possible and clearly has not been ruled out. Supporting this is the observation of type B reactions with regenerated cellulose or cellulose acetate dialyzers, while type A reactions are only rarely noted with those dialyzers. Type B reactions are treated merely with symptomatic and supportive care. The rate of ultrafiltration is generally slowed. Since there is an association between the use of ACE inhibitors and first-use reactions, particularly with polyacrylonitrile (PAN) membranes, switching to another class of antihypertensive agents is reasonable.

Prevention includes detoxifying the potting material, avoiding ethylene oxide entrapment and alternative sterilization. The dialysis team can also intervene with one liter rinses and discards at set-up and immediately before use, reprocessing prior to first use, and extra large dialysate rinsing, > 10 l [15–17].

The increased incidence of neoplasia in patients on immunosuppressive therapy has been well documented. It seems logical then that the patient with renal disease and immune compromise would be susceptible to neoplasia since tumor surveillance may be compromised in these patients. The incidence of neoplasia in hemodialysis patients is higher than in the general population, as opposed to CAPD patients in whom the risk is no higher. This may reflect better immune responsiveness with respect to tumor surveillance in the CAPD patient as compared to the predialysis or hemodialysis patient. Thus, standard preventive screening measures should be adopted in this patient population.

## 10.16 GASTROINTESTINAL

Azotemia results in changes in the gastrointestinal mucosa (e.g. gastritis) which predispose to the loss of blood. This is complicated by regular heparin in HD patients. Increased levels of serum gastrin also contribute to the severity of disease. Diagnosis can be made by endoscopy. Telangiectatic lesions of the lower gastrointestinal tract may be responsible for obscure anemia in renal failure. Conjugated estrogens may be beneficial in this setting (Section 10.8). CAPD may rarely predispose to the development of pancreatitis, due to the irritant effects of the dialysate on the surface of the pancreas and, possibly, the presence of hypertriglyceridemia.

Hemoperitoneum is unique to PD. It may result from menstruation or ovulation, or may signal more ominous events such as a leaking abdominal aortic aneurysm, ischemic bowel or cancer. Clinical correlation is needed to determine the significance of the bloody dialysate. A cell count, Gram stain and culture should be obtained. Chyloperitoneum, the appearance of high-density lipoproteins and chylomicrons in the peritoneum, is a second event unique to CAPD. This have been reported after trauma to the abdomen, lymphatic obstruction due to neoplasia or the presence of the Tenckhoff catheter. Dialysis ascites is a rare problem associated with hemodialysis. The recurrent accumulation of an exudative fluid (fluid protein/serum albumin ratio >0.72) has long been recognized. Treatment has been disappointing. Ultrafiltration during hemodialysis has resulted in hypotension. Intraperitoneal steroid therapy has not been consistently successful. PD has been used as a treatment for the ascites. One drawback to this solution is the loss of protein, which may aggravate the tendency to ascites, due to decreased plasma oncotic pressure. The placement of a peritoneovenous shunt may decrease the accumulation of ascitic fluid, but only at the risk of infection and shunt obstruction [18, 19].

## 10.17 NEUROLOGICAL

Uremic encephalopathy is characterized by confusion, asterixis, myoclonus and seizures. In the predialysis patient the rate of progression may be gradual in contrast to the rate noted in acute renal failure. Decreased cognition is an early sign; the patient seems disoriented, easily distracted and irritable. Myoclonus may affect the fact and proximal muscle groups, sometimes resembling partial seizures. Generalized motor seizures are a manifestation of advanced uremia.

In the patient on dialysis, aluminum toxicity is a well-recognized cause of dementia. Aluminum can cross the blood–brain barrier as a glutamate complex. Deposition in the grey matter leads to dystrophic changes. Early expressions of aluminum neurotoxicity include intermittent speech disturbances (e.g. hesitancy), and dyspraxia, while later manifestations include more constant speech disturbances, myoclonic jerks, seizures, personality change and global dementia. Sources of aluminum in this population include dialysate (in untreated water with high aluminum content) and aluminum-containing phosphate binders.

In patients with symptoms of aluminum (Al) toxicity, a serum aluminum concentration over 100 μg/l should be followed by a DFO challenge test. DFO chelates aluminum thereby releasing aluminum from the body stores. DFO at a dose of 40 mg/kg should be given intravenously over two hours in hemodialysis patients; intraperitoneal in the overnight dwell of patients on CAPD. An increase in the serum aluminum level of greater than 200 μg/l suggests significant aluminum accumulation. The use of reverse osmosis to deionise the water supply used as dialysate and render it virtually free of aluminum is now standard procedure, and considered mandatory in most HD centres in the Western world. It is recommended that dialysis water should be analyzed periodically to ensure that it is not a source of exogenous aluminum. The treatment of aluminum toxicity obviously includes the discontinuation of aluminum-containing medications and dialysate, and the subsequent removal of aluminum from the body by the administration of DFO.

Treatment consists of DFO 10 mg/kg intravenously over the last two hours of hemodialysis three times weekly, or 40 mg/kg in one dwell weekly in CAPD patients until the basal aluminum level drops to below 100 μg/l, or the rise in the serum aluminum level after DFO is less than 20 μg/l. The side effects of DFO include retinal degeneration leading to blindness, hypotension, cataract formation and rarely, mucormycosis.

Peripheral neuropathy is a manifestation of advanced CRF, and rarely complicates acute renal failure. It is usually sensorimotor, with a symmetric, distal distribution. Nerve conduction studies suggest demyelination. Adequate dialysis is the key to prevention as well as management. The symptoms of sensory neuropathy improve with adequate dialysis; however, the motor component is thought to improve only partially, due to the compensation of the remaining innervated muscle fibers. Other factors which may contribute to neuromyopathy include osteomalacia, drugs and vitamin deficiency.

Intracranial bleeding may occur as a consequence of hypertension in the setting of anticoagulation. The additional risk of intracranial aneurysm exists in the patient with polycystic kidney disease. In addition to hemorrhagic stroke, subarachnoid hemorrhage and subdural hematoma must be kept in mind. These problems are particularly encountered when continuous anticoagulation with heparin is employed for continuous hemofiltration – a technique now frequently used to treat acutely ill patients with renal failure, in intensive care units. The diagnostic study of choice for these conditions is the computed tomography scan. After the event, management of the dialysis regimen is critical. The goals are adequate dialysis, without the concomitant intracerebral shift of fluid, and minimal complications of dialysis-related anticoagulation. It is now well recognized that short dialysis (up to four hours) can be readily undertaken without the need for heparin or any other form of anticoagulation.

## 10.18 DIALYSIS DYSEQUILIBRIUM

This common but poorly defined neurovascular syndrome has a multifactorial etiology. Due to the more rapid removal of urea from the plasma and brain as compared to the cerebral spinal fluid (CSF), net movement of water into the CSF occurs with resultant increase in pressure. The rise in CSF $PCO_2$ during dialysis with a subsequent fall in the pH may be contributory. The presentation ranges from headache and agitation to disorientation and seizures. Prevention of these problems includes slowing the clearance of urea in very azotemic patients by using a smaller dialyzer, reducing the time of dialysis or reducing the blood or dialysate flow rate. Administration of osmotically active solutes such as mannitol or the use of a high sodium bath may help to reduce the fluid shifts that occur with clearance of urea.

## 10.19 ACCESS PROBLEMS

### 10.19.1 Hemodialysis

Vascular access may be lost due to thrombosis, infection or stenosis, and aneurysm formation is common. Thrombosis occurs in patients with AV fistulae as well as interposition grafts, the venous anastomosis being a common site of thrombus formation. Loss of the bruit and thrill, and inability to access the graft are signs of thrombosis. Thrombectomy has been the standard therapy for this, but thrombolytic therapy and mechanical thrombolysis have shown initial success. Doppler ultrasound may be useful for the evaluation of graft anatomy and flow.

The immunocompromised state of these patients coupled with repeated punctures predisposes the access to infection, particularly the foreign material of the interposition graft. Strict adherence to sterile technique as well as a high index of suspicion for infection can prevent loss. Treatment of graft infection depends on the clinical setting. The most common organism is *Staphylococcus aureus*. Localized infection without bacteremia may require only local care as opposed to the patient with positive blood cultures who should be treated with intravenous antibiotics, particularly in patients with synthetic grafts, who should be treated with prolonged courses, as for endocarditis. Removal of the graft may be required, with the use of a temporary catheter until blood cultures are negative for two weeks.

Ischemia due to steal of blood supply from distal extremities by fistulae or interposition grafts is not uncommon. Symptoms and signs include decreased temperature, pallor and pain. In the immediate postoperative period, the extremity may be cool; however, loss of neurologic function or persistent pain demand attention. Return of adequate flow to the extremity is crucial. This may mean removal of the fistula, or narrowing the lumen to a degree that restores adequate flow. Unfortunately, the narrowing of the lumen may compromise flow to the shunt in such a way as to limit adequacy of dialysis or precipitate thrombosis of the shunt [20].

### 10.19.2 Peritoneal dialysis

The loss of the peritoneal membrane surface area for CAPD can occur due to the development of fibrous adhesions as the result of peritonitis. A second mechanism of loss which may be independent of infection is the development of sclerosing peritonitis, in which the peritoneum develops a fibrinous exudate that prevents dialysis and ultrafiltration.

With sclerosing peritonitis patients present with combined ultrafiltration and solute transport failure, intestinal adhesions and possible obstruction. Peritoneal irritants (acetate, chlorhexidine, beta-blockers, bacterial by-products such as endotoxins, antibiotics) and the damage of lining cells from prolonged or recurrent infections are implicated in the pathogenesis. A similar but more severe form of sclerosis is sclerosing encapsulating peritonitis, in which a thick-walled membrane cocoon entraps bowel loops causing obstruction, vomiting and malnutrition. Because lymphokines may be involved, verapamil therapy may be helpful, as deceased intracellular calcium may decrease lymphokine activity. The antiestrogen tamoxifen inhibits protein kinase C and has been successfully utilized in peritoneal sclerosis.

The most common more serious complication of peritoneal dialysis is infective peritonitis, almost always due to bacterial presence in the dialysate. The origin of the bacteria is from contamination of the inflow dialysate during connections, along the trans-cutaneous catheter tunnel tract, or from intra-abdominal sources such as the bowel or biliary system. A major problem is that of recurrent/relapsing peritonitis caused by the same organism; it is now recognized as being the consequence of bacterial (mostly staphylococcal) production of 'slime', which coats the catheter and sequestrates the bacteria from the effects of antibiotics.

Most of these infections are in some ways preventable. Selection of patients and/or partners who perform the exchanges, proper training and discipline, and certain connection technologies and strategies reduce the incidence of peritonitis. For example, the 'flush before fill' Y-set connectology decreases the infection rates across the board. In addition, the placement methodology and care of the catheter, its exit site and trans-cutaneous tunnel tract can reduce infections. An anchored catheter with healthy fibrous ingrowth at placement, a downward-directed tunnel and prophylactic antibiotics prior to insertion all have been show to decrease the infection rate. The avoidance of constipation and straining at stool, prophylactic antibiotics prior to sigmoidoscopy or colonoscopy and elective cholecystectomy for cholelithiasis may decrease the chance of transmural bacterial migration and subsequent peritonitis.

The treatment of microbial peritonitis associated with peritoneal dialysis has been described in detail by an *ad hoc* advisory committee. The treatment incorporates antibiotics and, occasionally, the removal or replacement of the catheters. Since *staphylococci* are the most frequent pathogens, prophylactic regimens to reduce the frequency of its infections have been devised. These include oral rifampin for five days every three months, intranasal and exit-site mupiricin ointment and trimethoprim/sulfamethoxazole orally thrice weekly. There is some evidence that intraperitoneal urokinase can help eradicate infection in refractory cases, possibly by disrupting the layer of slime which protects the bacteria.

Temporary failure of CAPD with poor drainage is often due to constipation, to which these people are susceptible. It is therefore important to anticipate this and ensure regular bowel motions by the use of stool-softening agents. Refractory failure of CAPD drainage may be due to omental wrapping around the catheter, or catheter displacement into one of the hypochondrial regions. In these cases it becomes necessary to resort to surgical correction (omentectomy/re-positioning).

## 10.20 RENAL OSTEODYSTROPHY

This term embraces a spectrum of pathological processes, including osteomalacia, osteitis fibrosa cystica, osteoporosis, osteosclerosis, adynamic bone disease and pathological fractures. The basic pathology may be aggravated by other factors like aluminum deposition and drugs such as corticosteroids.

The progressive loss of excretory renal function results in secondary hyperparathyroidism, due to impaired production of vitamin D and hyperphosphatemia. The three types of bone disease identified are hyperparathyroid bone disease with high turnover of bone, low-turnover uremic osteodystrophy and a mixture of the two. Diagnosis of the type of bone disease is difficult just using serum levels of calcium, phosphorus, or alkaline phosphatase. The most specific diagnostic test is the bone biopsy which allows histologic typing of the disease. Prevention is the key to avoidance of the loss of bone mass. A low phosphorus diet (800 mg per day) when the glomerular filtration rate approaches 25% and the addition of phosphate binders is appropriate. The type of phosphate binder chosen depends on the patient. Unfortunately, the most effective binder is an aluminum salt which can lead to aluminum accumulation. Various calcium salts are available including carbonate (which may be beneficial in patients with persistent acidosis), citrate (which can increase the adsorption of aluminum) and acetate, which may be more effective than carbonate or citrate as a phosphate binder. Sometimes the dose of calcium compounds required to control serum phosphate results in hypercalcemia. In this case, the only previously available method was to switch to aluminum salts; now it is possible to reduce serum calcium by decreasing dialysate calcium in HD as well as CAPD. The use of vitamin D has been shown to have a direct suppressant effect on PTH synthesis. Both 1,$\alpha$-hydroxy cholecalciferol (alfacalcidol) and 1,25-dihydroxy cholecalciferol (calcitriol) are effective in replacing the vitamin D deficiency, and the recommended starting dose is 0.25 µg/day. Recently, it has been suggested that intravenous calcitriol may be a more effective way of delivering vitamin D to the tissues;

intravenous calcitriol (0.01 μg/kg) can be administered during each hemodialysis treatment. Serum calcium and phosphorus levels should be measured regularly (every two weeks in the case of intravenous treatment). The intravenous calcitriol should be discontinued if serum phosphorus levels reach 6.0 mg/dl (2.0 mmol/l) or higher. The dose of vitamin D replacement should be titrated according to the serum calcium [21].

## 10.21 MALNUTRITION

Studies from Australia and Italy suggest that the progression of renal disease can be slowed by dietary protein restriction (DPR) [22, 23]. The recent MDRD (Modification of Diet in Renal Disease) study however calls into question the benefit of DPR; this is discussed in greater detail in Chapter 2. Of concern is the potential price paid for this restriction with regard to nutritional status as the patient approaches dialysis or is transplanted. Protein energy malnutrition is evident in 20–60% of HD patients, and is a risk factor for increased morbidity and mortality in these patients. For obvious reasons, DPR must not be undertaken in patients once they have reached the end-stage. An exception may be made when patients are put onto strict DPR for short periods (up to four weeks) as a holding measure, say, between catheter changes for recurrent peritonotis. Protein and energy requirements in dialysis patients are not different from normals, at 35–45 kcal/kg/day and 1 g/kg/day respectively. Malnutrition in dialysis patients is due to a number of factors as follows.

1. Inadequate intake
   - Uremic anorexia – inadequate dialysis
   - Gastric problems – peptic ulcer, esophageal reflux, gastroparesis
   - Distasteful medication – phosphate binders
   - Psychosocial and economic problems
2. Increased catabolism
   - Inadequate dialysis
   - Metabolic acidosis
   - Blood–membrane interaction
   - Drugs, e.g. corticosteroids
3. Protein loss
   - Proteinuria
   - Aminoacid losses in HD/CAPD

The treatment of malnutrition in this setting is to first address the underlying cause. Thus, an evaluation of the gastrointestinal system is indicated along with a careful dietary history and counseling. At this time the intensity of dialysis should be increased, by lengthening the

HD treatment times or the number of exchanges in PD. There is some evidence that switching from a complement-activating cuprophan to a more biocompatible and permeable membrane will improve abnormal protein metabolism, especially with increasing the dose of dialysis by urea kinetic modeling.

The reversal of malnutrition and weight loss by oral supplements, enriched food or feeding tubes often fails because of the inconvenience, cost, palatability, anorexia, dysgeusia, lack of motivation, depression and non-compliance with such a difficult regimen. Thus, intradialytic parenteral nutrition (IDPN) evolved. A typical regimen consists of 250 ml of 50% dextrose plus 0.5–1 l of amino acids (13–15 g nitrogen/l) plus 250 ml of 20% lipid emulsion administered continuously by infusion pump during the HD treatment into the venous drip chamber of the circuit. Insulin is sometimes required and weekly parenteral vitamins are advised. Tolerance trials are necessary to individualize the formulation. Serum glucose, $Na^+$, $k^+$, phosphorus and lipids must be measured regularly, and urea kinetic modeling should be performed to assess the adequacy of dialysis as well as protein catabolic rate. Snacks must be ingested post-HD to avoid rebound hypoglycemia. A minimum trial period is about three months with IDPN administered at each treatment. While costly, this approach is often effective. If hospitalizations are prevented and quality of life improved, the treatment is worthwhile [24]. Appetite returns and routine nourishment takes over. The use of growth factors such as growth hormone or insulin-like growth factor is under investigation.

## 10.22 ADEQUACY OF DIALYSIS

The treatment goal of dialysis is to replace excretory renal function. Because of cost constraints (equipment, supplies, space and labor) and patient non-compliance, many dialysis treatments may be inadequate. Much of the preceding section described the complications of inadequate dialysis. The simplest solution to many of those problems is to increase the intensity of dialysis. There are a number of ways to achieve this. Dialyzer parameters which affect clearance include surface area, membrane type, geometry and reuse. Dialysate and blood flow, recirculation, ultrafiltration and duration of dialysis treatment also influence clearance. Manipulation of one or more of these variables may correct the inadequacy of the treatment. Virtually all aspects of dialysis care will improve with better membranes and longer (or more frequent) treatment times, but, unfortunately, this important parameter is often compromised by non-compliant patients and cost-conscious providers.

Crude measures of the adequacy of dialysis include late manifestations such as refractory anemia, bleeding, pericarditis, peripheral neuropathy, itching and skin manifestations, and malnutrition. Recently, urea kinetic modeling (UKM) and protein catabolic rate (PCR) determination have been employed in both HD and PD to assess dialysis requirement, efficiency and nutritional status. Urea spontaneously dissociates in plasma to form isocyanic acid which ultimately results in carbamylation of such molecules as hemoglobin. Protein carbamylation may therefore be used as an index of uremic toxicity, analogous to diabetes mellitus where hyperglycemia causes glycosylation of proteins and the formation of advanced glycosylation end products.

The use of urea kinetic modeling to individualize the dialysis prescription is based on the underlying differences of body habitus, endogenous generation of urea, diet and pathophysiologic basis for end stage renal disease in patients requiring renal replacement therapy. Urea is a representative solute for small solutes, particularly those that result from protein catabolism. Sargent and Gotch proposed the use of urea kinetics to prescribe dialysis in terms of solute removal.

The therapy prescription index $Kt/V$ is a dimensionless measurement of the amount of dialysis prescribed or delivered. $K$ is the dialyzer clearance, $t$ is treatment time and $V$ is the volume of distribution of urea. The second component of the urea kinetic model is the generation of urea in terms of the PCR that serves as an indicator of protein intake. In general, a $Kt/V$ of 1.2 three times a week is considered adequate dialysis. It is important to note that a target or prescribed $Kt/V$ of 1.4 may be a better goal since the prescribed amount of dialysis is rarely delivered, given the potential for error in the true clearance of the dialyzer, time on dialysis and changes in blood flow rates. The amount of residual renal function also contributes to the $Kt/V$. It is important to quantitate the residual renal function, since the loss of this residual capacity will deteriorate with time, necessitating a change in the dialysis prescription.

Small dialyzable toxins are largely responsible for uremic symptoms, as clearly shown by the National Cooperative Dialysis Study (NCDS) and subsequent studies. Urea itself is at worst only slightly toxic. However, it is an easily measured, easily manipulated breakdown product of protein metabolism. Since it quantitatively accounts for nearly all of protein nitrogen elimination, its accumulation and elimination are a measure of protein metabolism. Since protein catabolism is the most important determinant of dialysis need, urea levels can be used to assess both dialysis need *and* its efficiency. UKM provides data useful for dietary counseling and lends itself well to quality improvement monitoring. Thus, urea is an acceptable surrogate marker for the other end products of protein metabolism.

Underdialysis causes patients to lose their appetite and, as nutrition deteriorates, so does general health. This observation was clearly shown in the NCDS, and in other studies. The patients who do best on dialysis are well nourished *and* well dialyzed. As nutrition deteriorates, blood urea nitrogen (BUN) may fall, misleading the doctor into thinking that less dialysis is needed. Since patients consistently request reduction in dialysis time, the easy way out is to shorten dialysis time (i.e. deliver less dialysis therapy). This results in worsening uremia, anorexia, further malnutrition and a further decrease in BUN, thus setting up a vicious cycle. The patient effectively 'shrinks' to meet the inadequate therapy. Increasing the dose of dialysis through UKM has been shown to improve PCR in both HD and PD patients. By combining UKM with PCR determinations, one can evaluate the efficiency of therapy and nutritional status [25–27].

## REFERENCES

1. Golper, T.A. (1992) Management of hyperlipidemia in chronic dialysis patients, in: *Dialysis Therapy*, 2nd edn (eds A. Nissenson and R.N. Fine), Hanley and Belfus, Philadelphia.
2. Kudoh, Y. and Limura, O. (1987) Study on the atherosclerosis mechanism in chronic hemodialysis. *Jpn. Circ. J.*, **51**, 631–41.
3. Ritz, E., Rambausek, M., Mall, G. *et al.* (1990) Cardiac changes in uraemia and their possible relationship to cardiovascular instability on dialysis. *Nephrol. Dial. Transplant*, **5** suppl 1, 93–7.
4. Parfrey, P.S., Harnet, J.D., Griffiths, S.M. *et al.* (1990) The clinical course of left ventricular hypertrophy in dialysis patients. *Nephron*, **55**, 114–20.
5. Furukawa, A., Miyamoto, T., Tamura, M. *et al.* (1992) Study of factors related to hypotension in hemodialysis patients. *Nippon Jinzo. Gakkai. Shi.*, **34**, 417–22.
6. Peer, G., Korzets, A., Hochhauzer, E. *et al.* (1987) Cardiac arrhythmia during chronic ambulatory peritoneal dialysis. *Nephron*, **45**, 192–5.
7. Cardoso, M., Vinay, P., Vinet, B. *et al.* (1988) Hypoxemia during hemodialysis: a critical review of the facts. *Am. J. Kidney Dis.*, **11**, 281–97.
8. Golper, T.A. (1992) The effect of recombinant erythropoietin on the early hematocrit rise after CAPD initiation. *Perit. Dial. Int.*, **12**, 37–9.
9. Stivelman J.C. (1989) Resistance to recombinant human erythropoietin therapy: a real clinical entity. *Semin. Nephrol.*, **9**, suppl 2, 8–11.
10. Anastassiades, E., Howarth, D., Howarth, J. *et al.* (1993) Influence of blood volume on the blood pressure of predialysis and peritoneal dialysis patients treated with erythropoeitin. *Nephrol. Dial. Transplant*, **8**, 621–5.
11. Becker, B.N. and Koury, M.J. (1993) Resistance to erythropoietin in dialysis patients: factors that decrease erythropoietin responsiveness. *Dial. Transplant.*, **22** 686–90.
12. Marsen, T.A., Pollok, M. and Baldamus, C.A. (1992) Influence of various hemofilter membranes in elimination of B2 microglobulin during dialysis treatment. *Dial. Transplant.*, **21**, 788–805.
13. MacDougall, M.L. (1993) Acquired cystic kidney disease, in *Dialysis Therapy* (eds A.R. Nissenson and R.N. Fine), Hanley and Belfus, Philadelphia, pp. 315–7.
14. Vanherweghem, J.L., Tielemans, C., Goldman, M. and Boelaert, J. (1991) Infections in chronic hemodialysis patients. *Semin. Dial.* **4**, 240–4.

15. Stephens, G.W., Bernhard, D.B., Idelson, B.A. *et al.* (1985) Anaphylaxis: an unusual complication of hemodialysis. *Clin. Nephrol.*, **24**, 99–102.
16. Daugirdas, J.T. and Ing, T.S. (1988) First-use reactions during hemodialysis: a definition of subtypes. *Kidney Int.*, **33**, supp 24, S37–S43.
17. Rockel, A., Klinke, B., Hertel, J. *et al.* (1989) Allergy to dialysis materials. *Nephrol. Dial. Transplant.*, **4** 646–52.
18. Bargman, J. and Oreopoulos, D. (1989) Complications other than peritonitis or those related to the catheter and the fate of uremic organ dysfunction in patients receiving peritoneal dialysis, in *Peritoneal Dialysis*, (ed. K.D. Nolph), Kluwer Academic, Dordrecht, pp. 289–318.
19. Keane, W.F., Everett, E.D., Golper, T.A. *et al.* (1993) Peritoneal dialysis related peritonitis treatment recommendations, 1993 update. *Perit. Dial. Int.*, **13**, 14–28.
20. Golding, A.L. (1986) Complications of vascular access for chronic hemodialysis, in *Dialysis Therapy*, (eds A.R. Nissenson and R.N.Fine), Hanley and Belfus, Philadelphia, pp. 9–13.
21. Malluche, H.H. and Faugere, M.C. (1990) Renal bone disease 1990: an unmet challenge for the nephrologist. *Kidney Int.*, **38**, 193–211.
22. Ihle, B.U., Becker, G.J., Whitworth, J.A. *et al.* (1989) The effect of protein restriction on the progression of renal insufficiency. *N. Engl. J. Med.*, **31** 1773–7.
23. Locatelli, F., Alberti, D., Graziani, G. *et al.* and the Northern Italian Cooperative Study Group (1991) Prospective, randomised, multicentre trial of effect of protein restirction on progression of chronic renal insufficiency. *Lancet*, **337** 1299–304.
24. Foulks, C.J., Goldstein, D.J., Kelly, M.P. and Hunt, J.M. (1991) Indications for the use of intradialytic parenteral nutrition in the malnourished hemodialysis patient. *J. Renal Nutr.*, **1** 23–33.
25. Keshaviah, P. (1995) Kinetics of hemodialysis, in *Textbook of Nephrology*, 3rd edn (eds S.G. Masry and R.J. Glassock), Williams and Wilkins, Baltimore, pp. 1513–9.
26. Sargent, J.A., Gotch, F.A. (1989) Principles and biophysics of dialysis, in *Replacement of Renal Function*, 3rd edn (ed. J.F. Maher), Kluwer Academic, Dordrecht, pp. 87–143.
27. Golper, T.A. and Ward, R.A. (1995) Prescription hemodialysis, in *Textbook of Nephrology*, 3rd edn (eds S.G. Masry and R.J. Glassock), Williams and Wilkins, Baltimore, pp. 1536–41.

# 11

# Acute renal failure

*P.A. Kalra*

## 11.1 INTRODUCTION

Ever since Bywaters and Beal's [1] first detailed description of people with crush injuries suffering acute loss of kidney function during the London 'Blitz' of the Second World War, acute renal failure (ARF) has continued to provide a major challenge to clinical medicine and to nephrological research. It has been repeatedly stated that despite major advances in nutritional support, membrane technology and dialytic techniques, the mortality of ARF patients who require dialysis remains in excess of 50% [2]. Increased patient age and co-morbidity confer a poorer prognosis, as the aetiology of ARF is often multifactorial in the elderly.

The majority of cases of ARF ultimately result from renal hypoperfusion and consequent intra-renal ischaemic damage, the histological correlate being acute tubular necrosis (ATN) [3]. Many such patients have circulatory abnormalities that culminate in ARF, but pass through a phase of potentially reversible prerenal oliguria, during which renal physiological mechanisms aimed at restoring the extracellular fluid volume are maximally stimulated. Early recognition and prompt, appropriate treatment of these prerenal factors can prevent progression to established ARF, with the genuine prospect of improved patient morbidity and mortality.

This chapter will predominantly concentrate on ischaemic acute renal failure: the epidemiology, its complicated pathophysiology, the importance of preventative therapy in the early management of some patients

*Renal Disease*. Edited by G. Venkat Raman. Published in 1998 by Chapman & Hall, London. ISBN 0 412 45700 8.

as well as renoprotective strategies, whether established, putative or experimental. ARF due to severe parenchymal diseases and obstructive nephropathy will not be considered in this chapter.

## 11.2 EPIDEMIOLOGY OF ACUTE RENAL FAILURE

European surveys indicate that dialysis-requiring ARF occurs with an annual incidence of 60–70 patients per million population [2]. The importance of age-related predisposition cannot be overstated; in an audit of biochemical results in two Devon health districts, severe ARF was identifiable in 140 cases per million per annum but 72% of these patients were older than 70 years [4]. A more remarkable statistic was that age-related annual incidence increased from 17 per million in adults under 50 years to 949 per million in the 80–89 age group. Case note review revealed that only 51 patients per million had been referred for a nephrological opinion, whereas an estimated appropriate referral rate was nearer 70 per million.

In our own unit, which has a catchment population of 1.2 million, there were 124 ARF admissions in 1995 and 58 (47%) of these patients had ischaemic prerenal ARF or ATN (Figure 11.1); about a fifth of these ARF patients required intensive care unit (ICU) management due to co-morbid illness or complicating sequelae, most often sepsis. An additional 43 patients, whose ARF had occurred as a component of multi-organ failure, were referred to the ICU from non-nephrological sources, so that the overall proportion of ischaemic ARF was 60%. The figure highlights the fact that patients with ARF due to acute parenchymal disease (acute glomerulonephritis, systemic vasculitis and inter-

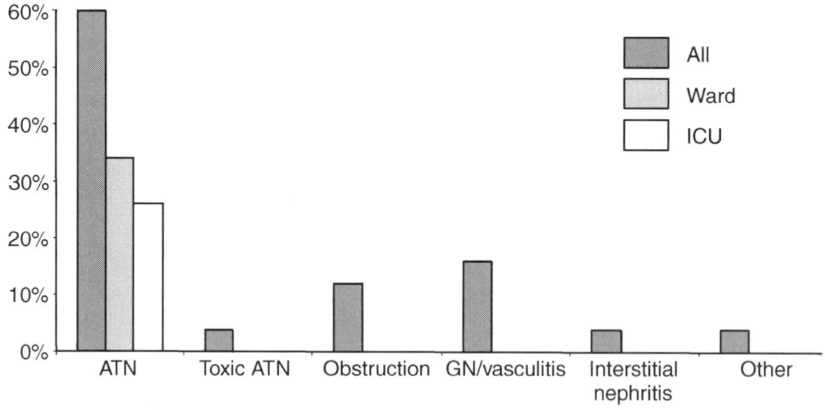


**Figure 11.1** Acute renal failure at Hope Hospital 1995 (167 cases including ICU).

stitial nephritis) or obstructive uropathy were in the minority. Other European studies of ARF have indicated a similar preponderance of cases with ischaemic renal damage [3, 5]. The epidemiology of ARF differs in the Third World, with almost 15% of cases resulting from obstetric complications (a proportion similar to that observed in the UK 30–40 years ago [6]), with tropical infections and even snake bites being well represented. Ischaemic ATN is also of major clinical importance in the setting of renal transplantation. At present approximately 10% of live-related donor grafts and 25–75% of cadaver renal allografts [7, 8] may be affected by primary non-function; post-transplant ATN may have an influence on long-term graft function.

## 11.3 CLASSIFICATION OF ACUTE RENAL FAILURE

The majority of patients with ARF primarily have an ischaemic insult that results in ATN [3].This may result from a diversity of systemic and intra-renal circulatory stresses (Table 11.1) including acute loss of blood

**Table 11.1** Classification of acute renal failure

| |
|---|
| **Prerenal factors leading to renal hypoperfusion and ATN (45%)** |
| Reduced circulating volume – blood loss; excess gastrointestinal losses; burns |
| Low cardiac output states – toxic or ischaemic myocardial depression |
| Systemic sepsis |
| Drugs inducing renal perfusion shutdown, e.g. angiotensin-converting enzyme inhibitors; non-steroidal anti-inflammatory drugs |
| **Toxic ATN (5%)** |
| Rhabdomyolysis with urinary myoglobin |
| Drugs, e.g. gentamicin |
| Radiocontrast nephropathy |
| Intravascular haemolysis |
| **Structural abnormalities of renal vasculature (10%)** |
| Large vessel occlusion (renovascular disease) |
| Small vessel occlusion, e.g. accelerated-phase hypertension; disseminated intravascular coagulation; haemolytic–uraemic syndrome; thrombotic thrombocytopenic purpura; pre-eclampsia; systemic sclerosis |
| Acute cortical necrosis |
| **Acute glomerulonephritis and vasculitis (15%)** |
| Idiopathic crescentic glomerulonephritis |
| ANCA positive vasculitis |
| Goodpasture's syndrome |
| Proliferative glomerulonephritis |
| **Interstitial nephritis (5%)** |
| Idiopathic immunologically mediated |
| Drug-induced hypersensitivity |
| Infection, e.g. pyelonephritis, leptospirosis |
| **Myeloma/tubular cast nephropathy (5%)** |
| **Urinary tract obstruction (15%)** |

and extracellular fluid, low cardiac output states such as following ischaemic or toxic myocardial damage, renovascular occlusion (following aortic surgery, thrombosis or embolus) and even from drug-induced renal perfusion shutdown (ACE inhibitors, non-steroidal anti-inflammatory agents). Many cases of ARF have a multifactorial aetiology (e.g. post-surgical sepsis with hypovolaemia, hypotension and injudicious antibiotic use), and these patients, who often have other organ failure, fit into the poorer prognostic category.

The above classification of ARF is not all-encompassing, but it indicates the approximate relative frequencies of those aetiological factors and renal pathologies most often encountered. Acute deterioration of renal transplant function, commonly seen with acute rejection, ATN, obstruction, urinary leakage or infarction, is excluded from this classification, as are the many patients who develop an acute decline of function on the background of pre-existing chronic renal impairment.

## 11.4 PATHOPHYSIOLOGY OF ISCHAEMIC ACUTE RENAL FAILURE

### 11.4.1 Animal models

The diverse nature of the aetiology of clinical ARF dictates that few human studies of its pathophysiology have taken place. Animal models enable accurate assessment of the changes in glomerular filtration rate (GFR), renal blood flow (RBF) and of pathological renal damage that result from ischaemic injury, but most differ significantly from the conditions that arise in human clinical practice. *In vivo* experimental work has usually involved a reproducible period of warm renal ischaemia followed by reperfusion of blood, as in the following models:

1. renal artery occlusion (RAO) by reversible clamping;
2. controlled haemorrhagic hypotension;
3. intra-renal arterial infusion of noradrenaline.

The most frequently used RAO model necessitates total interruption of RBF for a finite period, hence providing a massive single insult. Although a similar injury would be expected to occur during planned aortic or renal artery surgery (when aortic cross-clamping is necessary) in man, as stated previously, most human post-ischaemic ARF has a multifactorial aetiology. Renal pathological changes reflect this discordance between the pathogenesis of ARF in humans and in animal models [9], with more severe damage occurring in the proximal tubules and the thick ascending limb of the rat than the scanty ATN often seen in renal biopsies of human ARF. *In vitro* studies have involved isolated perfused whole organs, and renal tubular micropuncture and cell culture techniques, that have sought to elucidate the mechanisms of hypoxic and oxygen free radical-mediated cellular injury.

Post-ischaemic ARF often complicates human transplantation, and the above models have been extrapolated to transplant research; studies of cold preservation of allografts have also established the benefits of particular renoprotective regimes [10].

Despite their drawbacks, animal models have greatly augmented our understanding of the nature of post-ischaemic ARF and its underlying pathophysiology and the account given below is largely derived from such animal research.

### 11.4.2 Important renal physiological principles

The kidneys receive a generous blood supply (20% of the cardiac output although they only represent 0.5% of the total body mass) and so it is surprising that they are more susceptible to ischaemic damage than most other organs (including brain, heart and liver). The explanation for this lies in the regional variation of blood flow and oxygen supply within the kidney – those areas required to do the greatest work, and hence having the highest oxygen consumption, are, remarkably, the most frugally supplied with oxygenated blood.

*Renal blood flow (RBF)*

The blood flow to the outer cortex may be 20 times greater than to the inner medulla, as the medullary flow accounts for only 10–15% of the total RBF [11]. The medullary blood supply is derived entirely from efferent arterioles of the inner cortical glomeruli, these vessels passing into the medulla and dividing into the descending vasa rectae, which further descend in vascular bundles that supply the adjacent peritubular capillary plexi. The ascending vessels that drain the medulla are thin-walled and are most susceptible to compression by swollen renal tubules [12].

Renal arteriolar tone is influenced by several vasoactive systems which include renin–angiotensin, the prostanoids, endothelium-derived relaxing factor (EDRF, alias nitric oxide) and endothelin, and together these mediators help control the GFR and intra-renal blood flow. Autoregulation allows the RBF and GFR to remain constant despite major alterations in perfusion pressure; this capacity is lost when ATN supervenes.

*Intra-renal oxygen delivery*

The renal medulla has been shown to have a strikingly low oxygen tension – $PO_2$ values of 10 mm Hg have been demonstrated *in vivo*; this oxygen gradient between renal cortex and medulla is probably due to countercurrent diffusion from arterial to the venous branches of the hairpin loops of the vasa rectae. The poor medullary oxygenation is very close to a level in which mitochondrial cytochromes may, even in normal conditions, be partially or completely reduced, and thus at which mitochondrial and cellular function might be disorganized [13] – hence the particular vulnerability of certain renal tubular cells to ischaemic stress.

### 11.4.3 Pathophysiological events

*Alterations in renal blood flow following ischaemia*

Following an episode of renal ischaemia important changes occur in the glomerular and medullary circulations that are relevant to the pathogenesis of ARF and the resulting renal dysfunction. Thus after 60 min of RAO the total RBF is depressed to about 50% during reperfusion, and its return to normal may take several days [14]; the fall in total RBF is consequent upon an increase in renal vascular resistance that is due particularly to afferent arteriolar vasoconstriction [9]. Several mechanisms are thought to contribute to this increased preglomerular tone, which is partly responsible for loss of GFR, and ischaemic vascular endothelial damage may be of paramount importance. Endothelin is a potent vasoconstrictor peptide secreted by the endothelium, and studies have shown an upregulation of its secretion following renal ischaemia [15] as well as the beneficial effects upon GFR and RBF following its inhibition with antibodies [16] or specific antagonists. The severe renal vasoconstriction is probably also attributable to other circulating endocrine and paracrine agents, as well as mediators of inflammation – such as catecholamines, angiotensin II, peptidyl leukotrienes generated by activated leucocytes and potent vasoconstrictor arachidonic acid metabolites produced by oxygen free radicals (OFRs). The importance of the depletion of locally acting vasodilators, such as prostacyclin ($PGI_2$) and EDRF, the latter stripped from the endothelium by OFRs during reperfusion, is recognized, and there is a hypersensitivity to renal nerve stimulation that can exacerbate the vasoconstriction [17].

In addition to the initial fall in total RBF, a major redistribution of intra-renal blood flow is observed after renal ischaemia. Studies involving laser Doppler flow [18] or radiolabelled microspheres [19] have shown that the outer medullary region of the kidney suffers the most severe reduction in blood perfusion after ischaemia, whilst intra-renal shunting ensures that the inner medulla is spared. This perfusion defect is thought to result from vascular obstruction by aggregates of red cells in the medullary vasa rectae, secondary to haemoconcentration produced by the leakage of plasma and proteins from the vascular space following ischaemia [19]. A further insult to the already vulnerable tubular cells situated in the outer medulla results, and necrosis is consequently most noticeable in the $S_3$ portion of the proximal tubule and the medullary thick ascending limb (mTAL) of Henle's loop.

However, despite these alterations in vascular flow during the initiation phase of ischaemic ARF, they are not solely responsible for the resulting loss of renal function, and several other factors, both glomerular and tubular, have been shown to be of importance.

### *Renal tubular obstruction*

Tubular cell injury results from calcium-mediated processes during, and free radical-induced damage (see below) after, ischaemia. This manifests as cellular swelling, necrosis, detachment from the tubular basement membrane and then shedding into the tubular lumen [20]. The cellular debris creates a blockage to the flow of tubular fluid and intratubular pressure increases; glomerular filtration ceases when the intratubular pressure is equivalent to the hydrostatic pressure acting across the glomerular basement membrane (which is itself diminished by preglomerular vasoconstriction). These obstructed, distended proximal tubules, together with the local interstitial oedema, further exacerbate tubular cell ischaemia by compressing the neighbouring thin-walled vasa rectae and capillaries that drain the medulla. Thus tubular obstruction appears to be important in the maintenance phase of ARF in animal models, but there is less evidence for this in man [21].

### *Backleak of tubular filtrate*

The oliguria of the maintenance phase of ischaemic ARF is also partly due to backleakage of tubular filtrate through the damaged tubular wall and into the renal interstitium. Studies with microinjected inulin have shown that as much as 30% of the tubular filtrate may leak across into the medullary parenchyma in this way [22] and this has actually been demonstrated in patients developing ARF after cardiac surgery.

### *Tubuloglomerular feedback*

In the early stages after ischaemic damage the resorptive capacity of the tubular cells declines and an increased sodium load in the tubular fluid is presented at the macula densa. Angiotensin II is released and this exacerbates glomerular hypoperfusion by increasing afferent arteriolar tone [14] – negative tubuloglomerular feedback. This mechanism may contribute further to renal dysfunction in ARF as angiotensin provokes mesangial cell contraction, which decreases the effective glomerular capillary surface area available for filtration, and hence the coefficient of permeability, $K_f$.

The important pathophysiological events involved in ischaemic ARF are summarized schematically in Figure 11.2.

### 11.4.4 Specific mechanisms involved in tubular cell injury

The mechanisms which result in cellular injury, and ultimately necrosis, are not fully understood, but there is compelling evidence that calcium has an important role. Also, the paradox of high RBF under normal conditions, and yet a marked susceptibility of the kidney to ischaemic damage has been alluded to previously. A further explanation suggests that much of the cellular injury may occur during reperfusion, with the return of oxygenated blood and generation of free radicals.

*Oxygen free radicals*

OFRs are species with one or more unpaired electrons, rendering them highly reactive and capable of causing severe tissue damage. Their important role in the pathophysiology of ischaemic ARF has been shown by the amelioration of injury in experiments in which either OFR formation is prevented or OFR scavengers are administered [23, 24].

During ischaemia, continuing cellular metabolism provides substrates and an enzyme system ideal for the formation of OFRs when molecular oxygen is re-introduced to the tissue. The xanthine oxidase enzyme is synthesized as the dehydrogenase (type D), 90% of the enzyme being in this form in healthy tissue; the dehydrogenase converts hypoxanthine to xanthine without generating OFRs. The increased intracellular calcium concentration within ischaemic cells activates a calmodulin-regulated protease which converts xanthine dehydrogenase to the oxidase (type O) form by peptide cleavage [25]. Xanthine oxidase cannot interact with $NAD^+$ and so molecular oxygen, returning during reperfusion of the tissue, acts as the electron acceptor (Figure 11.3). By sequential univalent reduction of the oxygen the free radicals superoxide and peroxide are generated (Figure 11.4); hydroxyl, the most highly reactive radical of all, is formed by an iron-catalysed reaction between the above radicals. As well as this enzymic alteration major changes in the content of available substrate for the oxidase enzyme occur during ischaemia, which again favours the formation of OFRs. The production of mitochondrial ATP declines during ischaemia, and as ATP stores are depleted, the AMP concentration is elevated concomitantly. AMP is catabolysed to hypoxanthine (Figure 11.3) and the latter may increase by 300-fold following 60 min of renal ischaemia.

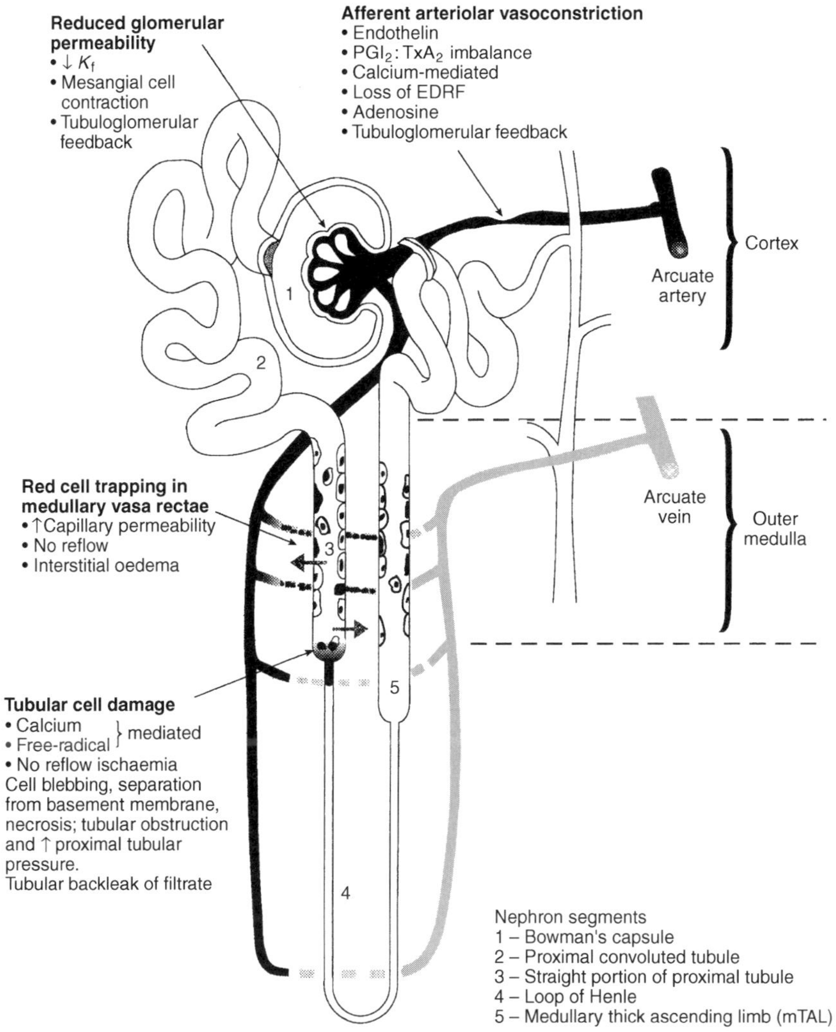


**Figure 11.2** Schema summarizing the pathological events involved in ischaemic acute renal failure.

During reperfusion oxygenated blood will, therefore, return to tissue containing an enzyme specialized in generating free radicals, and also large quantities of its favoured substrate. OFRs may also be released by polymorphonuclear leucocytes that infiltrate ischaemic tissue, but this source is only thought to be of importance two hours or more after reperfusion.

OFRs are highly reactive and can lead to massive cellular damage

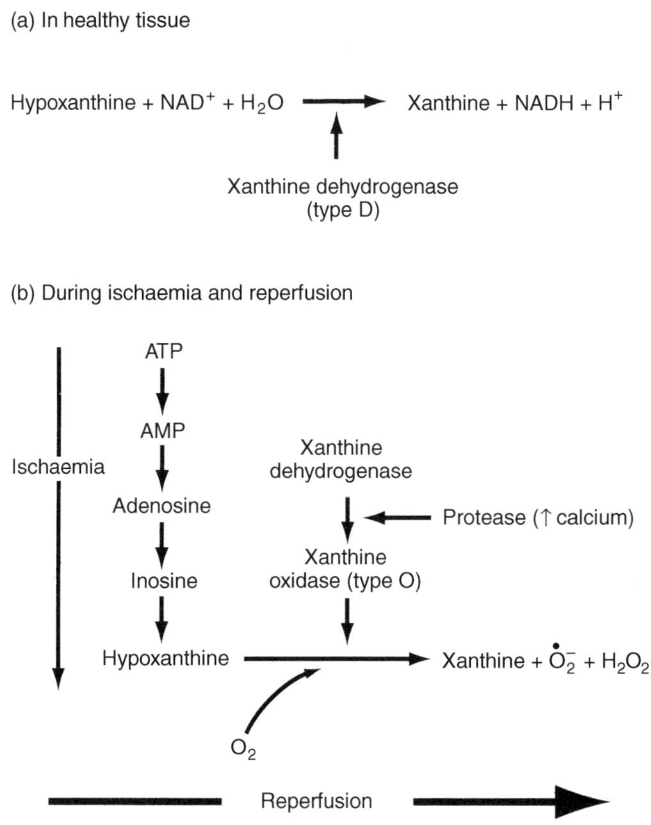


**Figure 11.3** Hypoxanthine metabolism under normal conditions (a) and the altered metabolism during ischaemia/reperfusion that results in superoxide radical generation (b) (modified from ref. 10).

mediated largely by the peroxidation of cellular and mitochondrial membrane lipids [26]. Peroxidation involves abstraction of a hydrogen atom from an unsaturated fatty acid of a membrane phospholipid, so creating an organic free radical; chain reactions of OFR damage are then propagated. The native scavenger systems, which exist in order to limit unwanted peroxidative damage due to OFRs generated under normal conditions, are likely to be overwhelmed by excess OFR, and so it is that reduced glutathione diminishes in concentration during ischaemia [24] and superoxide dismutase is consumed in the reperfusion phase. The overall result of OFR-induced membrane damage is an alteration of the molecular arrangement of membrane lipid bilayers with accompanying increases in membrane permeability, particularly to sodium and calcium, and impairment of enzymatic processes and ion-pump systems

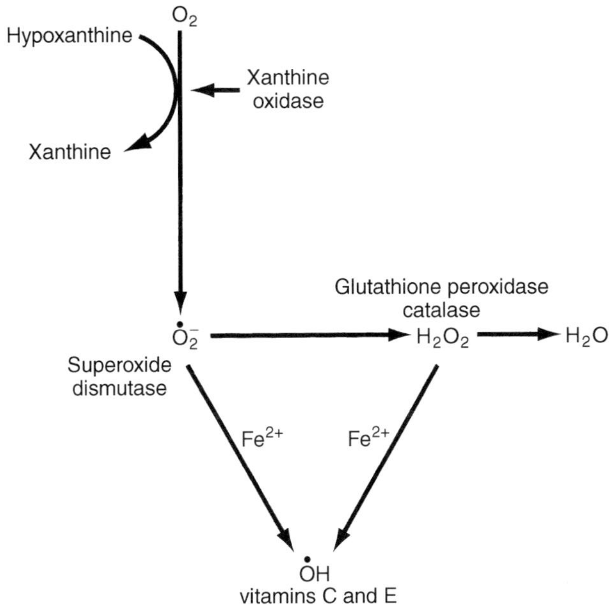


**Figure 11.4** Pathways of generation of oxygen free radicals (superoxide, peroxide and hydroxyl). Native antioxidant defences are also indicated.

[27]. Enhanced movement of sodium into injured cells, coupled with a loss of cellular volume regulatory mechanisms, encourages swelling; cell lysis may then occur due to the membrane damage which is further exacerbated by phospholipases activated by calcium.

*Role of calcium*

Calcium is an ubiquitous intracellular messenger that has a critical role in coupling membrane-associated stimuli with cellular response. The intracellular concentration of free ionized calcium is normally many thousand times less than that of the extracellular compartment; this gradient is maintained by an intrinsically low membrane permeability to calcium and by energy-dependent calcium extrusion [28]. With ischaemia, cellular processes that require energy become inefficient, membrane permeability increases, and the trans-membrane gradient cannot be preserved; intracellular calcium levels increase dramatically and contribute towards the pathophysiology of cell damage by stimulating cellular energy consumption, uncoupling oxidative phosphorylation within mitochondria and activating phospholipases (Figure 11.5). Studies with cell culture have emphasized the critical involvement of

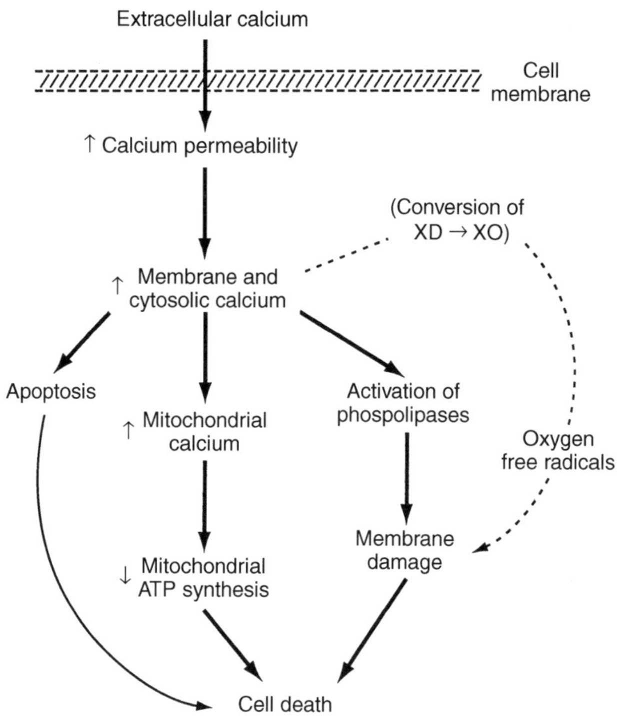


**Figure 11.5** Potential schema of pathophysiological events during ischaemia/reperfusion that involve calcium (modified from ref. 28).

calcium in the mediation of reperfusion injury – calcium greatly potentiates the damaging action of OFRs on renal mitochondria, with progression to cellular death often the end result [29].

### 11.4.5 Histopathological changes in ARF

As previously described, a pattern of selective vulnerability to ischaemic damage exists in the cells of the renal tubules, those at greatest risk being the most metabolically active and yet having the poorest blood supply. Short periods of RAO in the rat lead to necrosis only of cells in the pars recta, whereas 60 min of renal ischaemia induces necrosis along the entire length of the proximal tubule, with accompanying irreversible renal failure [9]. The ultrastructural changes that lead to tubular obstruction have also been detailed. Within minutes of reperfusion after 60 min of ischaemia, blebs of the plasma membrane are formed and shed successively into the tubular lumen [9]. These blebs swell and impact in the straight segments of the proximal tubules, resulting in obstruction of most tubules; although after several hours the blebs have lysed, they are replaced by casts composed of necrotic cells and protein which can maintain the tubular obstruction for a further week. As might be expected, with shorter occlusive periods the obstruction is more transient.

Vascular pathological changes are also prominent; the importance of congestion and obstruction of the medullary vasa rectae to the pathogenesis of tubular cell damage has already been emphasized, and vascular endothelial cell swelling may contribute to this. Areas of focal arterial necrosis also follow complete RAO, and this pathology may exacerbate the reduction in RBF seen in the maintenance phase of ischaemic ARF [30].

In contrast, the histopathological changes in human ischaemic ARF are less severe and correlate poorly with functional impairment. ATN is usually focal, or limited to clusters of cells, but effacement of the brush border of proximal tubules is a consistent finding [31].

### 11.4.6 Recovery from ischaemic ARF

*Recovery of blood flow and renal function*

By 24 hours of the maintenance phase the trapped erythrocytes of the medullary vasa rectae have been washed out and the medullary blood flow is restored. Afferent arteriolar vasoconstriction is prominent in the early stages after the ischaemic injury, and may be further increased by tubuloglomerular feedback. At one week after 45 min of RAO glomerular filtration resumes, albeit at only 10% of normal, as at this stage the capillary hydrostatic pressure is increased by efferent arteriolar vasoconstriction [32]. Tubular factors are important in maintaining oliguria during the first week or two after the injury; tubular backleak has completely resolved by two weeks, at which stage tubular obstruction by cellular debris has also fully cleared. RBF returns to normal by one month and GFR to about 50% of control; restoration of the GFR between two and eight weeks is brought about by a gradual relaxation of the intense preglomerular vasoconstriction. It is unclear exactly what happens to glomerular capillary surface area and $K_f$ during recovery.

The pattern of recovery from human ARF is far more variable, reflecting the heterogeneity of its aetiology. Oliguria may have resolved after only 24 hours, or can persist for up to six weeks, depending on the severity of the original renal ischaemic insult and upon the patient's subsequent clinical course.

*Tissue repair and regeneration*

Within 24 hours of renal ischaemia, intense regenerative activity is observed in tubular cells; there is an interstitial inflammatory infiltrate and the tubules are dilated. Those necrotic cells shed into the tubular lumen are replaced with a flattened epithelium lacking in microvilli [9]. With a severe injury, such as 60 min of RAO, most nephrons will be irreversibly damaged and interstitial fibrosis then becomes evident.

Previous attention to ischaemic cell death has been focused on necrosis, but the importance of apoptosis ('programmed cell death') in the tissue response to ischaemia has recently been recognized. Apoptosis refers to cell death that is finely controlled by active processes, and it has been demonstrated in post-ischaemic renal tissue. Ischaemia and reperfusion are accompanied by the induction of various genes that encode for proteins implicated in cellular proliferation, repair and apoptosis; these markers can be detected within 48 hours of injury [33]. Growth factors such as insulin-like growth factor (IGF-1) and epidermal growth factor (EGF) are delivered to renal epithelial cells from local and systemic sources and are thought to orchestrate the proliferative repair of the nephron after ATN [34]. An intact tubular basement membrane is crucial to the healing process as it provides a structural framework for proliferating cells.

However, despite major advances in molecular and cell-signalling biology, the control mechanisms that determine whether a cell dies by apoptosis or proliferates to replace adjacent dead cells have yet to be elucidated.

## 11.5 PATHOPHYSIOLOGY OF MULTIORGAN FAILURE

Many patients develop ARF as a component of multiple organ damage. This often follows a very severe precipitating illness in which multiple aetiological factors combine to cause organ dysfunction, or the patient may have pre-existing co-morbid disease. The pathophysiology of the ARF is accordingly complex – for example, it would be extremely difficult to distinguish the relative injurious contributions of coexistent hypotension, systemic sepsis, hypoxaemia and prolonged therapy with nephrotoxic antibiotics to the ultimate organ dysfunction that develops in a patient at risk of multiorgan failure (MOF). Nevertheless, the fundamental abnormalities of the intra-renal circulation, as well as tubular cell metabolism and injury, that have been described in the previous sections are still likely to be important in the pathogenesis of the acute renal dysfunction in such a patient.

The additional mechanisms which may contribute to the development of renal dysfunction in patients with multiorgan failure include abnormalities of regional blood flow, endotoxaemia, and undesirable stimulation of coagulation or cytokine release. Only a brief account of these is appropriate within the remit of this chapter.

One factor that may be central to the pathogenesis of MOF is splanchnic hypoperfusion, and this occurs with all types of 'shock' state [35]. The increased permeability of the gut mucosal barrier may then allow translocation of Gram negative bacteria and endotoxin into the systemic circulation. Endotoxin, or in other patients tissue trauma, can lead to a massive activation of inflammatory cells with the generation of cytokines such as tumour necrosis factor (TNF), interleukin-1 (IL-1) and nitric oxide; intravascular thrombosis and disseminated coagulation can also be triggered by the release of thromboplastins and platelet-activating factor [36]. It has been hypothesized that these mediators and rheological abnormalities predispose to further hypotension and impaired perfusion of vital organs, creating a vicious cycle; thus within the kidney, endothelin and angiotensin will be stimulated, thromboxanes predominate over prostacyclin ($PGI_2$), and the intense afferent arteriolar vasoconstriction described previously would supervene. A contributory role for OFR-induced damage in the development of the resulting oliguric ARF is readily visualized. Similar pathophysiological mechanisms are likely to be important in the hypoperfusion and damage that probably occurs in other organs during the initiation of MOF.

Although at this stage of our understanding the above sequence of events is largely speculative, abnormalities can be detected in patients with MOF that do lend support to the hypothesis. Endotoxaemia can be identified in ICU patients, and bursts of TNF have also been demonstrated. Recent studies have indicated that exogenous antiendotoxin antibodies may confer a benefit to specific morbidities and survival in patients with MOF [37].

## 11.6 BASIC CLINICAL MANAGEMENT

Many patients who later develop ischaemic ARF first pass through a potentially reversible phase of renal hypoperfusion; if these systemic and intra-renal circulatory abnormalities are corrected at an early stage, then progression towards oliguric ARF can be prevented, with the expectation of improved patient morbidity and survival. The following account, which is based on clinical experience and the current literature [38, 39], is not intended to provide a comprehensive guide to the management of ARF, but seeks to highlight common pitfalls and fundamental principles in the recognition and management of these patients.

### 11.6.1 Early diagnosis

Transient renal dysfunction may complicate up to 5% of all medical and surgical admissions, but is much greater in the acutely unwell; this indicates the size of population at risk of developing ARF. The clinician must remain alert to the potential for complications in these patients, and diligent attention to daily weight and fluid balance, coupled with daily assessment of renal biochemistry, is essential, including over the weekend period.

Several common pitfalls may delay diagnosis of incipient renal failure in the acutely unwell.

1. Fluid balance – accurate assessment may be hindered unless it is appreciated that insensible losses may increase three-fold during fever (i.e. 1.5 l/day); this emphasizes the importance of assessing daily weight.
2. Serum creatinine – renal functional reserve ensures that serum creatinine only exceeds the normal range in previously fit patients when GFR is reduced to less than 50%; this problem is exaggerated in patients with diminished muscle mass, such as the elderly and malnourished, in whom GFR may drop as low as 25% before renal impairment is signalled by a 'raised' serum creatinine.
3. Hypercatabolism – the acutely ill patient may lose 0.5 kg/day of flesh weight, and this will impact upon serum creatinine and fluid balance estimations. **The importance of early and intensive nutritional support for patients with ARF, which undoubtedly has an impact upon prognosis, must be emphasized** here, but further detailed consideration is beyond the scope of this account (see Chapter 13).
4. Chronic renal failure – patients with pre-existing chronic renal disease are particularly vulnerable to acute deterioration in function during intercurrent illness.
5. Nephrotoxic drugs – ARF is more likely to follow therapy with angiotensin-converting enzyme inhibitors and non-steroidal anti-inflammatory agents when given to patients with renal hypoperfusion. Other nephrotoxic agents, such as gentamicin and amphotericin, require careful dosage adjustment and monitoring in patients with renal impairment, otherwise acute decline in function may result.

### 11.6.2 Specific diagnosis of ARF

Once the diagnosis of ARF is established, its aetiology must be defined at the earliest opportunity so that preventative measures and specific therapy can be instituted. A detailed history directed at the identification of a precipitating cause for ARF is essential, and particular regard should be given to concurrent medications. Analysis of urinary sediment for casts, red cells and protein, though often overlooked, may provide a clue to acute glomerulonephritis. An ultrasound scan of the urinary tract should be performed within 24 hours of diagnosis in order to assess renal size and exclude obstruction, but it is noteworthy that pelvicalyceal dilatation may not always be apparent in the early stages after obstruction, and renography may then be necessary in cases of unexplained anuria.

The case for percutaneous renal biopsy in patients with a clinical picture of glomerulonephritis or systemic vasculitis, abnormal urinary sediment or positive specific autoimmune antibodies will be clear to all physicians. However, renal biopsy should also be seriously considered in patients with normal-sized kidneys in whom a precipitating cause for ARF is not readily apparent; acute interstitial nephritis is one example of an eminently treatable pathology which may have few clinical hallmarks.

### 11.6.3 Differentiation of prerenal impairment and established ATN

We have already established that the majority of patients with ARF have renal hypoperfusion, and that this renal ischaemia can result from many factors. However, some patients pass through a phase of oliguria, during which intra-renal physiological mechanisms are manifestly normal, before established ATN ensues. The early identification of these patients with prerenal uraemia is important, as prompt correction of circulatory abnormalities and consequent restoration of renal perfusion may reverse the condition; a normal haemodynamic state is also desirable in ATN but is most unlikely to rapidly improve renal function.

The characteristic urinary biochemical picture of prerenal uraemia reflects the physiological response of the kidney to hypovolaemia and hypoperfusion; stimulation of the renin–angiotensin–aldosterone axis increases sodium reabsorption, whereas antidiuretic hormone (ADH) activity maximizes urinary concentrating power. Thus, the urinary sodium content is typically $<20\,\text{mmol/l}$, urine:plasma urea concentration $>10{:}1$, and urinary osmolality at least 30% greater than that of plasma. The plasma urea is disproportionately increased compared to creatinine in these patients, a fact well recognized. This is explained by the clearance of creatinine being better preserved than that of urea at lower levels of renal function, due to both tubular secretion of creatinine into urine and increased urea reabsorption and backdiffusion.

In practice, it is not advisable to delay treatment whilst waiting for biochemical confirmation of ATN or prerenal uraemia. Correction of haemodynamic abnormalities should be equally expedient in both clinical situations, and the response to this initial therapy will then retrospectively clarify the diagnosis as well as determining further management.

### 11.6.4 Prevention of ARF

In order to avoid the development of ARF in acutely ill patients, the following key points are worthy of re-emphasis:

1. maintenance of an optimal circulating volume and blood pressure;
2. careful monitoring of renal function, with regular biochemical analysis and accurate fluid balance;
3. nephrotoxic agents should be avoided, or where their use is essential, monitored carefully.

These principles are also particularly applicable to those patients susceptible to ARF as a result of surgery. For example, the avoidance of hypovolaemia and maintenance of high urine flow is essential in jaundiced patients undergoing biliary tract surgery or in those requiring aortic aneurysm resection.

*Optimizing the circulation*

Unfortunately there is no *in vivo* method for repeated measurement of renal perfusion, and reliance upon basic bedside assessment of volume status and circulatory function is necessary; more invasive techniques are required in certain patients. Signs of fluid depletion (postural hypotension, reduced tissue turgor, low or undetectable jugular venous pressure) or overload should be actively sought. The value of intravascular catheter placement for central venous pressure (CVP) measurement is sometimes overrated. Patient morbidity is common when the operator is inexperienced and there are further potential pitfalls when relying on CVP readings.

1. CVP will only be a useful guide for optimizing the circulation when cardiac and lung function is normal – higher filling pressures may be needed in patients with chronic heart or lung disease.
2. Hypoalbuminaemic patients may have peripheral or pulmonary oedema in association with a contracted intravascular space.

In the above patient groups the relationship between right and left-sided cardiac filling pressures is inconsistent and optimal management will necessitate invasive monitoring of such parameters as pulmonary capillary wedge pressure (PCWP) with a pulmonary artery catheter.

*Nature of replacement fluid*

Fluid depletion is detectable in many patients with prerenal uraemia or ATN; the deficit should be estimated and rapidly corrected with an intravenous (IV) replacement fluid **appropriate to the aetiology of the hypovolaemia**. This point deserves further emphasis as:

1. dextrose solutions will distribute throughout the total body water; only about 9% will remain in the vascular space after equilibration, and its use should be restricted for cases of water depletion;
2. 0.9% saline equilibrates into the extracellular space, and so about a quarter will remain in the vascular space; many cases of prerenal oliguria are due to salt and water depletion;
3. colloid solutions or blood should be infused in patients with acute blood loss or severe hypotension, as these products will largely remain within the intravascular compartment.

If the patient's circulatory volume is indeterminate, a cautious fluid challenge may be justifiable, e.g. 100–250 ml over five minutes, with careful clinical observation and repeat of the infusion if well tolerated.

*Encouragement of urine flow*

A urinary catheter will aid the assessment of urine flow and hence response to treatment. Although there is scant evidence to suggest that loop diuretics and dopamine confer renoprotection in human ARF, conversion to a non-oliguric condition will provide obvious advantages in the fluid and nutritional management of a patient. The following is a protocol commonly used to encourage urine output in ARF.

1. After repletion of intravascular volume, administer a loop diuretic, e.g. frusemide 80 mg or bumetanide 2 mg IV.
2. If no increase in urine flow, commence dopamine infusion at a rate of 2.5 $\mu$g/kg/min and continue for several hours; concurrently give a high dose of diuretic e.g. bumetanide 5 mg/h for two hours.
3. Continue the dopamine infusion if urine output responds; withdraw the therapy if the patient remains oligo-anuric.
4. Further IV replacement fluid should then match urine output, with a daily allowance made for insensible losses; ideally, the sodium input should be similar to that excreted in urine, for example, if urine sodium is 75 mmol/l, then 50% of the replacement fluid should consist of 0.9% saline (155 mmol/l).

A clinical algorithm for the management of patients with ARF is shown in Figure 11.6.

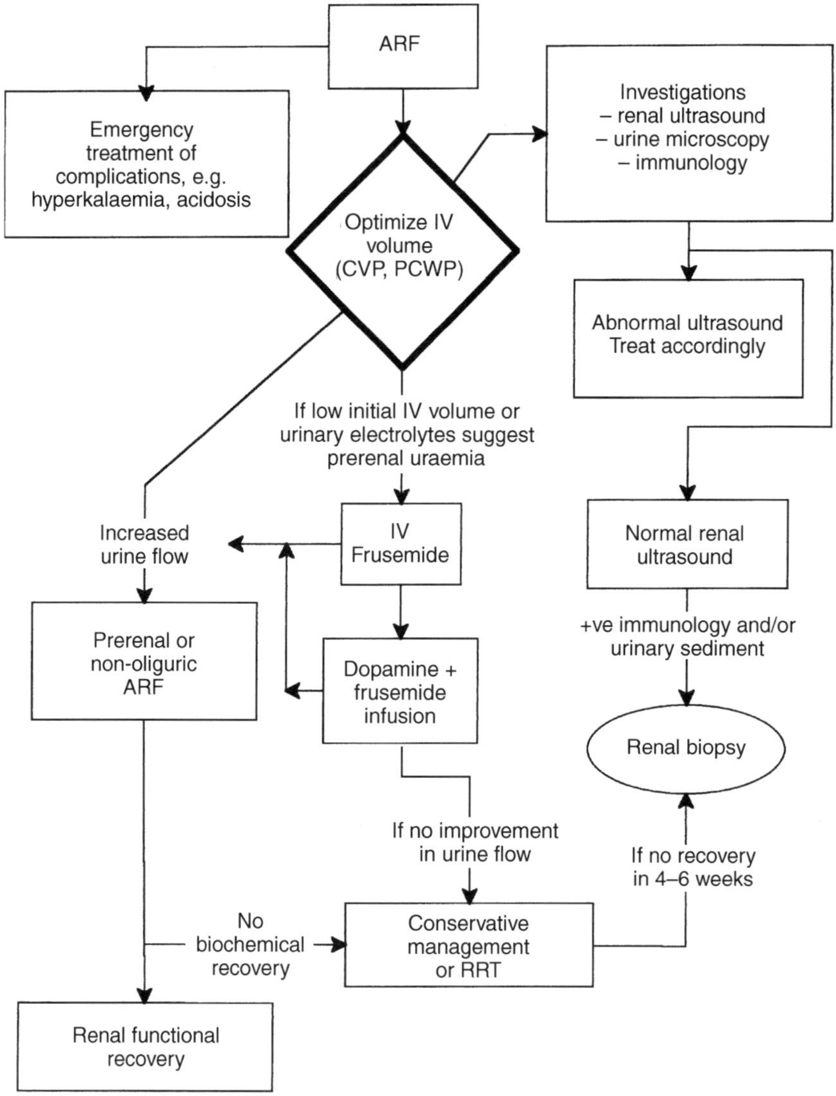


**Figure 11.6** Algorithm for optimal management of ARF.

### 11.6.5 Immediate treatment of life-threatening complications

Hyperkalaemia, severe uraemia, acidosis, pulmonary oedema and uraemic pericarditis all indicate the need for urgent renal replacement therapy in patients with ARF. Adjunctive measures are still essential and increase the chance of survival, particularly during inter-hospital patient transfer or whilst awaiting commencement of dialysis.

*Hyperkalaemia*

ECG changes of 1st-degree block, broadening of the QRS complex and peaked T waves constitute a more reliable indication of cardiotoxicity than the absolute serum potassium concentration. Nevertheless, when the potassium exceeds 6 mmol/l the following measures should be taken.

1. 10 ml calcium gluconate IV over 1–2 min, with continued observation of a cardiac monitor for arrhythmia, to provide myocardial cellular protection.
2. 50 ml dextrose 50% solution administered IV over 10 min, with an accompanying 10 unit bolus of soluble insulin, to drive potassium into the intracellular compartment; the blood glucose concentration should be monitored for several hours thereafter.
3. A 50–100 mmol infusion of a sodium bicarbonate solution will also help control the potassium concentration, by combating acidosis and driving potassium into the cells. This may be particularly applicable as a component of the fluid replacement in patients with hypovolaemic prerenal uraemia.

*Pulmonary oedema*

Diuretics are of little value in the treatment of pulmonary oedema in patients with ARF. The majority of cases require fairly prompt dialysis; the principles of non-dialytic therapy are to maximize oxygenation by ensuring an upright posture and giving high-flow oxygen, and reducing cardiac preload with IV opiates or nitrate infusion. Immediate venesection of 200–500 ml of blood remains a potentially life-saving measure for patients *in extremis*.

### 11.6.6 Prevention of secondary complications of ARF

Acutely ill patients with ARF are at increased risk of local or systemic sepsis and gastrointestinal haemorrhage. Reduced gastric mucosal blood flow and non-specific gastritis are likely contributors to stress ulcer formation; prophylactic therapy with $H_2$-antagonists or antacids is recommended.

*Sepsis*

Infection is still the leading cause of death in patients with ARF. Infective complications should be anticipated and daily chest physiotherapy performed in all acutely ill patients. As Gram negative bacteraemia commonly complicates, or can exacerbate, MOF, gut sterilization protocols have been introduced for vulnerable patients in some ICUs. If sepsis is suspected in a patient with ARF, then the following should be considered:

1. regular microbiological surveillance is essential;
2. check and/or remove and replace all intravascular catheters;
3. frequent chest radiography;
4. in patients with likely abdominal sepsis, regular ultrasound should be performed, and a low threshold for surgical exploration may improve prognosis in this high-mortality patient group.

## 11.7 RENAL REPLACEMENT THERAPIES FOR ARF

Many patients with ARF can be managed without dialysis. In our own unit, 63% of non-ICU-managed patients with ATN (equivalent to 35 ARF patients) were treated without replacement therapy in 1995. Conservative management is particularly applicable to the following groups:

1. prerenal uraemia;
2. non-oliguric ARF;
3. patients who invariably have suffered a limited renal insult resulting in a milder form of ATN with only a brief oliguric phase.

When it becomes clear that renal replacement therapy will be necessary, then it should be commenced without delay. Early correction of uraemia (e.g. when urea $<30$ mmol/l and creatinine 500–700 $\mu$mol/l) can be expected to improve outcome as it will facilitate patient nutrition and indirectly help minimize extra-renal complications, such as pneumonia, gastrointestinal bleeding and pressure-area damage. Extrapolation of this rationale is responsible for replacement therapy being commenced at considerably lesser degrees of uraemia in patients with MOF on the ICU. Intermittent haemodialysis remains the standard modality of first choice for ARF in renal units. Peritoneal dialysis is less popular, though still valuable in certain clinical and resource-limited circumstances.

### 11.7.1 Continuous replacement therapies

Although intermittent haemodialysis (HD) has traditionally been the principal renal replacement therapy (RRT) in ARF, there is evidence that continuous replacement therapies, such as haemofiltration (HF) and haemodiafiltration (HDF), may provide advantages to the critically ill patient with ARF. One ICU study found that patients treated with HDF had almost twice the likelihood of survival as a well-matched retrospective group who had received peritoneal or HD [40]. However, a more recent prospective multicentred ICU study showed that continuous RRT increased the likelihood of renal functional recovery yet provided no survival advantage over conventional HD [41]. There are several possible explanations for these findings. Critically ill patients treated with continuous replacement therapies benefit from improved cardiovascular stability, optimal circulatory volume regulation and enhanced nutritional replacement; techniques that involve a component of haemofiltration may also remove cytokines and other inflammatory mediators from the circulation. Lastly, the impaired renal autoregulation that accompanies ARF may make the kidneys vulnerable to further ischaemic injury during episodes of HD-related hypotension [17], an effect which can extend the duration of ARF and its attendant complications.

### 11.7.2 Biocompatibility in dialysis

There is increasing awareness of the advantages conferred by biocompatible dialysis membranes to patient well-being. Cytokines such as TNF and IL-1 are released during standard cuprophane dialysis, and the complement system is activated. These inflammatory mediators may exacerbate tissue damage and the hypoperfusion of kidneys and other organs in patients with ARF; their potential role in the pathogenesis of MOF has already been discussed, and they may also help prolong the oliguric period in some patients treated with HD. Newer membranes, such as polyacrylonitrile, polysulphone and polycarbonate, are more appropriate for the dialysis or HF/HDF of patients with ARF as they do not appear to stimulate cytokine release [42] and may even adsorb complement components and cytokines from the circulation [43], a contention supported by the recent finding that improved renal functional recovery in ARF patients accompanied HD with polymethyl methacrylate as opposed to conventional cuprophane membranes [44].

It is also now accepted that bicarbonate dialysate should be used in preference to acetate, as the latter is far more likely to provoke cardiovascular lability and impaired oxygenation in patients with ARF.

## 11.8 RENOPROTECTIVE STRATEGIES IN ISCHAEMIC ACUTE RENAL FAILURE

### 11.8.1 Putative strategies used in clinical practice

Several agents which, theoretically at least, possess renoprotective properties are regularly used in human clinical ARF. The evidence for their roles in ameliorating the course of ischaemic ARF is briefly reviewed below.

### *Mannitol*

This osmotic diuretic encourages filtrate flow and might be expected to clear the cellular casts and other intratubular obstructive debris that result from ATN; as a hydroxyl radical scavenger, mannitol could also directly reduce post-ischaemic cellular injury. Thus in animal models, mannitol reduces endothelial and tubular cell swelling, improves renal function by increasing urine flow, but it does not limit ATN [45]. The evidence for mannitol limiting human ARF is weak and its application in clinical practice is reserved for:

1. use as a component of renal transplant preservation solutions, as it probably diminishes cellular swelling during the cold ischaemic phase of storage and so reduces post-transplant ATN;
2. prophylactic maintenance of urine flow in high-risk surgical patients, e.g. the jaundiced during biliary operations or those undergoing aortorenal surgery.

### *Frusemide and other loop diuretics*

As with mannitol, it would be anticipated that loop diuretics attenuate ARF by increasing urine flow and clearing tubular obstruction; their natriuretic effect may also reduce tubular cell injury after ischaemia by preventing the cellular energy consumption that normally accompanies sodium reabsorption [46]. *In vivo* studies in the rat have shown that frusemide can limit ARF when given before and after RAO. However, the evidence for a protective effect in human ARF is again lacking, perhaps because these diuretics act on the loop of Henle which is distal to much of the intratubular obstructing debris. The clinical value of loop diuretics is hence limited to:

1. conversion of oliguric ARF to a non-oliguric state;
2. maintenance of urine flow during surgery in high-risk patients, as for mannitol.

### *Dopamine*

The possible renoprotective effects of dopamine have been debated in the literature for many years. Its action upon specific dopamine receptors within the kidney results in a dose-dependent increase in RBF due to intrarenal vasodilatation, within an infusion range of 1–10 $\mu$g/kg/min; it also stimulates natriuresis, and angiotensin-induced mesangial cell tone may be relaxed. Dopamine provides no unequivocal survival advantage in animal models of ARF [47], but benefits of prophylactic treatment seem to be enhanced by combination with mannitol or a loop diuretic. Although dopamine is frequently used in 'renal dose' (2.5–5 $\mu$g/kg/min) in human ARF, no conclusive benefit to post-ischaemic renal function is recognized. In practice the clinical usefulness of dopamine is probably limited to a natriuretic, and hence diuretic, action which may convert oliguric to non-oliguric ARF.

*Calcium channel blockers (CCBs)*

The pivotal role of calcium in the pathophysiology of ischaemia–reperfusion injury has already been described, and the advantages of calcium channel-blocking agents have been demonstrated in both *in vitro* cell culture and in many animal studies of ARF [48]. Their theoretical benefits include attenuation of ischaemic cellular damage, OFR formation and of the increased afferent arteriolar tone that accompanies the early stages of ARF [28]. The finding in some animal studies that post-ischaemic administration of calcium blockers can still improve ARF may have important implications for human disease [49].

In contrast to dopamine and the osmotic or loop diuretics, there is evidence that the calcium blockers can ameliorate the course of ATN in certain clinical situations. Hence, pretreatment of both renal allografts and transplant recipients with diltiazem will reduce primary non-function after transplantation, an effect which may have longer-term consequences for graft survival as patients with initial ATN have poorer one-year allograft function [50]; similar effects have been observed with other calcium channel blockers. These agents have also been shown to be protective against radiocontrast-induced nephrotoxicity. Although the clinical value of CCBs in the treatment of ARF is still under investigation, their future application is quite possible in protocols that involve:

1. pretreatment of cadaveric allografts and transplant recipients;
2. renoprotection by intra-renal infusion of calcium blockers during elective warm ischaemia;
3. post-injury administration to patients at risk of developing ARF or MOF.

### 11.8.2 Experimental strategies in renoprotection

In clinical practice, preventative measures during the ischaemic period may limit the insult to the kidneys, provided that the hypoperfusion injury has not progressed to ATN. However, most patients who develop ischaemic ARF present after the insult, and so recent research has concentrated on the attenuation of ARF by influencing pathogenetic events that occur early in the phase after restoration of renal blood supply, during reperfusion.

*Scientific basis for renoprotection*

The previous account of the intricate pathophysiology of ARF indicates that renoprotection may potentially be provided by any of the following.

1. Increasing or redistributing intra-renal blood flow.
2. Relieving renal vasoconstriction.
3. Diminishing tubular cell work after ischaemia.
4. Clearing intra-tubular obstructive debris.
5. Buffering acidosis and cellular swelling.
6. Interacting with calcium metabolism.
7. Reducing oxygen free radical-mediated damage.
8. Stimulating tubular repair and recovery.

*Summary of experimental findings*

Innumerable animal and *in vitro* experiments have sought to determine the protective value of various agents in attenuating the structural or functional damage that follows renal ischaemic injury, and a wealth of literature has resulted. It is beyond the scope of this chapter to provide anything other than a brief overview of the essential findings.

The intense afferent arteriolar vasoconstriction characteristic of the maintenance phase of oliguric ARF can be attenuated by inhibition of the local effects of endothelin with specific antagonists or antibodies [16], and with calcium channel blockers [28], adenosine antagonists and vasodilator prostaglandins such as $PGI_2$ [51] or $PGE_1$. The resulting increase in RBF is usually associated with improvement in post-ischaemic GFR. Intra-renal shunting of blood away from the medulla is partly due to increased vascular permeability and erythrocyte trapping in medullary capillaries; strategies such as reducing an animal's haematocrit before ischaemia, or infusing hyperoncotic albumin solutions, will limit both the perfusion defect and tubular cell injury and improve renal function [52].

The benefits of reducing tubular cell reabsorptive work with loop diuretics, or clearing intratubular obstruction by the increase in urine flow that accompanies treatment with these agents or mannitol, have already been considered. Mannitol will also limit cellular swelling in ARF, an effect observed with other osmotic agents including sucrose; the cellular protective action of lower pH solutions (e.g. pH 7 instead of pH 7.4) has also been documented [53]. Calcium channel blockers have several likely beneficial effects in ARF [28] and will improve post-ischaemic RBF, renal function and ATN [48, 49], as discussed previously.

Prevention of the damage associated with oxygen free-radical release can be conferred in many ways. Allopurinol reduces OFR generation by inhibition of xanthine oxidase and limits ARF after RAO [24] as well as ATN in pig allografts [23]; exogenous OFR scavengers, such as superoxide dismutase, have similar effects. Further, an increase of the activity of native scavenger systems can also yield cytoprotection – glycine, a component amino acid of glutathione, protects tubular cell cultures during hypoxia–reoxygenation [54]. Cytoprotection may involve stabilization of the cytoskeletal elements in cellular membranes and maintenance of membrane fluidity, and the latter may be important in the protective effects of $PGI_2$ [51] and misoprostil [55].

More recent research has evaluated the importance of cell adhesion molecules in the pathogenesis of ARF [56]; antibody against ICAM-1 in particular will improve post-ischaemic renal function. The important role of growth factors, such as IGF-1 and EGF, in stimulating tissue repair and recovery in ARF [34] has been alluded to in a previous section.

*Comparison of the renoprotective effects of several agents*

It would be invidious to attempt comparison of the renoprotective effects of these varied therapeutic strategies, as the models of ischaemic ARF have differed widely with respect to the experimental animal and the nature of ischaemic injury. The author therefore investigated the protective effects of several agents, all differing in their putative mechanisms of action, within the same rat model of ischaemic ARF [57]. Renal ischaemia was effected with 30 min of bilateral renal artery occlusion and the protective agents were pre-infused, or administered at the time of clamp release, in dosages considered to be optimal in previous experiments. Renal function was assessed at 24 hours and seven days after ischaemia, and a distinct pattern of protection was observed. During the maintenance phase GFR was only improved by $PGI_2$ and dopamine (Figure 11.7); a concomitant increase in RBF, as assessed by laser Doppler flow, was observed with both of these agents. In the early recovery phase, GFR was improved by all renoprotective agents (Figure 11.8), but particularly by those possessing cytoprotective actions (mannitol, allopurinol, calcium channel blocker and non-specific OFR scavenger). Acute tubular necrosis was only attenuated by allopurinol and felodipine. These findings have led to the hypothesis that alleviation of intra-renal vasoconstriction may improve renal function to a greater extent than cellular damage, in the early stages of ARF, whereas cytoprotective agents manifest their benefit later after ischaemic injury, at which stage the effects of cellular injury predominate in maintaining the renal dysfunction.

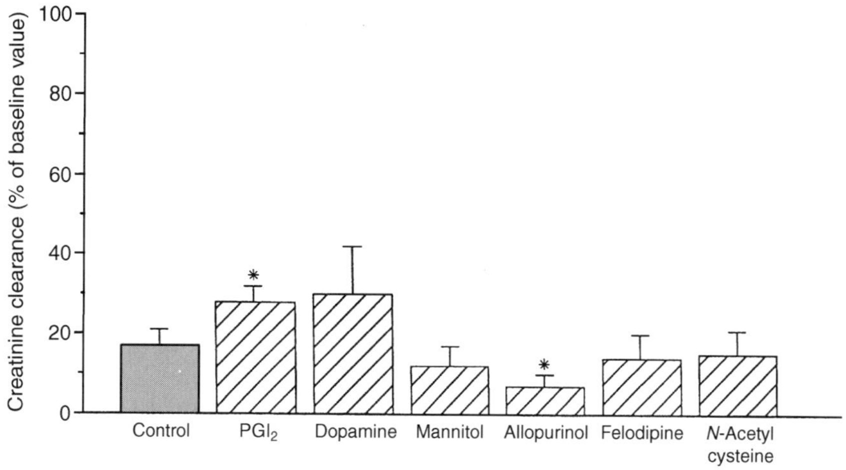


**Figure 11.7** Renal function at day 1 after 30 min bilateral RAO and treatment with different renoprotective agents (mean ± SEM). *$P < 0.05$ compared to control group.

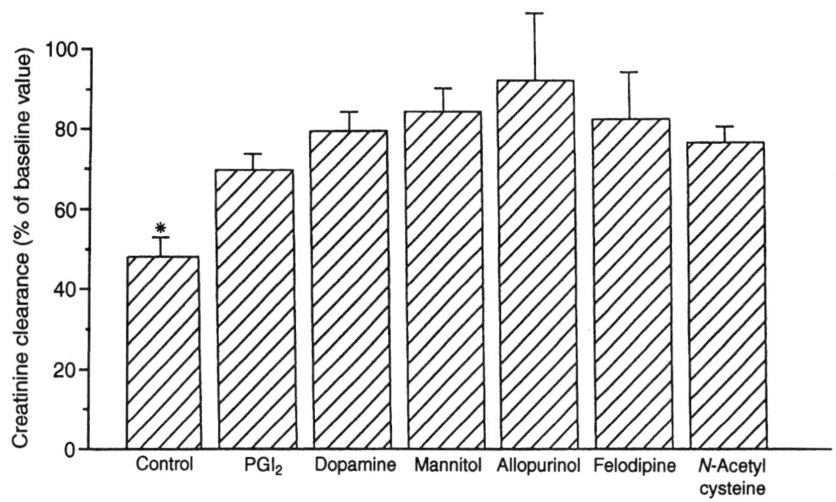


**Figure 11.8** Renal function at day 7 after 30 min bilateral RAO and treatment with different renoprotective agents (mean ± SEM). *$P < 0.05$ compared to all other groups.

## 11.9 PROGNOSIS OF ISCHAEMIC ACUTE RENAL FAILURE

Despite major advances in the management of patients with ARF, such as improved nutrition (considered in detail in Chapter 13) and renal replacement therapy, the mortality rate remains alarmingly high. A single-centre review of all patients with severe ARF, that spanned three decades in Leeds, found that overall survival had increased from 49% in the 1950s to only 58% in the late 1980s [6]. Mortality is increased in patients with sepsis and in the elderly – a 70% fatality was observed in patients older than 65 years of age.

Other investigators have looked specifically at critically ill patients with ARF managed in ICUs. In Leicester, overall survival was 35% in all categories of ICU patient with ARF, but survival fell to 27% if ventilatory support had been necessary [58]; in some surgical ICUs mortality may be as great as 88%. Such depressing statistics for outcome of ARF are due to the fact that many ICU patients develop ischaemic ATN as a complication of (or part of) another systemic disease process and they often have MOF, which itself carries a far poorer prognosis. Patients tend to die from their multiple pathology rather than renal failure *per se,* a fact borne out by European Dialysis Transplant Association (EDTA) data that has shown ARF patient survival being determined by the nature and number of other associated organ failures [2]; mortality was 8% for ARF in isolation, 65% if there was failure of a second organ (either pulmonary, hepatic, circulatory failure or uncontrolled sepsis) and an overall mortality of 98% if a third organ was involved [5].

However, to end on a more positive note, the long-term renal functional outcome is good for patients who survive the episode of ischaemic ARF. At least 60% of patients have full recovery of renal function, about 30% will have mild to moderate chronic renal impairment and only 6–10% remain with dialysis-requiring end stage renal failure [59].

## REFERENCES


1. Bywaters, E.G.L. and Beal, D. (1941) Crush injuries with impairment of renal function. *Br. Med. J.*, **i**, 427–33.
2. Wing, A.J., Broyer, M., Brunner, F.P. *et al.* (1983) Combined report on regular dialysis and transplantation in Europe, XIII, 1982. Acute (reversible) renal failure. *Proc. Eur. Dial. Transplant. Assoc.*, **20**, 64–71.
3. Kleinknecht, D. (1990) Epidemiology of acute renal failure in France today, in *Renal Failure in the Intensive Therapy Unit* (eds D. Bihari and G. Neild), Springer-Verlag, Berlin, pp. 13–22.
4. Feest, T.G., Round, A. and Hamad, S. (1993) Incidence of severe acute renal failure in adults: results of a community based study. *Br. Med. J.*, **306**, 481–3.
5. Cameron, J.S. (1986) Acute renal failure – the continuing challenge. *Q. J. Med.*, **59**, 337–43.
6. Turney, J.H., Marshal, D.H., Brownjohn, A.M. *et al.* (1990) The evolution of acute renal failure, 1956–1988. *Q. J. Med.*, **74**, 83–104.
7. Canafax, D.M., Torres, A., Fryd, D.S. *et al.* (1986) The effects of delayed function on recipients of cadaver renal allografts. *Transplantation*, **41**, 177–81.

8. Parrott, N.R., Forsythe, J.L.R., Matthews, J.N.S. *et al.* (1990) Late perfusion: a simple remedy for renal allograft primary nonfunction. *Transplantation*, **49**, 913–5.
9. Venkatachalam, M.A., Bernard, D.B., Donohoe, J.F. and Levinsky, N.G. (1978) Ischemic damage and repair in the rat proximal tubule. Differences among the S1, S1, and S3 segments. *Kidney Int.*, **14**, 31–49.
10. Baker, G.L., Corry, R.J. and Autor, A.P. (1985) Oxygen free radical induced damage in kidneys subjected to warm ischemia and reperfusion. *Ann. Surg.*, **202**, 628–41.
11. Brenner, B.M., Zatz, R. and Ichikawa, I. (1986) The renal circulations, in *The Kidney*, 3rd edn (eds B.M. Brenner and F.C. Rector), W.B. Saunders, Philadelphia, pp. 93–123.
12. Kriz, W. (1982) Structural organization of renal medullary circulation. *Nephron*, **31**, 290–5.
13. Epstein, F.H., Balaban, R.S. and Ross, B.D. (1982) Redox state of cytochrome *aa*3 in isolated perfused rat kidney. *Am. J. Physiol.*, **243**, F356–F363.
14. Arendshorst, W.J., Finn, W.F. and Gottschalk, C.W. (1975) Pathogenesis of acute renal failure following temporary renal ischemia in the rat. *Circ. Res.*, **37**, 558–68.
15. Firth, J.D. and Ratcliffe, P.J. (1992) Organ distribution of the three rat endothelin messenger RNAs and the effects of ischaemia on renal gene expression. *J. Clin. Invest.*, **90**, 1023–31.
16. Kon, V., Yoshioka, T., Fogo, A. and Ichikawa, I. (1989) Glomerular actions of endothelin *in vivo*. *J. Clin. Invest.*, **83**, 1762–7.
17. Conger, J.D., Robinette, J.B. and Schrier, R.W. (1988) Smooth muscle calcium and endothelium-derived relaxing factor in the abnormal vascular responses of acute renal failure. *J. Clin. Invest.*, **82**, 532–7.
18. Hellberg, P.O.A., Kallskog, O. and Wolgast, M. (1991) Red cell trapping and postischemic renal blood flow. Differences between the cortex, outer and inner medulla. *Kidney Int.*, **40**, 625–31.
19. Mason, J., Torhorst, J. and Welsch, J. (1984) Role of the medullary perfusion defect in the pathogenesis of ischemic renal failure. *Kidney Int.*, **26**, 283–93.
20. Kreisberg, J.I. and Ventkatachalam, M.A. (1988) Morphological factors in acute renal failure, in *Acute renal failure*, 2nd edn, (eds B.M. Brenner and J.M. Lazarus), Churchill Livingstone, New York, pp. 45–65.
21. Myers, B.D. and Moran, S.M. (1986) Hemodynamically mediated acute renal failure. *N. Engl. J. Med.*, **314**, 97–105.
22. Donohoe, J.V., Ventkatachalam, M.A., Bernard, D.B. and Levinsky, N.G. (1978) Tubular leakage and obstruction after ischemia: structure–function correlations. *Kidney Int.*, **13**, 208–22.
23. Koyama, I., Bulkley, G.B., Williams, G.M. and Im, M.J. (1985) The role of oxygen free radicals in mediating the reperfusion injury of cold-preserved ischemic kidneys. *Transplantation*, **40**, 590–5.
24. Paller, M.S., Hoidal, J.R. and Ferris, T.F. (1984) Oxygen free radicals in ischemic acute renal failure in the rat. *J. Clin. Invest.*, **74**, 1156–64.
25. Roy, R.S. and McCord, J.M. (1983) Superoxide and ischemia: conversion of xanthine dehydrogenase to xanthine oxidase, in *Oxy Radicals and their Scavenger Systems, Volume 2, Cellular And Molecular Aspects*, (eds R. Greenwald and G. Cohen), Elsevier Science, New York, pp. 145–53.
26. McCord, J.M. (1985) Oxygen-derived free radicals in post-ischemic tissue injury. *N. Engl. J. Med.*, **312**, 159–63.

27. Vladimirov, Y.A., Olenev, B.I., Suslova, T.B., Cheremisina, Z.P. (1980) Lipid peroxidation in mitochondrial membrane. *Adv. Lipid Res.*, **17**, 173–249.
28. Schrier, R.W., Arnold, P.E., Van Putten, V.J., Burke, T.J. (1987) Cellular calcium in ischemic acute renal failure: Role of calcium entry blockers. *Kidney Int.*, **32**, 313–21.
29. Malis, C.D., Bonventre, J.V. (1986) Mechanism of calcium potentiation of oxygen free radical injury to renal mitochondria. A model for post-ischemic and toxic mitochondrial damage. *J. Biol. Chem.*, **261**, 14201–8.
30. Kashgarian, M., Siegel, N.J., Ries, A.L. *et al.* (1976) Hemodynamic aspects in development and recovery phases of experimental postischemic acute renal failure. *Kidney Int.*, **10**, S160–S168.
31. Solez, K., Morel-Maroger, L. and Sraer, J.D. (1979) The morphology of 'acute tubular necrosis' in man: analysis of 57 renal biopsies and a comparison with the glycerol model. *Medicine*, **58**, 362–76.
32. Wolgast, M., Karlberg, L., Kallskog, O. *et al.* (1982) Hemodynamic alterations in ischemic acute renal failure. *Nephron*, **31**, 301–3.
33. Witzgall, R., Brown, D., Schwarz, C. and Bonventre, J.V. (1993) Localization of PCNA, vimentin, clusterin, and c-*fos* in post-ischemic kidneys. Evidence for a large pool of mitotically active and dedifferentiated cells (abstract). *J. Am. Soc. Nephrol.*, **4**, 747.
34. Toback, F.G. (1992) Regeneration after acute tubular necrosis. *Kidney Int.*, **41**, 226–46.
35. Harris, C.E., Griffiths, R.D., Freestone, N. *et al.* (1991) Intestinal permeability in the critically ill. *Intensive Care Med.*, **18**, 38–41.
36. Wardle, E.N. (1982) Acute renal failure in the 1980s: the importance of septicaemia and endotoxaemia. *Nephron*, **30**, 193–200.
37. Greenberg, R.N., Wilson, K.M., Kunz, A.Y. *et al.* (1992) Observations using anti-endotoxin antibody (E5) as adjuvant therapy in humans with suspected serious gram-negative sepsis. *Crit. Care Med.*, **20**, 730–35.
38. Firth, J.D. and Winearls, C.G. (1995) Acute renal failure, in *Oxford Textbook of Medicine*, (eds D.J. Weatherall, J.G.G. Ledingham and D.A. Warrell), 3rd edn, Oxford Medical Publications, **20**, 179–94.
39. Brenner, B.M. and Lazarus, J.M. (eds) (1988) *Acute Renal Failure*, 2nd edn, Churchill Livingstone, New York.
40. Bellomo, R., Farmer, M., Parkin, G. *et al.* (1995) Severe acute renal failure: a comparison of acute continuous haemodiafiltration and conventional dialytic therapy. *Nephron*, **71**, 59–64.
41. Mehta, R.L., McDonald, B., Gabbai, F. *et al.* (1996) Continuous versus intermittent dialysis for acute renal failure (ARF) in the ICU: results from a randomized multicenter trial (abstract). *J. Am. Soc. Nephrol.*, **7**, 1457.
42. Ghysen, J., De Plaen, J.F. and van Ypersele de Strihou, C. (1990) The effect of membrane characteristics on tumour necrosis factor kinetics during haemodialysis. *Nephrol. Dial. Transplant.*, **5**, 270–4.
43. Pascual, M. and Schifferli, J.A. (1993) Adsorption of complement factor D by polyacrylonitrile dialysis membranes. *Kidney Int.*, **43**, 903–11.
44. Hakim, R.M., Wingard, R.L. and Parker, R.A. (1994) Effect of the dialysis membrane in the treatment of patients with acute renal failure. *N. Engl. J. Med.* **331**, 1338–42.
45. Zager, R.A., Mahan, J. and Merola, A.J. (1985) Effects of mannitol on the postischemic kidney. Biochemical, functional and morphological assessments. *Lab. Invest.*, **53**, 433–42.

46. Brezis, M., Rosen, S., Silva, P. and Epstein, F.H. (1984) Transport activity modifies thick ascending limb damage in isolated perfused kidney. *Kidney Int.*, **25**, 65–72.
47. Mann, H.J., Fuhs, D.W. and Hemstrom, C.A. (1986) Acute renal failure. *Drug Intell. Clin. Pharm.*, **20**, 421–38.
48. Burke, T.J., Arnold, P.E., Gordon, J.A. *et al.* (1984) Protective effect of intrarenal calcium membrane blockers before or after renal ischemia. *J. Clin. Invest.*, **74**, 1830–41.
49. Wait, R.B., White, G. and Davis, J.H. (1983) Beneficial effects of verapamil on postischemic renal failure. *Surgery*, **94**, 276–82.
50. Neumayer, H.-H., Kunzendorf, U. and Schreiber, M. (1992) Protective effects of diltiazem and the prostazycline analogue iloprost in human renal transplantation. *Renal Failure*, **14**, 289–96.
51. Finn, W.F., Hak, L.J. and Grossman, S.H. (1987) Protective effect of prostacyclin on postischemic acute renal failure in the rat. *Kidney Int.*, **32**, 479–87.
52. Mason, J., Welsch, J. and Torhorst, J. (1987) The contribution of vascular obstruction to the functional defect that follows renal ischemia. *Kidney Int.*, **31**, 65–71.
53. Ferwana, O.S., Pirie, S.C. and Potts, D.J. (1989) Effect of phosphate-buffered sucrose flush solution upon the initial phase of ischaemic acute renal failure in the rat. *Clin. Sci.*, **77**, 77–84.
54. Weinberg, J.M., Davis, J.A., Abarzua, M. and Rajan, T. (1987) Cytoprotective effects of glycine and glutathione against hypoxic injury to renal tubules. *J. Clin. Invest.*, **80**, 1446–54.
55. Paller, M.S. and Manivel, J.C. (1992) Prostaglandins protect kidneys against ischemic and toxic injury by a cellular effect. *Kidney Int.*, **42**, 1345–54.
56. Simon, E.E. (1993) Cell adhesion molecules in acute renal failure, in Proc. 3rd Int. Satel. Symposium on ARF, Halkidiki, Greece (eds M. Papadimitriou and E. Alexopoulos), University Studio Press, Thessalonika, pp. 7–18.
57. Kalra, P.A. (1995) An investigation of the effects of prostacyclin and other renoprotective agents in a model of ischaemic acute renal failure. M.D. thesis, Cambridge University.
58. Wheeler, D.C., Feehally, J. and Walls, J. (1986) High risk acute renal failure. *Q. J. Med.*, **61**, 977–84.
59. Bonomini, V., Stefoni, S. and Vangelista, A. (1984) Long-term patient and renal prognosis in acute renal failure. *Nephron*, **36**, 169–72.

# 12

# Drugs and the kidney

*D.G. Waller and C.F. George*

The interactions between drugs and the functions of the kidney will be dealt with in three major sections. The first section outlines the key processes involved in drug absorption, distribution, metabolism and elimination. The kidneys play a central role in the elimination of many drugs from the circulation and their role is examined in detail and the mechanisms of renal drug handling highlighted. The contribution of the kidneys to drug metabolism is also considered. The second section outlines the effects that impaired renal function can have on drug pharmacokinetics. The principles underlying dose modification in renal failure and renal dialysis are described. The third section examines the harmful effects that drugs can have on the kidney. The mechanisms involved in the genesis of nephrotoxicity are described and the effects of important nephrotoxic drugs discussed in more depth.

## 12.1 PRINCIPLES OF PHARMACOKINETICS

### 12.1.1 Drug absorption

The commonest method of delivery of drugs is still by the oral route, though they can be administered for systemic delivery by other routes such as subcutaneous, intramuscular, intravenous, trans-cutaneous, rectal or by inhalation. Little drug absorption occurs from the stomach, due to its small surface area. If the drug is acidic, e.g. acetylsalicylic acid (aspirin), it will be in a lipid soluble form at gastric pH and some absorption will occur. However, most absorption, even for aspirin, will be from the larger surface area of the small bowel. The rate of gastric

*Renal Disease.* Edited by G. Venkat Raman. Published in 1998 by Chapman & Hall, London. ISBN 0 412 45700 8.

emptying has little influence on the amount of drug absorbed, but may delay the onset of absorption – important if rapid delivery is required, for example for the treatment of acute pain. Once in the small bowel, rapid intestinal transit can reduce overall absorption, particularly if the drug is in a modified-release formulation which depends on slow delivery of the agent from an inert matrix.

### 12.1.2 Drug distribution

Once a drug has reached the systemic circulation, it will gain access to a variety of tissues. The extent of distribution to these tissues will be determined by several factors, the most important of which are protein binding and lipid solubility. A highly protein-bound drug will be retained largely in the circulation if it has a high affinity for binding sites on plasma proteins such as albumin (for acidic drugs) or $\alpha_1$-acid glycoprotein (for basic drugs). Examples include the non-steroidal anti-inflammatory drugs, warfarin, phenytoin and the sulphonylureas. Other drugs avidly bind to tissue proteins, e.g. amiodarone. These will selectively concentrate in the tissues and are only slowly released, prolonging their residence in the body. If protein binding of a drug is low, its distribution will be determined by lipid solubility. A highly lipid soluble drug readily crosses cell membranes and will also be selectively concentrated in adipose tissue. By contrast, water-soluble molecules are largely confined to extracellular fluid spaces. The apparent volume of distribution of a drug ($V_d$) is a measure of the extent of tissue distribution. When the amount of drug reaching the circulation is known, $V_d$ can be calculated by assuming that the measured concentration of the drug in plasma is equivalent to its concentration in the tissues. Thus, a drug that is selectively concentrated in extravascular tissues will have a low blood concentration and a high apparent volume of distribution. Changes in the volume of distribution will therefore affect the amount of drug in the circulation and the concentration to which the target tissue is exposed.

### 12.1.3 Metabolism

Metabolism is the main process which enables the body to eliminate lipid-soluble chemicals, converting them to a water-soluble derivative which can then be excreted. Drug metabolism reactions are separated into two phases. Many drugs undergo sequential transformation by reactions in both phases while others may undergo only a phase I or a phase II reaction. These processes of biotransformation can be complex. The chemical entity produced by metabolism frequently has very different pharmacological or toxicological properties from the parent compound.

Metabolism usually decreases the therapeutic activity of the parent drug. However, certain drugs which are active in the parent form are also metabolized to active molecules which contribute a useful therapeutic effect and often prolong the duration of action of the parent drug, e.g. diazepam and amitriptyline. Other compounds are formulated as pro-drugs, which have little or no therapeutic activity in their own right. These overcome problems of palatability or absorption of the active compound. They are metabolized before reaching the systemic circulation to highly effective derivatives, e.g. enalapril to enalaprilat.

Excessive production of a metabolite can be responsible for drug toxicity, e.g. the hepatotoxic and nephrotoxic metabolite of paracetamol in overdose, and the central nervous system toxicity produced by metabolites of lignocaine.

### *Phase I reactions*

During phase I reactions, the drug undergoes either oxidation, reduction or hydrolysis. These processes may add or reveal active chemical groups which are then available to undergo phase II or conjugation reactions.

Drug oxidation is carried out by mixed function oxidases collectively known as cytochrome P450. Members of this family of enzymes are found in many body tissues, the highest concentrations being in the liver. Extrahepatic enzymes contribute little to overall metabolism but may contribute to the expression of drug toxicity [1].

Many isoenzymes involved in drug metabolism show genetic or ethnic variation in activity. Occasionally this variation may be substantial, e.g. cytochrome P45011D6 (CYP2D6) which is responsible for the metabolism of debrisoquine (and about 20 other known chemical entities) is deficient in some 5–10% of Caucasians who therefore metabolize debrisoquine very slowly. This enzyme deficiency is inherited as an autosomal recessive. Similarly, the oxidation of nifedipine by cytochrome P450IIIA4 (CYP3A4) is slower in South Asians. Poor metabolizers have higher plasma concentrations of parent drug which produces exaggerated pharmacological effects and may predispose to drug toxicity.

Enzyme systems other than cytochrome P450 are also involved in oxidation reactions, including a mono-oxygenase in the endoplasmic reticulum and specific enzymes such as alcohol dehydrogenase, aldehyde dehydrogenase and monoamine oxidase.

Reduction reactions are also performed by cytochrome P450 and various cytosolic enzymes, but are less common than oxidation reactions. Sulindac is an example of a drug metabolized by this process. Hydrolysis reactions are important for some drugs; these occur in plasma and several extrahepatic tissues, mediated by esterases and amidases. Procaine, lignocaine and physostigmine are among the drugs which are metabolized in this way.

### *Phase II reactions*

Phase II or conjugation reactions usually involve the synthesis of a high-energy substrate which is then attached to the drug. Examples of these, each of which is produced by the action of a specific enzyme, include glucuronide, glycine, sulphate or mercapturic acid. For comparatively few compounds methylation or acetylation produces the conjugate. The products of conjugation are usually more water soluble and less toxic than the substrate compound but this is not always the case [2]. The enzymes involved in conjugation are found in several tissues other than the liver, including the gut wall and kidney.

### *First-pass metabolism*

After absorption from the gastrointestinal tract, drugs enter the portal venous circulation and pass to the liver. Lipid-soluble drugs such as lignocaine and glyceryl trinitrate are almost completely absorbed from the gut, but undergo extensive extraction during first passage through the liver. Extensive first-pass metabolism (or more correctly presystemic elimination) then substantially reduces systemic bioavailability of these drugs, transforming them to inactive derivatives [3]. For some drugs, such as propranolol or glyceryl trinitrate, the metabolism is saturable; increasing the size of the dose can overcome the limited bioavailability. For others, such as lignocaine, it is not saturable and increasing concentrations of the metabolite, monoethylglycinerylidide, can produce convulsions before therapeutic concentrations of lignocaine are achieved. To achieve a therapeutic effect lignocaine must therefore be given parenterally to avoid first-pass metabolism.

For other drugs, first-pass metabolism generates active compounds which contribute substantially to the overall activity of the drug. Examples are tricyclic antidepressants, such as amitriptyline and isosorbide dinitrate which is converted to the longer-acting isosorbide 5-mononitrate. First-pass metabolism is responsible for the activation of pro-drugs such as nabumetone and enalapril. The process of first-pass metabolism can occur in the gut lumen or gut wall, but the majority occurs in the liver. If hepatic metabolism predominates then processes involved in first-pass metabolism are usually the same as those responsible for the elimination of the drug from the circulation.

### 12.1.4 Renal drug elimination

There are several potential routes for drug elimination from the body, either as the parent compound or as a metabolite. Some elimination occurs through biliary excretion into the gut. For gaseous anaesthetics, exhalation in expired air is a major route. However, for many compounds the kidney is the principal route of elimination, and the processes involved will be considered in more detail.

The amount of drug removed by the kidney is dependent on its water solubility. Large amounts of water-soluble or polar drugs can be removed by renal elimination. Four processes are involved in drug handling in the kidney: glomerular filtration, passive back-diffusion from the proximal renal tubule, active tubular secretion and active tubular reabsorption [4].

*Glomerular filtration*

This is a passive process that delivers up to 125 ml of ultrafiltrate each minute to the proximal tubules of the nephrons. Since the glomerular membrane acts as a selective filter, smaller macromolecules pass more readily into the filtrate. The passage of neutral molecules is much greater than that of charged molecules of similar size. Drug molecules cross the glomerular membrane through extracellular pathways; the principal physical barriers are the capillary basement membrane of the endothelial cell layer and the epithelial filtration slits.

The driving force for ultrafiltration, the glomerular capillary hydrostatic pressure, is generated by the perfusion pressure in the afferent renal artery. Since the capillary bed in the glomerulus links two arterioles, there is no significant fall in hydrostatic pressure across the capillary. This contrasts with most other capillaries in which there is a progressive fall in pressure along their length.

Excretion of drugs which are able to cross the glomerular membrane is dependent on their rate of delivery, which in turn is determined by renal plasma flow. Drugs can only undergo ultrafiltration if they are dissolved in plasma water. Proteins responsible for binding drugs in plasma (mainly albumin and $\alpha_1$ acid glycoprotein) are too large to be filtered, and bound drug dissociates too slowly for significant ultrafiltration to occur. Plasma clearance of a drug by glomerular filtration will, therefore, be inversely related to the degree of protein binding. As a consequence, if a drug is not protein bound and does not undergo secretion or reabsorption from the renal tubule, then its plasma clearance will be close to that for glomerular filtration. For drugs that are protein bound, anything that alters the extent of their protein binding, e.g. reduced binding in nephrotic syndrome or competition between two drugs for binding sites, will increase the free drug fraction and the rate of renal excretion.

Many compounds gain access to the glomerular ultrafiltrate as the parent drug and this represents their major route of elimination from the body. Examples include digoxin, atenolol and tubocurarine. For others, biotransformation must first occur to produce a water-soluble derivative that is then eliminated by the kidney. The anaesthetic agent propofol is an example of a drug that is eliminated as its inactivated conjugated metabolite by ultrafiltration.

### *Passive backdiffusion*

Isosmotic reabsorption of most of the filtered water occurs from the proximal tubule. Ionized drugs are poorly lipid soluble and their backdiffusion from the proximal tubule is minimal. The extent to which a molecule is ionized is determined by the pH of the urine and the $pK_a$ of the drug. Acidic compounds such as aspirin have a low $pK_a$ and alkalinization of urine favours ionization. Thus alkaline diuresis can be used to enhance aspirin elimination following overdose.

If a drug is mainly non-ionized within the physiological range of urinary pH, then its reabsorption will be independent of urinary pH and determined by its inherent lipophilicity and the concentration gradient across the tubular membrane. The latter will vary according to the amount of water reabsorbed and, therefore, the urine flow rate. Highly lipid-soluble drugs undergo almost complete reabsorption independently of variations in urine flow rate while highly water-soluble drugs are hardly reabsorbed under any condition. However, most water-soluble drugs have some lipophilicity and their rate of elimination will vary directly with urine flow rate.

### *Active tubular reabsorption*

Specific carrier-mediated mechanisms are found in the proximal tubule to facilitate conservation of essential organic compounds such as glucose, amino acids, vitamin C and urate. Few drugs appear to be handled by these carriers although lithium probably undergoes some active reabsorption. Its urinary excretion is directly related to sodium balance and is enhanced by a high sodium intake.

Endocytosis is responsible for reabsorption of some compounds.

Gentamicin binds to proximal tubular cells and is carried into the cells in vesicles formed from the brush border membrane.

*Active tubular secretion*

Drugs can act as substrates for secretory processes in the proximal renal tubule designed for the elimination of various endogenous molecules. Specific pathways exist for organic anions or cations. Micropuncture studies have defined three functional regions in the proximal tubule: $S_1$, $S_2$ and $S_3$. Cation transport is concentrated in $S_1$ and $S_2$ while anion transport principally occurs in $S_2$ Both mechanisms handle most compounds irrespective of their degree of protein binding, in contrast to the process of glomerular filtration. This may be because the exposure of plasma to the tubular excretory pathways is sufficiently prolonged (usually several seconds) to allow dissociation of the drug–protein complex and subsequent transport of free drug. In a few situations, however, protein binding does appear to impair tubular secretion, for example, with frusemide.

The anion transport carrier is located on the basolateral tubular membrane adjacent to the capillary. The driving force for anion transport is the trans-membrane sodium gradient which produces a substantial intracellular concentration of anions. Transfer of anions across the brush border membrane into the tubular lumen is by passive facilitated diffusion down their electrochemical gradients. This may involve either an anion exchange mechanism or a gated channel. Both basolateral and brush border transport systems are competitively inhibited by probenecid. Examples of drugs secreted by the anion transport system are shown below.

1. Acetazolamide
2. Cephalosporins
3. Loop diuretics (e.g. frusemide, bumetanide)
4. Methotrexate
5. Non-steroidal anti-inflammatory drugs
6. Penicillin
7. Probenecid
8. Salicylates
9. Spironolactone
10. Thiazides

The cation transport carrier is at the luminal brush border membrane. At the basolateral membrane, cations pass by facilitated diffusion. The driving force for the carrier is probably hydrogen ion counter transport secondary to a proton gradient produced by a sodium–hydrogen antiport system. The cation carrier mechanism is competitively inhibited by cimetidine. Examples of drugs secreted by the cation transport system are shown below.

1. Amiloride
2. Cimetidine
3. Disopyramide
4. Dopamine
5. Isoprenaline
6. Metformin
7. Morphine
8. Pindolol
9. Quinine
10. Ranitidine
11. Triamterene

The location of the active transporters has important implications for potential drug toxicity. Anions such as cephalosporins can be selectively concentrated in proximal tubular cells where they may have a local nephrotoxic action. By contrast, significant intracellular concentration of cationic drugs is unlikely to occur.

## 12.2 PHARMACOKINETICS IN RENAL FAILURE

Drug handling is often altered in patients with significant impairment of renal function [5, 6]. However, in addition to the expected changes in renal drug excretion, other less obvious effects can occur.

### 12.2.1 Absorption

There are few clinically significant problems with drug absorption in renal impairment. Nevertheless, uraemia may delay gastric emptying in some patients and delay the onset of action of some drugs. Advanced renal failure can be associated with vomiting, diarrhoea or gastrointestinal oedema which could reduce overall drug absorption.

### 12.2.2 Distribution

Several alterations in body composition in renal failure can alter the apparent volume of distribution ($V_d$) of drugs. Changes in total body water will only influence drugs with a small volume of distribution, i.e. those which are not selectively concentrated in certain body tissues such as fat. For such drugs (usually those with $V_d$ less than 50 l) dehydration will reduce the $V_d$ while oedema or ascites will increase it. Examples of drugs for which this might be important are lithium and aminoglycoside antimicrobials.

Changes in plasma protein binding are important for drugs that are highly protein-bound in plasma. Acidic drugs bind to low-affinity sites on albumin and plasma albumin may be decreased, particularly in nephrotic syndrome. In addition, accumulation of metabolites and uraemic toxins in plasma can either displace drugs from albumin binding sites or cause configurational changes that reduce drug binding. If protein binding is decreased, then the free (active) fraction of drug will be increased. However, free drug is also available for metabolism or elimination and at steady-state (achieved after an interval of four or five half-lives) the free fraction will be at the concentration that would have been achieved if protein binding were normal. Thus, the active fraction of drug will be unaffected at steady-state, even though the total plasma drug concentration (bound plus free drug) will be lower than usual.

There are two important clinical implications of decreased protein binding. First, if the drug is highly protein-bound and has a narrow therapeutic index, then the initial higher free concentration before steady-state is reached could produce toxicity. Examples of drugs for which this is important include phenytoin, warfarin, morphine and theophylline. For other drugs, such as diazepam or penicillins, a short-lived increase in the plasma free-drug concentration will have little clinical importance. Secondly, if total plasma drug concentrations are measured for therapeutic monitoring, then the usual 'therapeutic reference range' cannot be applied. Increasing drug dosage to achieve the same total plasma drug concentration as for patients with normal protein binding will risk producing toxicity.

By contrast with albumin, the plasma concentration of $\alpha_1$ acid glycoprotein, which carries high-affinity binding sites for basic drugs, can be increased up to three-fold in uraemic patients. Increased protein binding to $\alpha_1$ acid glycoprotein will reduce the active free-drug fraction; this has been reported for clindamycin. Tissue drug binding may be reduced in uraemic patients, which will reduce the volume of distribution. This occurs with digoxin which is displaced from skeletal muscle in renal failure; such patients will need a smaller loading dose of digoxin than those with normal renal function.

Predicting the effects of renal dysfunction on protein binding of drugs is not straightforward. The plasma urea concentration at which these effects occur differs widely among patients, presumably due to variations in the concentrations of other accumulated metabolites and toxins.

### 12.2.3 Metabolism

Hepatic biotransformation of drugs can be altered by renal failure. Most oxidative reactions are unaffected, but the rates of some in the hepatic endoplasmic reticulum can actually be accelerated; the mechanism behind this effect is poorly understood. Examples of drugs showing increased metabolism are phenobarbitone, phenytoin and propranolol. Conjugation reactions are usually unaffected, but reduction, acetylation and ester hydrolysis reactions are usually slower in renal failure. Uraemic metabolites may inhibit drug transport into the hepatocyte, or inhibit drug metabolism either by competing for enzyme binding sites or by feedback inhibition [7]. Fortunately, most of these changes in enzyme activity do not have important clinical consequences.

The kidney also has metabolizing enzymes for many drugs, but usually contributes only a small amount to the total metabolic capacity [8]. However, the kidney is a major site of metabolism for insulin. The requirement for insulin is, therefore, often reduced in diabetic patients who develop renal failure. The kidney is also involved in the activation of dietary vitamin D. 25-Hydroxylation occurs in the liver, but 1α-hydroxylation takes place in the kidney and is required for full efficacy. Vitamin D supplements are often required to prevent bone disease in chronic renal failure; these should be given either as 1,25-dihydroxy cholecalciferol or 1α-hydroxy cholecalciferol.

### 12.2.4 Renal elimination

Impaired kidney function slows the clearance of many drugs or their metabolites. For most drugs which undergo renal elimination, the rate of excretion is proportional to the glomerular filtration rate (GFR) [9] and reflects the number of remaining functional nephrons (Figure 12.1). Reduction in the dosage of drugs in renal failure should take into

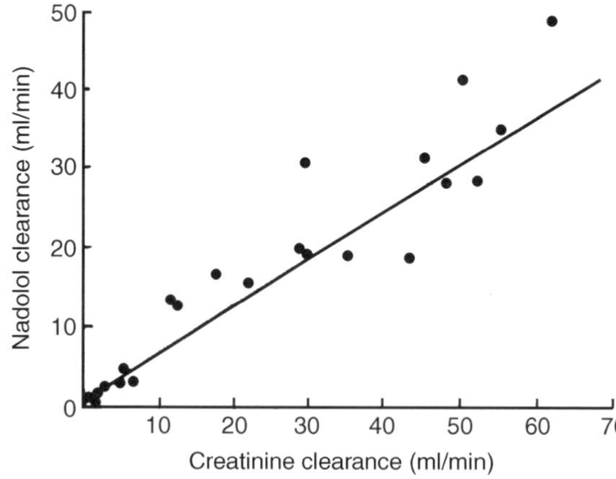


**Figure 12.1** The urinary clearance of nadolol in 24 patients with different degrees of impaired renal function following an oral dose of 80 mg [10].

**Table 12.1** Classification of the severity of renal impairment in the 'average' patient

| | GFR (ml/min) | Approximate serum creatinine ($\mu$mol/l) |
|---|---|---|
| Mild | 20–50 | < 300 |
| Moderate | 10–20 | 300–700 |
| Severe | < 10 | > 700 |

account two factors: the degree of reduction of GFR and the fraction of the drug excreted by the kidney (as against other routes). Several drugs use more than one pathway for elimination. For these, the non-renal route of elimination may partially compensate for the reduced renal excretion, for example doxycycline.

Renal impairment can be arbitrarily divided into three degrees of severity (Table 12.1). At the less pronounced levels of renal insufficiency dose modification is not necessary for drugs with a wide therapeutic index even if they are mainly eliminated in the kidney, e.g. penicillins. However, it is important to reduce the dose of drugs with a narrow therapeutic index, for example aminoglycoside antimicrobials, digoxin and lithium.

Other factors can modify the effects of reduced GFR on drug elimination. The urinary concentration of acidic drugs, such as amphetamine, is dependent on urinary pH. Patients taking a low-protein diet usually have a high urinary pH, and acidic drugs will remain non-ionized, resulting in considerable tubular reabsorption and prolonged effects. For this reason, urinary screening for amphetamine should include an estimate of urinary pH, since almost no drug will appear in the urine if the pH is above 6. Diet can influence tubular reabsorption of other drugs. Oxypurinol, the active metabolite of allopurinol, has a reduced clearance in renal insufficiency. This is further reduced if a low-protein diet is used, leading to a greater risk of toxicity, with desquamative skin rash, fever, eosinophilia and progressive deterioration in renal function. An increase in tubular oxypurinol reabsorption is the most likely explanation.

The processes of tubular anion and cation secretion are saturable [11] and drugs which undergo elimination by this route may show concentration-dependent renal clearance. If less than 20% of drug is eliminated by this route, then changes in tubular secretion are unlikely to produce clinically important changes in plasma drug concentration. However, if the amount is greater, then as the plasma drug concentration is increased, renal clearance will progressively decrease once the secretion mechanism becomes saturated. This could have important clinical consequences. First, agents such as diuretics, the uricosuric drugs probenecid and sulphinpyrazone, and the antimicrobial nitrofurantoin have an intratubular site of action. Impaired secretion may make them less effective, particularly if the agent is highly bound to plasma proteins and not readily filtered at the glomerulus. Secondly, competition for transport may occur. This can affect endogenous substances: for example, many diuretics inhibit tubular uric acid secretion, contributing to the development of gout. Alternatively, competition between two drugs may produce severe toxicity: for example, the excretion of methotrexate is substantially reduced by the concurrent use of non-steroidal anti-inflammatory drugs.

### 12.2.5 Drug toxicity and efficacy in renal impairment

Altered tissue sensitivity to drugs can enhance the toxicity of several compounds in patients with renal impairment. This occurs even if the concentration of the drug is unaffected by renal dysfunction. Important examples include the higher prevalence of gastrointestinal bleeding in patients receiving oral anticoagulants or non-steroidal anti-inflammatory drugs (NSAID). The blood–brain barrier may also be more permeable to hypnotics and sedatives leading to exaggerated effects.

In the case of other agents, renal failure may impair their efficacy. One example is the thiazide diuretics, which have reduced hypotensive and diuretic actions, particularly when GFR falls below 20 ml/min (Figure 12.2).

### 12.2.6 Dosage adjustment in renal failure

The pharmacokinetic and pharmacodynamic changes that occur in renal failure are complex and not always readily predictable. Although precise recommendations for dosage adjustment are not possible, certain general principles can be applied [13]. The most important issues are the margin of safety or therapeutic index of the drug and the importance of achieving adequate plasma concentrations rapidly. In many situations, e.g. treatment of hypertension, a cautious approach with the initial use of small doses and gradual titration will allow identification of the minimum effective dose and limit the risk of toxicity. However, for other conditions such as the treatment of serious infections, the attainment of effective drug concentrations is more critical. If the chosen drug has a narrow therapeutic index then dosage adjustment should be guided by measurement of plasma drug concentrations to minimize toxicity. Good examples are aminoglycoside antibiotics, since the clinical outcome is determined by both the maximum plasma concentration and the area under the plasma concen-

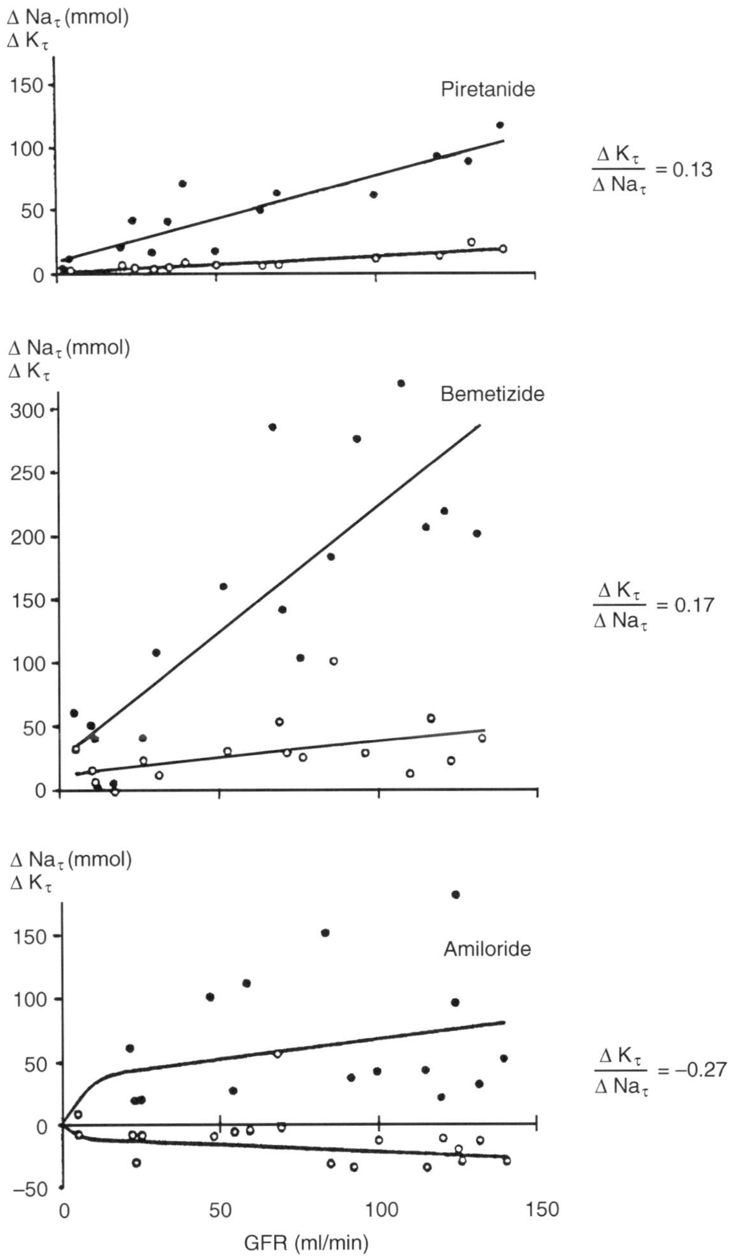


**Figure 12.2** Diuretic-induced excretion of sodium (●) and potassium (○) produced by oral administration of the loop diuretic piretanide (6 mg), the thiazide diuretic bemetizide (20 mg) and the potassium-sparing diuretic amiloride (5 mg) at different levels of renal function [12].

tration–time curve, but both peak and trough plasma concentrations are related to toxicity [14, 15]. Nomograms can be used to guide initial dosage adjustment at varying levels of renal function. For other antibiotics such as the penicillins and cephalosporins, the wide therapeutic index, and in many cases compensatory extra-renal elimination, makes dosage reduction less important, except in advanced renal impairment [16].

Dosage reduction can be achieved in two ways. The first is to use a standard maintenance dose, but to increase the interval between doses. The dosage interval will be determined by an estimate of the prolongation of the elimination half-life of the drug. The second is to reduce the dose but to maintain dosage intervals. This approach may be less convenient if standard dosage forms are not easily divided, and there is a potential risk of toxicity if trough plasma concentrations are related to adverse effects. Both methods will maintain the same average plasma drug concentrations, but the latter will produce less fluctuation between peak and trough plasma concentrations. Loading doses are usually unchanged in renal impairment, unless the volume of distribution of the drug is likely to be reduced, e.g. digoxin.

Formulae have been published to derive dosage adjustments for drugs affected by renal impairment [9]. A widely used example equates the dosing frequency to the degree of renal dysfunction:

$$\text{daily dosing in renal failure} = \text{normal daily dosage} \times [(1 - F_u) + (F_u \times \text{RF})]$$

where $F_u$ is the fraction of drug excreted in the urine and RF is the degree of renal impairment. The latter is calculated from the patient's creatinine clearance divided by the ideal creatinine clearance (usually taken as 120 ml/min). Creatinine clearance is most readily derived using the serum creatinine and a formula which considers the patient's age and weight. The equation published by Cockcroft and Gault (1976) [17] is most widely employed and well validated [18]:

$$\text{Creatinine clearance (ml/min)} = \frac{1.23 \times (140 - \text{age in years}) \times (\text{weight in kg})}{\text{Serum creatinine } \mu\text{mol/l}}$$

For women, the value should be multiplied by 1.04 rather than 1.23. Such equations do, however, become unreliable if renal function is rapidly changing, and some doubt exists over their accuracy when there is coexistent hepatic impairment.

The use of a formula to predict creatinine clearance is strongly recommended rather than relying on the serum creatinine concentration. The rate of creatinine formation is dependent on muscle mass, which differs not only between men and women but, importantly, with age. In the elderly, muscle forms a smaller proportion of total body weight and a serum creatinine within the laboratory reference range may misleadingly suggest that renal function is normal. For example, using the equation above, a serum creatinine of 120 $\mu$mol/l in a 20-year-old 80 kg male reflects a creatinine clearance of 98 ml/min. The same serum creatinine in a 50 kg, 80-year-old woman corresponds to a creatinine clearance of 26 ml/min.

### 12.2.7 Dosage adjustment during dialysis

Several factors will influence the extent of drug removal during haemodialysis [19]. The concentration gradient across the membrane will determine the passage of unbound, ultrafiltrable drug. Drugs with a molecular weight above 500 D (e.g. insulin and heparin) do not readily pass across most membranes and compounds with a large volume of distribution or high-protein binding will not be dialysed in significant quantities.

Factors relating to dialysis, such as blood and dialysate flow rates and the intrinsic properties of the dialysis membrane, may also be relevant. Because many of these variables are not readily determined, the exact clearance of a drug during dialysis is usually difficult to predict. In addition, many of the estimates for drug removal in the literature were made during dialysis with older machines and may not accurately reflect the situation with current haemodialysis methods, or indeed with ambulatory peritoneal dialysis.

Those drugs that are significantly removed by haemodialysis may be more appropriately given after dialysis on dialysis days. If treatment is essential before dialysis, a supplementary dose may be required after dialysis is complete.

## 12.3 NEPHROTOXICITY

The kidneys are vulnerable to functional and structural damage from a wide variety of both direct and indirect actions of drugs. Different forms of renal disease can occur and most are reversible if the offending drug is withdrawn early in their course. Even so, recovery of function may not necessarily indicate complete recovery of structural damage. The intrinsic renal reserve and the considerable ability of the kidney to compensate for toxic insults may mask the extent of nephron loss. The patterns of drug-induced disorders are shown below.

1. Functional effects on renal blood flow
2. Renal vascular damage
3. Acute tubular necrosis

4. Glomerulonephritis
5. Interstitial nephritis
6. Ureteric obstruction
7. Retroperitoneal fibrosis
8. Papillary necrosis

Determinants of the patterns of toxicity include structural and functional differences between cortical and juxtamedullary nephrons and the distribution of intra-renal concentrations of the drug or its metabolites [20]. The proximal tubule of the nephron, especially segments $S_1$ and $S_2$, is particularly vulnerable to drug-induced injury [21] due to the large osmotic gradient across the cell and the presence of tubular transport mechanisms. The $S_3$ segment has a greater amount of drug-metabolizing enzymes such as cytochrome P450 and mixed function oxidases, which may produce reactive and potentially nephrotoxic intermediate metabolites. In the renal medulla there is a higher concentration of cyclo-oxygenases, which are responsible not only for prostaglandin production, but are also involved in co-oxidation of drugs, producing intermediates that must be conjugated with glutathione to protect the cells from oxidative stress. Depletion of reduced glutathione may, therefore, contribute to cellular injury. Drugs can also influence intracellular signal transduction and the generation of second messengers. Loss of intracellular calcium regulation or modulation of enzyme activity may then produce functional changes in the cell or lead to cell death.

The renal cortex relies heavily on aerobic metabolism and is, therefore, vulnerable to hypoxic injury. However, ischaemia is even more likely to enhance drug toxicity in the medulla, which is characterized by low blood flow, relative hypoxia due to the counter-current exchange of oxygen and the high metabolic requirements of the ascending limb of the loop of Henle. The following discussion uses examples of important nephrotoxins to illustrate the range of clinical problems that can occur and their pathogenesis.

### 12.3.1 Nephrotoxic drugs (See also Chapter 8)

*Non-steroidal anti-inflammatory drugs (NSAIDs)*

Most drugs from this class can produce several types of renal disorder [22]. The most frequent serious consequence is acute renal failure due to a critical reduction in renal perfusion. Several prostaglandins are synthesized by the kidney, including the vasodilators $PGD_2$, $E_2$ and $I_2$. Inhibition of cyclo-oxygenase by NSAIDs has little effect in the normal kidney, but in the presence of high renin production, prostaglandins are required to counteract the vasoconstrictor action of angiotensin II. At-risk groups include the elderly, those with congestive cardiac failure or cirrhosis with ascites, patients with pre-existing renal disease or systemic lupus erythematosus, those with salt and water depletion or patients concurrently treated with angiotensin-converting enzyme (ACE) inhibitors. The loss of vasodilator prostaglandins leads to an abrupt fall in renal blood flow and, as a consequence, glomerular filtration rate. This type of toxicity is dose-related and usually produces a reversible decline in renal function, although end stage renal disease has been reported following NSAID-induced acute renal failure. Some reports suggest that sulindac may spare renal prostaglandin production, but the evidence is inconsistent.

Inhibition of renal prostaglandin synthesis also predisposes to electrolyte disturbances even in patients who do not develop renal failure. NSAIDs can cause salt and water retention due to the loss of the inhibitory action of prostaglandins on the tubular hydro-osmotic effect of ADH and loss of their modulatory action on tubular chloride transport. This may be particularly important in patients with hypertension or those with a pre-existing tendency to fluid retention. Prostaglandins also stimulate renin release and NSAIDs can cause hyperkalaemia by inhibiting renin (and therefore aldosterone) release and by reducing sodium delivery to the distal tubule thus decreasing sodium:potassium exchange. Hyperkalaemia is most common in diabetics, patients receiving other drugs that retain potassium (such as potassium-sparing diuretics and ACE inhibitors) and those with pre-existing renal disease.

The nephrotoxic effects of other agents such as aminoglycosides and radiocontrast agents may also be enhanced by concurrent use of NSAIDs.

Less commonly, NSAIDs can produce an idiosyncratic acute allergic tubulo-interstitial nephritis. This initially presents with proteinuria, defective tubular acidification and sometimes with acute renal failure (often of the polyuric variety). The pathogenesis is believed to involve the release of cytokines, such as interleukins 1, 2 and 6, and growth factors from renal macrophages. These interact with circulating hormones such as vasopressin to stimulate release of further cytokines, including transforming growth factor $\beta$ and platelet-derived growth factor, from interstitial and tubular epithelial cells. The consequence is activation and proliferation of fibroblasts which produce interstitial collagen [23].

Chronic tubulo-interstitial nephritis may also develop with NSAIDs and tends to produce a distal nephron dysfunction. Slow progression to chronic renal failure may result from, in addition to progressive fibrosis and scarring, raised intra-renal ammonia concentrations and activation of the alternative complement pathway. These processes can lead to progressive renal damage even after the initiating insult is withdrawn.

Alternatively, recurrent subclinical episodes of acute interstitial nephritis could eventually produce end stage renal disease.

Chronic analgesic nephropathy, classically caused by metabolites of phenacetin (usually in combination with other analgesics), may also be associated with NSAID use [24]. Excessive use over a period of years is required and the effects are believed to be due to prolonged prostaglandin synthesis inhibition within the renal medulla and reduction in medullary blood flow. Papillary necrosis occurs and impairment of tubular function with reduced urine concentrating ability, acidification defects and salt wasting.

*ACE inhibitors* (See also Chapter 3)

Modest increases in plasma creatinine and urea are not uncommon after the initiation of ACE inhibitor treatment, when congestive cardiac failure has already reduced renal perfusion. ACE inhibitors produce a further reduction in perfusion pressure but the renal impairment often stabilizes or recovers with continued treatment, as cardiac function improves. However, more serious renal failure may arise if cardiac failure is severe and the ACE inhibitor is given together with potent diuretics in a salt-depleted patient. Reducing the diuretic dose may improve renal function in this situation.

In the presence of renal artery stenosis, ACE inhibitors produce a severe fall in GFR in the affected kidney(s). This phenomenon has been used as a challenge test during renography in patients suspected of having the condition. If the condition is unilateral, compensation by the normal kidney means that there is little overall effect on renal function. However, in bilateral renal artery stenosis, rapid progression to renal failure is often the result. Patients at greatest risk from unsuspected renal artery stenosis are the elderly hypertensives with peripheral vascular disease [25]. The mechanism relates to a loss of angiotensin II-mediated vasoconstriction of the efferent glomerular arteriole, which maintains glomerular perfusion pressure in the face of reduced glomerular perfusion pressure.

Captopril has specifically been reported to cause a membranous nephropathy. This may be related to the presence of a sulphydryl group, which is not found in most other drugs in this class. It has usually been related to very high dosage, not employed these days and therefore rarely seen now.

*Cyclosporin A*

Nephrotoxicity with cyclosporin A (CsA) is dose-related and produces functional and structural changes in the kidney [26]. The most common initial effect is renal vasoconstriction, which reduces both effective renal plasma flow and GFR, without disturbing the filtration fraction. This occurs within the first week of treatment and is often accompanied by a rise in blood pressure. It probably reflects interference with vasoactive intra-renal hormones. The most plausible explanation is the reduced production of the vasodilator kinins [27], although increased synthesis of endothelin-1 and the vasoconstrictor thromboxane $A_2$ has also been implicated. CsA also enhances intracellular free calcium release from vascular smooth muscle, a process that could enhance the sensitivity to other vasoconstrictor influences such as endothelin-1. In this respect the observation that calcium antagonists may protect against the vasoconstriction could be relevant. In renal transplant recipients, survival of the graft does not seem to be affected by the vasoconstriction.

A more chronic form of toxicity is also recognized with cyclosporin, which is associated with morphological changes in the kidney and a significant rise in serum creatinine. It usually occurs during the first six months of treatment. Several different features have been found histologically (see Chapter 15). Renal arterial damage includes intimal proliferation and hyaline degeneration of the arteriolar wall, changes which have been reported in association with a haemolytic uraemic-like syndrome. Diffuse interstitial fibrosis is also found, with tubular atrophy. Animal models suggest that tubular toxicity is most marked initially in the $S_3$ segment of the proximal tubule, where cells develop vacuolation and giant mitochondria. Metabolism of CsA by the mixed function oxidases found in these cells may be inhibited by CsA itself. Ischaemia of this region of the kidney as a consequence of the action of CsA may also be important.

A variety of effects of cyclosporin on intracellular regulatory processes have been reported, leading to inhibition of microsomal protein translation and altered protein conformation. The relative importance of these to the nephrotoxic actions of the drug is poorly understood. The chronic toxicity associated with CsA is dose-related and may be reversible (often with dose reduction rather than stopping treatment), unless marked interstitial fibrosis has occurred.

Concomitant use of other nephrotoxic drugs greatly enhances the risk of CsA nephrotoxicity, e.g. aminoglycosides, amphotericin, or NSAIDs, as will pre-existing renal impairment. It is also important to recognize that concurrent treatment with macrolide antibiotics, such as erythromycin, azole antifungal agents, such as ketoconazole, and the calcium antagonists diltiazem and verapamil can all lead to a significant increase in the plasma CsA concentration, with a greater risk of nephrotoxicity.

*Radiological contrast media*

Intravascular use of iodinated radiocontrast agents has long been associated with nephrotoxicity, usually presenting as a rise in serum creatinine within 48 hours of their use [28]. At risk groups include those with pre-existing renal impairment, particularly from diabetic nephropathy. There is also a higher incidence in congestive heart failure, in the presence of hypovolaemia and in patients with multiple myeloma. Concurrent use of ACE inhibitors or NSAIDs may also increase the risk. In high-risk groups, a significant rise in serum creatinine occurs in about 15%. Newer low-osmolality agents have reduced, although not eliminated, the risk, particularly if the pre-investigation serum creatinine is elevated. The reactions are dose-related and more common after intracardiac injection.

The mechanism is unclear, but probably reflects a combination of renal vasoconstriction (possibly due to vasopressin release) leading to regional hypoxia and direct tubular toxicity. However, it is uncertain whether agents that increase renal blood flow alter the extent of toxicity. Calcium antagonists are likely to offer protection in this situation. There is also evidence to suggest that low-dose dopamine and atrial natriuretic peptide are protective in non-diabetic patients. However in diabetics, despite an improvement in renal blood flow, toxicity was unaffected. Frusemide and mannitol have been shown to be ineffective. Hydration with saline before and after radiocontrast use is strongly recommended in patients at risk.

*Aminoglycosides*

Clinical disturbance of renal function is common during aminoglycoside therapy occurring in up to one third of patients. Although it usually produces a transient rise in serum creatinine, the longer the drug is given the greater the risk of permanent damage. Gentamicin has been implicated most often and recovery may be slow.

Aminoglycoside toxicity is most clearly seen in proximal tubular cells [29]. About 5% of the filtered drug is reabsorbed at this site, but selective intracellular concentration and retention of the drug occurs in the $S_1$ and $S_2$ segments following uptake by active transport. Binding to phospholipids in the luminal membranes triggers pinocytosis and transfer to intracellular lysosomes. Inhibition of intracellular phospholipases by the drug prevents phospholipid metabolism, and reduces the release of the intracellular second messenger inositol triphosphate. Cell damage is probably the end result of disturbed intracellular regulation with inhibition of microsomal protein synthesis. Altered membrane transport functions may also reduce the capacity for cell repair.

Tubular proteinuria and enzymuria are early evidence of aminoglycoside toxicity, but subsequently non-oliguric acute renal failure can occur if acute tubular necrosis develops. Both trough and peak plasma drug concentrations correlate with the extent of damage and since aminoglycosides are eliminated principally by the kidney, dose reduction in renal impairment and close monitoring of drug concentrations are essential. However, even if the plasma concentration is carefully controlled the more prolonged the duration of treatment, the higher is the risk of toxicity. The elderly are at greatest risk, and nephrotoxicity is also more common in patients with liver disease. Toxicity is enhanced if other nephrotoxic drugs are used concurrently, particularly frusemide, cisplatin, amphotericin and methoxyflurane.

The relative nephrotoxicity of different aminoglycosides is not well documented. Neomycin has the greatest potential, but limiting its use to topical or oral administration means that little is absorbed, and toxicity is unlikely except in patients with pre-existing chronic renal failure. Most other agents appear to have a similar toxicity, although direct comparative studies, or studies with comparable diagnostic criteria, are lacking. There are suggestions that some members of this class, such as netilmicin, may be less nephrotoxic than gentamicin, but firm evidence is lacking.

### *Cisplatin*

Cisplatin, like aminoglycosides, is selectively toxic to the proximal tubules, although in this case to the $S_3$ segment. It is a cytotoxic agent that acts by inhibition of nuclear DNA synthesis. Functional changes are often delayed for up to three days after the structural damage begins. Subtle early changes in electrolyte handling may progress to produce hypomagnesaemia, hypocalcaemia and hypokalaemia. With more pronounced toxicity, renal blood flow and glomerular filtration rate fall and are associated with evidence of acute tubular necrosis. Polyuria with reduced renal concentrating ability is common.

The mechanism is incompletely understood. There is an increase in renal vascular resistance producing a fall in renal blood flow, but intracellular production of toxic metabolites in the proximal tubule is believed to be responsible for morphological and functional changes. The platinum molecule may not be the major problem since carboplatin is less nephrotoxic than cisplatin. It is believed that the structure of cisplatin leads to a greater concentration in the nuclei of renal tubular cells with consequent inhibition of DNA synthesis. Interference with cell respiration may then promote tubular cell death.

Cisplatin nephrotoxicity can be reduced by ensuring adequate hydration before, during and after administration. In small studies other specific agents such as intravenous thiosulphate or ethiofos have been reported to protect the kidneys.

### *Gold*

Membranous nephropathy is a well-recognized complication of gold therapy, but is not clearly dose-related. Clinically, it usually presents within six months of starting treatment as proteinuria, and sometimes microscopic haematuria. Occasionally the renal lesion, on histology, has turned out to be minimal change disease.

Proteinuria is common during gold therapy (between 1 and 7% in one review) and does not always require cessation of therapy. However, if it exceeds 1 g/day, treatment should be stopped, after which the proteinuria usually recovers within a few months [30]. In renal biopsies, gold is deposited in glomerular mesangial cells and sometimes in proximal tubular cells. Gold is believed to induce an immune complex nephritis, and possession of the class 2 major histocompatibility antigen DR3 may confer greater susceptibility. If patients develop proteinuria with gold, they are more likely to do so with penicillamine as well, suggesting a genetic link. Oral gold appears to be less likely to produce glomerular disease, but severe proteinuria has also been reported with this preparation.

### *Penicillamine*

Membranous glomerulonephritis is well recognized during treatment with penicillamine; the risk appears to be greater than with gold (about 12%) and is dose-related. The onset of proteinuria may be delayed for up to 18 months after the start of treatment, and on withdrawal of the drug takes several months to disappear [30].

### *Lithium*

Up to 80% of lithium filtered at the glomerulus is reabsorbed in the proximal tubule, creating a high concentration gradient in the kidney. The most frequent effect of lithium on the kidney is nephrogenic diabetes insipidus [31]. The mechanism is not fully understood, but relates to functional inhibition of the distal and collecting tubular actions of the antidiuretic hormone (ADH). Various intracellular biochemical abnormalities are recognized, including changes in inositol triphosphate release and reduced protein kinase C activity. The consequence may be altered regulation of membrane adenylate cyclase activity and reduced intracellular generation of cyclic AMP in response to ADH.

The clinical sequel to these effects is impaired maximum urine concentrating ability, but only a minority of patients develop severe polyuria. There is a relationship between the severity of the concentrating defect and the duration of therapy as well as the cumulative dose of lithium received, but not with the daily dosage. Some authors have suggested that polyuria is more common if the plasma concentration is maintained with sustained-release formulations of lithium. Recovery, although incomplete, is seen after several months' cessation of lithium treatment. Polyuria *per se* is not a reason to stop treatment although this may be necessary if frank nephrogenic diabetes insipidus develops. A mild urinary acidification defect is also common, but of little clinical importance.

There is little evidence that lithium produces a progressive deterioration in glomerular filtration rate, despite observations suggesting that this can occur in some patients. However, recurrent and subclinical episodes of acute lithium toxicity may contribute to progressive renal impairment in a small subgroup of patients.

Histological changes in the kidney during lithium therapy include principally, enlarged convoluted and distal tubular cells with vacuolation of the apical membranes. Areas of interstitial fibrosis are also found. However, their relationship to the severity of polyuria is uncertain and although they can progress with continuing treatment, recovery is usual on withdrawal of lithium. A contributory nephrotoxic action from the other psychotropic drugs often used with lithium has been suggested by some authors.

Lithium has been reported to induce a nephrotic syndrome, as a rare complication, due to minimal change glomerulonephritis, which recovers on withdrawal of the drug. Acute lithium toxicity can cause acute renal failure due to tubular necrosis. Such toxicity can be precipitated by salt and water depletion, which promotes avid proximal tubular reabsorption of lithium from the glomerular filtrate. Thus, the polyuria of chronic lithium nephrotoxicity can predispose to acute lithium toxicity unless hydration is well maintained.

### *Amphotericin*

Amphotericin is toxic to distal tubular cells, producing hypokalaemia, hypomagnesaemia, impaired urine concentrating ability and distal tubular acidosis [29]. If exposure continues, then acute tubular necrosis can develop, leading to non-oliguric renal failure. Toxicity is dose-related and usually reversible; it can usually be minimized by ensuring adequate hydration. Recent formulation developments of colloidal or liposomal amphotericin appear to minimize the extent of renal damage in high-risk patients.

*Obstructive uropathy*

In addition to direct renal damage, renal impairment can result from obstruction within the renal tubules, calyces or ureter. Examples include tubular blockage by light-chain proteinuria reported on rare occasions during rifampicin therapy or as a consequence of myoglobin release into the plasma due to rhabdomyolysis. Filtered myoglobin is converted to ferrihaeme which blocks the tubule. Drugs causing rhabdomyolysis include cocaine, major tranquillizers (neuroleptic malignant syndrome), and various lipid-lowering agents (particularly certain fibric acid derivatives and the HMG CoA reductase inhibitors). Combinations of lipid-lowering drugs, especially when given with cyclosporin, carry a greater risk of rhabdomyolysis [32].

Crystalluria can also produce obstructive uropathy. Examples are uric acid deposition in patients taking uricosuric agents or during lysis of soft tissue tumours with cytotoxic drugs. Acyclovir can crystallize in the urine, especially after intravenous use.

Retroperitoneal fibrosis produces ureteric obstruction. This condition is most commonly associated with the use of methysergide for migraine prophylaxis, but has also been suspected as a rare complication of $\beta$-blocker therapy. Regression is usual if the drug is withdrawn, but surgery is often necessary.

## REFERENCES


1. Gram, T.E., Okine, L.K. and Gram, R.A. (1986) The metabolism of xenobiotics by certain extrahepatic organs and its relation to toxicity. *Ann. Rev. Toxicol.*, **26**, 259–91.
2. Atio, A. (ed.) 1978 *Conjugation Reactions in Drug Biotransformation*, Elsevier, Oxford.
3. George, C.F., Shand, D.G. and Renwick, A.G. (1982) *Presystemic Drug Elimination*, Butterworth Medical, London.
4. Hewitt, W.R. and Hook, J.B. (1983) The renal excretion of drugs, in (eds J.W. Bridges and L.F. Chasseaud), *Prog. Drug. Metab.*, Vol. 7. John Wiley and Sons Ltd, Chichester, pp. 11–56.
5. Fillastre, J.-P. and Singlas, E. (1991) Pharmacokinetics of newer drugs in patients with renal impairment (Part 1). *Clin. Pharmacokinet.*, **20**, 293–310.
6. Singlas, E. and Fillastre, J.-P. (1991) Pharmacokinetics of newer drugs in patients with renal impairment (Part 11). *Clin. Pharmacokinet.*, **20**, 389–410.
7. Gibson, T.P. (1986) Renal clearance and drug metabolism: an overview. *Am. J. Kidney Dis.*, **8**, 7–17.
8. Vree, T.B., Hekster, Y.A. and Anderson, P.G. (1992) Contribution of the human kidney to the metabolic clearance of drugs. *Ann. Pharmacother.*, **26**, 1421–8.
9. Dettli, L. (1976) Drug dosage in renal failure. *Clin. Pharmacokinet.*, **1**, 126–34.
10. Herrera, J., Vukovich, R.A. and Griffiths, D.L. (1979) Elimination of nadolol by patients with renal impairment. *Br. J. Clin. Pharmacol.*, **7**, suppl. 2, 227s–231s.

11. van Ginneken, C.A.M. and Russel, F.G.M. (1989) Saturable pharmacokinetics in the renal excretion of drugs. *Clin. Pharmacokinet.*, **16**, 38–54.
12. Knauf, I.T. and Mutschler, E. (1990) Pharmacokinetics of diuretics, in Proc. of Lasix 25th Anniversary Symposium, Media Medica, Chichester, pp. 41–53.
13. Talbert, R.L. (1994) Drug dosing in renal insufficiency. *J. Clin. Pharmacol.*, **34**, 99–110.
14. Drusano, G.L. (1988) Role of pharmacokinetics in the outcome of infections. *Antimicrob. Agents Chemother.*, **32**, 289–97.
15. Marian, F.A., Stone, W.J. and Alford, R.H. (1990) Adverse antibiotic effects associated with renal insufficiency. *Rev. Infect. Dis.*, **12**, 236–49.
16. St Peter, W.L., Redic-Kill, K.A. and Halstenson, C.E. (1992) Clinical pharmacokinetics of antibiotics in patients with impaired renal function. *Clin. Pharmacokinet.*, **22**, 169–210.
17. Cockcroft, D.W. and Gault, M.H. (1976) The estimation of creatinine clearance from serum creatinine concentration. *Nephron*, **16**, 31–8.
18. Waller, D.G., Fleming, J.S., Ramsay, B. and Gray, J. (1991) Creatinine clearance with and without urine collection as a measure of glomerular filtration rate. *Postgrad. Med. J.*, **67**, 42–6.
19. Lee, C.S. and Marbury, T.C. (1984) Drug therapy in patients undergoing haemodialysis: clinical pharmacokinetic considerations. *Clin. Pharmacokinet.*, **9**, 42–66.
20. Walker, R.J. and Fawcett, J.P. (1993) Drug nephrotoxicity – the significance of cellular mechanisms. *Prog. Drug. Res.*, **41**, 51–94.
21. Trump, B.F., Berezesky, I.K., Lipsky, M.M. and Jones, T.W. (1985) in *Renal Heterogeneity and Target Cell Toxicity* (eds P.H. Bach and E.A. Lock), John Wiley and Sons, Chichester, pp. 31–42.
22. Grand Round, (1994) Nephrotoxicity of non-steroidal antiinflammatory drugs. *Lancet*, **344**, 515–8.
23. Wolf, G. and Neilson, E. (1991) Molecular mechanisms of tubulointerstitial hypertrophy and hyperplasia. *Kidney Int.*, **39**, 401–20.
24. Perneger, T.V., Whelton, P.K. and Klag, M.T. (1994) Risk of kidney failure associated with the use of acetomirophen, aspirin and non-steroidal anti inflammatory drugs. *N. Engl. J. Med.*, **331**, 1675–9.
25. Hricik, D.E. (1985) Captopril-induced renal insufficiency and the role of sodium balance. *Ann. Intern. Med.*, **103**, 222–4.
26. McNally, P.G. and Feehally, J. (1992) Pathophysiology of cyclosporin A nephrotoxicity: experimental and clinical observations. *Nephrol. Dial. Transplant.*, **7**, 791–804.
27. Spragg, J., Weinblatt, M.E., Coblyn, J. *et al.* (1988) Effect of cyclosporine on urinary kallikrein excretion in patients with rheumatoid arthritis. *J. Lab. Clin. Med.*, **112**, 324–32.
28. Barrett, B.J. (1994) Contrast nephrotoxicity. *J. Am. Soc. Nephrol.*, **5**, 125–37.
29. Kaloyanides, G.J. (1994) Antibiotic-related nephrotoxicity. *Nephrol. Dial. Transplant.*, **9**, suppl. 4, 130–4.
30. Hall, C.L. (1989) The natural course of gold and penicillamine nephropathy a long-term study of 54 patients. *Adv. Exp. Med. Biol.*, **252**, 247–56.
31. Waller, D.G. and Edwards, J.G. (1989) Lithium and the kidney: an update. *Psychol. Med.*, **19**, 825–31.
32. Prendergast, B.D. and George, C.F. (1993) Drug-induced rhabdomyolysis – mechanisms and management. *Postgrad. Med. J.*, **69**, 333–6.

# 13

# Nutrition in renal disease

*H.A. Lee*

## 13.1 INTRODUCTION

There can be little doubt that nutritional support plays a pivotal role in the management of patients with renal failure [1]. In particular, in acute renal failure (ARF), whatever other management strategies are involved – circulatory and ventilatory support, cardiac monitoring, haemodialysis (HD), intermittent peritoneal dialysis (IPD), continuous arteriovenous haemofiltration (CAVH) – ultimately, unless these patients receive adequate nutritional support the mortality rate will and does remain high. Any effect on the mortality rate must be judged against the wider implications for the treatment of acute renal failure patients, particularly in the elderly, who two or three decades ago would not have been considered for such management. This chapter is largely focused on nutrition in 'acute' renal impairment, either as part of genuine ARF, or as part of a phase of acute impairment superimposed on chronic renal failure (CRF). Malnutrition is the common denominator in both situations.

## 13.2 OBJECTIVES OF NUTRITIONAL SUPPORT

As with so many other support treatments, so in acute renal failure the objectives of nutritional support are:

1. to reduce morbidity and mortality;
2. to ameliorate the consequences of associated problems, such as infection, surgery, drugs;
3. to compensate for the nutritional losses associated with dialysis therapy itself, be that haemodialysis, CAVH or even IPD.

*Renal Disease*. Edited by G. Venkat Raman. Published in 1998 by Chapman & Hall, London. ISBN 0 412 45700 8.

The following discussion will review the past thirty years, during which nutritional support has varied from very low oral protein intakes (aiming to decrease the urea appearance rate and the frequency of haemodialysis), to the current opinion that patients should receive, on assessment, whatever nutritional support they require and dialysis accordingly, by whatever modality considered most appropriate.

## 13.3 ACUTE RENAL FAILURE – A CATABOLIC EVENT

Acute renal failure *per se* is a well-known catabolic event irrespective of aetiology. Persike and Addis [2] were the first to describe acute renal failure as a catabolic event. Subsequently Sellers *et al.* [3] incubated liver slices from rats with acute renal failure and compared these to sham operated controls. Although the rats with acute renal failure were given 50% glucose, these still had higher liver urea appearance rates (UAR) than normal controls. These observations were further extended by Lacy [4, 5], who found that perfused livers of rats with acute renal failure, compared with sham operated controls, had increased hepatic urea synthetic rates and an increased amino acid uptake; furthermore, amino acids were removed at an accelerated rate from the perfusate, with the exception of the branched chain amino acids, leucine, isoleucine and valine (which are exclusively metabolized in skeletal muscle).

Frohlich *et al.* [6] showed in liver perfusion experiments, that rats with acute renal failure (compared with normal or sham operated ones) had increased rates of gluconeogensis and ureagenesis. This was attributed to the rapid uptake of amino acids by the liver. It was suggested that the glucose intolerance of acute renal failure could possibly be due to this increased rate of gluconeogensis. Bondy *et al.* [7], in rat experiments, studied the nephrectomized and adrenalectomized versus nephrectomized ones and found increased corticosteroid-dependent release of amino acids from extrahepatic tissue and suggested, in particular, that this could be from muscle. This observation would support the opinion that muscle wasting in patients with severe acute renal failure is as a result of amino acid release from muscle tissue. Further studies on catabolism in acute renal failure in animal models and in patients have been reviewed [8, 9].

The above observations are supported by Feinstein *et al.* [10], who showed that the 'catabolic drive' in humans with acute renal failure would be sufficient to cause abnormally high urea appearance rates in spite of adequate amino acid provision. They also considered that the amount of nitrogen required to offset this catabolic response might be totally impossible to administer. In my view such technicalities have long since been overcome and there is rarely, if ever, any indication to infuse more than 25 g of nitrogen a day to man; otherwise, the liver pathways for utilization of amino acids are overwhelmed and simply more urea synthesis takes place.

It has long been known that treatment with amino acids and glucose could reduce the rate of rise of urea and possibly hyperkalaemia, but it did little to alter the survival of acute renal failure patients [11]. Silva *et al.* [12] and Lee *et al.* [13] suggested that an aggressive nutritional approach could improve patient survival, although not proven by controlled trials.

Horl *et al.* [14, 15] showed increased proteolytic activity in 25% of acute renal failure patients. They also observed that alpha-2-macroglobulin could inhibit serum proteinase activity and this suggested the possibility of a pharmacological tool that could be used to inhibit the catabolic rate. Later Clowse *et al.* [15] described a 'circulating peptide' in sepsis and post-operative patients. It is known that interleukin-1 (IL-1) can cause fever, redistribution of essential biological elements, increased amino acid mobilization, increased amino acid oxidation, increased skeletal and collagen protein degradation, with a final common pathway of proteolysis in sepsis or fever. Interleukin-l is known to promote synthesis of prostaglandin $E_2$ in rat cardiac and skeletal muscle, resulting in increased tissue proteolysis, and this may well be a problem occurring in patients with ARF.

The catabolic events of acute renal failure are complex, influenced by the nature and severity of the primary injury, surgery and anaesthesia, associated infection, effects of drugs (such as steroids), but this can be offset by the delivery of nutritional support. Dialysis treatment itself increases the catabolic rate by almost 30% [17–20]. These studies showed that during haemodialysis the urea nitrogen appearance rate (UNA) could be increased by 27% and this was related to IL-1 release. When considering the preventative aspects of the consequences of ARF and the associated metabolic events it has been suggested [21] that the prostaglandin inhibitor indomethacin before and during haemodialysis might reduce the UNA rate. Such observations need to be extended and await confirmation. Other quests for a therapeutic tool to diminish the catabolic response to modern surgery or trauma have been unsuccessful [22].

## 13.4 MALNUTRITION IN ACUTE RENAL FAILURE

The consequences of inadequate nutritional support are increased morbidity, increased mortality, increased wound dehiscence, diminished threshold for ventilatory support (as a result of intercostal muscle wasting), increased risks of infection, overall muscle wasting and finally, general apathy and anorexia, further worsening malnutrition. With nutritional support cognizance is given to electrolyte provision, vitamin and essential biological element requirements and maintenance of circulating blood and plasma volume. Though it is not possible to counteract totally the catabolic effects of ARF, and the attendant complications, it can be ameliorated to a considerable extent, with attendant clinical benefit.

### 13.4.1 How to measure nutritional requirements

Central to the provision of nutritional support in ARF is the determination of patients' nitrogen losses and requirements. Over the past three decades a number of formulae have been put forward, but they do not always solve the specific and difficult problems of these patients. Lee and Hartley [23] described a method for determining daily nitrogen requirements in postoperative patients, one that has been modified over the years and more recently by Feinstein and Massry [9], but there are still assumptions.

A recent study [24] showed the dangers of making assumptions about nitrogen losses, emphasizing the widely differing catabolic rates in patients with ARF. Even though the study was undertaken in a unit where nutritional support was an essential part of management, nutritional support was grossly inadequate in many subjects. Thus, nutritional requirements are frequently underestimated, whilst accepting that to provide above 200 mg of nitrogen per kg of body weight [25] does not result in improved nutritional status.

### 13.4.2 Nutritional losses consequent upon dialysis treatment

Most authorities would now advocate either haemodialysis or haemofiltration as the preferred method of treatment for the management of acute renal failure patients, irrespective of injury or age of the patient. IPD, although useful in certain circumstances, is not optimal for the long-term management of ARF. Nutritional losses related to dialysis treatment itself are mainly in the form of amino acids:

1. 13–15 g amino acids/40 l peritoneal dialysis;
2. 20–30 g protein/40 l peritoneal dialysis [26];
3. 2–3 g amino acids/hour of haemodialysis.

## 13.5 NUTRITIONAL SUPPORT IN ACUTE RENAL FAILURE

Although aggressive nutritional support (enteral or parenteral) was advocated for improving outcome in ARF some three decades ago [12, 13], over the years the number of controlled trials with parenteral nutrition in ARF – investigating the use of essential amino acids, essential amino acids with non-essential amino acids, versus glucose only or minimal energy requirements – have been centred on 175 patients! In six studies [10, 27–31] over this period, no significant difference has been shown between those patients given essential amino acid support with energy compared with those given energy support alone. This is not surprising because the number of patients studied has been so small. None of the studies was comparable, strict measurement of nitrogen balance was not carried out and therefore outcomes cannot be compared. It is perhaps an indicator of the difficulty of measuring nitrogen balance in acute renal failure patients, who are so heterogeneous, that has complicated the whole issue of nitrogen requirements.

Borst [32] and Bull *et al.* [33] demonstrated that providing large amounts of carbohydrate (glucose) energy could reduce the UAR. Berlyne *et al.* [11] also showed in ARF patients, that a diet supplying 9.21 kJ (2200 kcal) and 2.6 g nitrogen per day as high-quality protein could reduce the UAR. However, this did not take into consideration their catabolic rates or indeed survival.

The debate continues about how to provide nitrogen for renal failure patients, i.e. should that be as essential amino acids alone or essential amino acids with non-essential amino acid components. Ang *et al.* [34] showed that there is a limit to the amount of nitrogen that can be utilized to improve negative nitrogen balance. These investigations showed that, at three different levels of nitrogen intake (7.9, 11.9 and 15.8 g nitrogen per day) as part of a total parenteral nutrition (TPN) regimen for malnourished patients, protein synthesis reached a plateau at 11.9 g nitrogen per day. Schizgal and Forse [35] gave TPN with different amounts of nitrogen to depleted hypercatabolic patients and found a positive correlation between nitrogen intake and nitrogen balance at intakes less than 204 mg of nitrogen/kg body weight per day. However, there was no improvement in nitrogen balance with higher intakes, and similarly Wolfe *et al.* [36] found that protein equilibrium was not improved with intakes above 224 mg of nitrogen per kg of body weight in patients with burns. Finally, Greig *et al.* [25] fed septic patients with 191 and 336 mg nitrogen per kg and found no significant difference in nitrogen balance between the two levels of intake after five days. This supports our current view [8] that providing more than 200 mg of nitrogen per kg of body weight will not improve the metabolic/nutritional response.

One can question how nutritional support should be given, enterally, nasogastrically (NG), nasoenterally or intravenously. However, there is a wide discrepancy between the nutrition prescribed and that received by the three common routes used (Table 13.1) [24]. Given all the other medical problems associated with ARF – surgery and anaesthesia,

**Table 13.1** Acute renal failure: nitrogen intake

| | % nitrogen received against nitrogen prescribed | | |
|---|---|---|---|
| | Mean | SEM | Number of patients |
| **Enteral** | | | |
| Oral | 52.4 | 6.1 | 5 |
| NG | 53.7 | 15.6 | 5 |
| All enteral | 53.0 | 7.9 | 10 |
| **Intravenous** | | | |
| IV only | 84.0 | 3.0 | 19 |
| IV and NG | 97.1 | 18.2 | 3 |
| All intravenous | 85.8 | 3.5 | 22 |

wound sepsis, etc. – nutritional support often becomes the 'Cinderella' of the management process. Therefore, there is a compelling argument to support the view [37] that all acute renal failure patients should be dialysed optimally and receive aggressive nutritional support, preferably as TPN. This is not to deny the commonly stated adage 'if the gut works use it', but Table 13.1 shows the potential shortcomings.

### 13.5.1 Types of nutritional support

It has been shown [9] that non-essential amino acids are a better source of non-specific nitrogen than urea nitrogen. Varcoe *et al.* [38] and Mitch *et al.* [39], showed that urea nitrogen recycling is of little nutritional value in chronic renal failure patients and there is no proof that such metabolic pathways have any significance in ARF either. Although leucine has been shown to be the probable branched chain amino acid (BCAA) regulator of muscle metabolism [40] the provision of solutions with increased BCAA content has not been shown to be superior. Attempts to control protein metabolism have focused on the role of leucine or its analogue alpha-ketoisocaproate and the effect on protein synthesis and degradation. Hence, Goldberg and Tischler [41] incubated rat diaphragms with leucine and found that protein synthesis was increased whilst degradation was decreased and concluded that leucine had a direct stimulatory effect on protein synthesis and its metabolites, and decreased protein degradation. Sapir and Walser [42] showed that the infusion of BCAA in starving obese human subjects decreased nitrogen wasting, and this report was confirmed by Mitch *et al.* [43] when they gave only alpha-ketoisocaproate to starving obese subjects. However, to date, there have been very few studies on the value of adding increased amounts of BCAA, or indeed ketoacid analogues, to nutritional regimens in ARF. Proeitti *et al.* [44] showed that TPN with a high BCAA:essential amino acids ratio given to acute renal failure patients resulted in a less negative nitrogen balance and a decrease in plasma urea concentration, but mortality was unchanged. The infusion of ketoacids showed no benefit on plasma urea concentration or survival when compared to essential amino acids in dogs made acutely uraemic by a bilateral nephrectomy [45]. It remains to be shown what is the real role, if any, of additional BCAA or ketoacid analogue additions to nutritional therapies in ARF.

A number of studies have shown that glutamine infusions can improve nitrogen balance in patients after surgery, injury, sepsis and steroids. Glutamine, however, is unstable in solution, undergoing rapid hydrolysis. Following infusions of glutamine–alanine dipeptide solutions into catabolic patients, Furst *et al.* [46] showed that this maintained the muscle glutamine pool and improved nitrogen balance compared to a control group given as isonitrogeneous isoenergetic TPN regimen. Therefore a possibility exists that acute renal failure patients who are similarly catabolic, protein depleted and assumed glutamine depleted, could benefit by receiving glutamine-containing dipeptide solutions. Low plasma glutamine concentrations have been found in ARF.

To what extent can the actual nitrogen losses in acute renal failure patients be covered? In some patients nitrogen losses may amount to as much as 40 g per day, but clearly one cannot provide an equivalent amount. This is because the metabolic capacity of the liver for the average 70 kg man cannot handle a daily load greater than 23 g of amino acid nitrogen. If this is exceeded the simple result is that excess amino acids are deaminated, increasing the urea nitrogen appearance rate and leading to increased dialysis requirements.

The measurement of nitrogen balance in ARF has been notoriously difficult to measure, because of the heterogeneity of the causes of acute renal failure, the various treatments they receive, the severity of the attendant conditions (such as sepsis, operative intervention, etc.), ventilatory support and drugs, such as corticosteroids. The nitrogen balance in a carefully studied series of thirty-three acute renal failure patients [24] was increasingly negative according to the catabolic rate index (CRI). It was also observed that with increasing CRI the actual nitrogen input did not increase. However, those studies showed that nitrogen balance does improve with increased nitrogen intake although 50% of the nitrogen intake goes towards the increased urea appearance rate. In these studies it was shown that up to 200 mg of nitrogen per kg body weight could be usefully metabolized in improving the nitrogen balance.

### 13.5.2 Energy provision

There is no consensus on the most suitable energy substrate for the critically ill patient. Wilmore [47] showed that the provision of exogenous non-protein energy decreases nitrogen excretion and this relates equally to the administration of both fat and carbohydrate sources. When energy (fat or carbohydrate, or both) is given with nitrogen to normal human subjects or animals both energy sources improve nitrogen retention. This applies equally to patients with sepsis who are not malnourished [48]. However, in hypercatabolic patients (the majority of patients with ARF) Woolfson *et al.* [49] showed a rapid decrease in nitrogen excretion with carbohydrate infusion. Wilmore [47] failed to show a similar response when fat was infused. These alternative observations are difficult to explain, though it may be that different metabolic responses occur as a result of different neurohormonal signals between normo- and moderately catabolic and hypercatabolic patients. In hypercatabolic patients the neurohormonal scenario is set to signal the 'request' for accelerated gluconeogenesis, with an overriding ability of the body to adapt its metabolism to various energy sources. Askanazi *et al.* [50] showed that the administration of excess carbohydrate as an energy source resulted in excessive carbon dioxide production, which in turn could lead to respiratory problems in patients requiring ventilation. It is my view that energy provision should be provided equally divided between fat and carbohydrate, irrespective of the route of administration. However, it is common practice to administer the majority of energy as carbohydrate (dextrose) in TPN, fat emulsion being given twice or thrice a week, to facilitate administration of fat-soluble vitamins. Enteral feeding supplementation will be largely governed by the products used.

Feinstein *et al.* [10] who studied a group of postoperative and trauma patients with ARF, suggested an energy requirement of 209 kJ (50 kcals) per kg body weight, but this figure has not been confirmed elsewhere. Glucose intolerance in acute renal failure patients is now thought to be primarily due to peripheral insulin resistance [51] whilst hepatic glucose uptake is normal [52], conflicting with earlier animal experiments. There is no real evidence to support the view that the infusion of a fat emulsion (triglycerides) promotes the generation of excess free fatty acids in serum causing cardiac arrhythmias. Indeed, some of the early observations may have been due to poor laboratory techniques [53].

### 13.5.3 Assessment of nutritional requirements

When assessing the nutritional requirements of any patient it is necessary to consider other requirements over and above nitrogen and energy. A comprehensive approach is required, providing nitrogen, energy, electrolytes, essential biological elements (EBE) or trace elements, vitamins and fluids. Clearly, with the current state of knowledge it is impossible to prescribe precise amounts of vitamins and EBE. However, every effort should be made to at least provide the basic normal daily requirements of vitamins and EBE. It is recommended that patients receive not more than 200 mg of nitrogen per kg body weight and between 30 and 50 kcal per kg body weight depending on the catabolic event. With adequate dialysis normal electrolyte provision can be maintained. Furthermore, although it is customary to reduce phosphate and/or potassium provision for such patients, if and when they enter the anabolic phase, failure to provide these elements will result in a loss of the optimum benefits from the nutritional support provided [26].

The modern view must be that ARF patients must receive aggressive nutritional support and dialysis, according to individual requirements. There is no longer any place for the earlier approaches [11, 27] which suggested the provision of small amounts of nitrogen aimed at decreasing the urea appearance rate or dialysis requirement. Those studies showed very convincingly that there was no improvement in survival, which is the goal. Equally, to match simply the nitrogen output in such patients by infusing large amounts of nitrogen would or could result in overload and increased urea appearance rate, again without benefit.

### 13.5.4 Outcome of nutritional support in acute renal failure

There is no evidence in the literature, either from animal work or human research, that nutritional support by itself increases the rate of recovery from renal failure. However, there can be little doubt that nutritional support can reduce the rate of infection, the rate of wound dehiscence, improve the rate of wound healing, decrease the length of time of ventilatory support, improve overall well-being and survival in such patients. Although it has been previously shown that the rate of discharge of postoperative patients is improved as a result of parenteral nutrition, no such figures are available for ARF patients. Kleinknecht *et al.* [54] studied the effects of late versus early haemodialysis. In 279 patients dialysed when the blood urea was higher than 350 mg/100 ml (58 mmol/l) there was a 42% mortality rate compared to 221 patients dialysed early with a blood urea concentration of less than 200 mg/100 ml (33 mmol/l), where the mortality rate was 29%. Conger [55] showed in patients where the blood urea concentration was maintained below 25 mmol/l that there was a 37% mortality rate compared with an 80% mortality rate in patients where the blood urea concentration was above 54 mmol/l. Abel *et al.* [27] selected 53 of 150 patients with acute renal failure for nutritional support, these patients being the least catabolic. In that study those who received amino acids and energy (glucose) had a mortality rate of 25%, whereas in those fed glucose only there was a 56% mortality rate.

Baek *et al.* [56] studied 129 postoperative patients with acute renal failure and compared one group receiving a fibrin hydrolysate with glucose versus a second group receiving glucose only. In the first group there was a 46% mortality rate versus a 70% mortality rate in the second group. Again, Rainsford [37] looked at three cohorts of patients where the underlying basic dialysis treatment had not changed but in the third group immediate comprehensive parenteral nutrition had been given. He found in the group given comprehensive total parenteral nutrition there was a 31.6% mortality rate whereas in those who received dialysis treatment alone it was 52.1% and in those given dialysis and some nutritional support it was 42.3%. Rainsford suggested that TPN should be given immediately to acute renal failure patients irrespective of gastrointestinal function and that there were no particular problems associated with TPN itself.

Elsewhere, Pelosi et al. [57] studied forty-six patients with ARF, all requiring haemodialysis. They undertook appropriate nitrogen balance studies in these patients and found them all to be in negative balance. They observed that those patients receiving full profile amino acid solutions plus glucose were in less negative nitrogen balance then those given isocaloric regimens with essential amino acids only. Shear *et al.* [58], using $C^{14}$-leucine-labelled amino acids, showed that protein synthesis was increased in the liver and also in heart muscle, but decreased in skeletal muscle in acute renal failure. These observations support the view of Feinstein *et al.* [10] who suggested that the 'catabolic drive' in man with acute renal failure would be sufficient to cause abnormally high urea appearance rates in spite of adequate amino acid provision. Feinstein *et al.* also suggested that the quantity of nitrogen required to offset this catabolic effect might be technically impossible to administer.

## 13.6 NUTRITIONAL SUPPORT IN CHRONIC RENAL FAILURE

As described by Lee [59] the patient with chronic renal failure who requires an operation, or who acquires a severe infection, should be treated as one with ARF. He/she should be treated by regular haemodialysis or CAVH; chronic peritoneal dialysis may have to be suspended for a time. It should be clear that dialysis time is nutrition time and the chronic renal failure patient in the acute situation is no different from the normal individual who suddenly acquires acute renal failure. Furthermore, as mentioned previously, there is no evidence to suggest that urea nitrogen recycling is of any nutritional value in acute renal failure, be that primary or secondary to chronic renal failure. Therefore in patients undergoing regular haemodialysis and/or chronic ambulatory peritoneal dialysis (CAPD) treatment, if they undergo an acute event which merits appropriate nutritional support then their method of dialysis should be adapted as for a patient with ARF.

A number of patients with CRF, either approaching end stage renal failure or on some form of dialysis, may be clinically malnourished. This is typically seen in patients with the nephrotic syndrome and rapidly progressive renal failure, failing kidney transplants, and in patients with complications such as CAPD peritonitis. They are not necessarily hypercatabolic, and do not in general require TPN. Enteral support, with oral and sip feeds, is usually successful and must be employed with the same degree of vigour as for TPN in ARF. It is important to note that in patients treated with CAPD before coming to renal transplantation, those who have a low serum albumin concentration have a poorer prognosis. The same applies equally to haemodialysis patients. Given the paucity of cadaveric organs available, it behoves all clinicians concerned with the management of chronic renal failure to ensure that their patients are in their best nutritional status when a transplant becomes available.

Following transplantation, the main nutritional problem in a successful renal transplantee is that of obesity, usually as a result of much improved appetite and quality of life, and steroid therapy. Nutritional restriction, rather than support becomes the order of the day!

## REFERENCES


1. Lee, H.A. (1980) Diet and renal failure, in *Recent Advances in Clinical Nutrition: 1* (eds A. Howard and I. MacLean Baird), John Libbey, London, pp. 159–69.
2. Persike, E.C. and Addis, T. (1949) Increased rate of urea formation following removal of renal tissue. *Am. J. Physiol.*, **158**, 149–58.
3. Sellers, A.L., Katz, J. and Marmosten, J. (1957) Effects of bilateral nephrectomy on urea formation in rat liver slices. *Am. J. Physiol.*, **191**, 345–9.
4. Lacy, W.W. (1969) Effect of acute uraemia on amino acid uptake and urea production by perfused rat liver. *Am. J. Physiol.*, **216**, 1300–5.
5. Lacy, W.W. (1970) Uptake of individual amino acids by perfused rat liver; effect of acute uraemia. *Am. J. Physiol.*, **219**, 649–53.
6. Frohlich, J., Scholmreich, J., Hoppe-Seyler, G. *et al.* (1974) The effect of acute uraemia on gluconeogenesis in isolated perfused rat livers. *Eur. J. Clin. Nutr.*, **46**, 1040–7.
7. Bondy, P.K., Engel, F.L. and Farrar, B. (1949) The metabolism of amino acids and protein in the adrenalectomized versus nephrectomized rat. *Endocrinology*, **44**, 476.

8. Lee, H.A. and Talbot, S.T. (1990) Nutrition in acute renal failure management, in *Acute Renal Failure* (eds D. Rainsford and P. Sweny), Farrand Press, London, pp. 245–55.
9. Feinstein, E.I. and Massry, S.G. (1988) Nutritional therapy in acute renal failure, in *Nutrition of the Kidney* (eds W.E. Mitch and S. Klahr), Little, Brown and Company, Boston, pp. 80–103.
10. Feinstein, E.I., Blumenkratz, M.J., Healy, M. *et al.* (1981) Clinical and metabolic responses to parenteral nutrition in acute renal failure. A controlled double blind study. *Medicine*, **60**, 124–37.
11. Berlyne, G.M., Bazzard, F.J., Booth, E.M. *et al.* (1967) The dietary treatment of acute renal failure. *Q. J. Med.*, **36**, 59–83.
12. Silva, H., Pomeroy, J., Rae, A.I. *et al.* (1964) Daily haemodialysis in 'hypercatabolic' acute renal failure. *Br. Med. J.*, **2**, 407–10.
13. Lee, H.A., Sharpstone, P. and Ames, A.C. (1967) Parenteral nutrition in acute renal failure. *Postgrad. Med. J.*, **43**, 81–90.
14. Horl, W.H., Grabner, E. and Heidland, A. (1978) Increased proteolytic enzyme activity in blood serum of patients with acute and chronic uraemia. 15th EDTA, abstract 332.
15. Horl, W.H. and Heidland, A., (1980) Enhanced proteolytic activity – cause of protein catabolism in acute renal failure. *Am. J. Clin. Nutr.*, **33**, 1423–7.
16. Clowse, G.H.A., George, B.C., Villee, C.A. and Saravis, C.A. (1983) Muscle proteolysis induced by a circulating peptide in patients with sepsis or trauma. *N. Engl. J. Med.*, **308**, 545–52.
17. Ward, R.A., Shirlow, M.J., Hayes, J.M. *et al.* (1979) Protein catabolism during haemodialysis. *Am. J. Clin. Nutr.*, **32**, 2443–9.
18. Port, F.K., van de Kerkhove, K.M., Kunkel, S.L. and Kluger, M.J. (1987) The role of dialysate in the stimulation of interleukin-1 production during clinical haemodialysis. *Am. J. Kidney Dis.*, **10**, 118–22.
19. Bingel, M., Lonneman, G., Shaldon, S. *et al.* (1986) Human interleukin-1 (IL-1) production during haemodialysis. *Nephron*, **43**, 161–3.
20. Bingel, M., Lonneman, G., Koch, K.M. *et al.* (1987) Enhancement of in-vitro human interleukin-1 production by sodium acetate. *Lancet*, **i**, 14–6.
21. Arisi, L., Garini, G., Paganelli, E. and Franco, V. (1989) Blunting of dialysis induced hypercatabolism (DIHC) by indomethacin (i). *Kidney Int.*, abstract. **32**, 204.
22. Jackson, J.M., Khawaja, H.T., Weaver, P. *et al.* (1984) Naftidrofuryl and the nitrogen, carbohydrate and lipid responses to moderate surgery. *Br. Med. J.*, **289**, 581–4.
23. Lee, H.A. and Hartley, T.F. (1975) A method of determining daily nitrogen balance. *Postgrad. Med. J.*, **51**, 441–5.
24. Talbot, S.T. (1990) A study of nitrogen requirements in acute renal failure in man. MPhil Thesis, University of Southampton, UK
25. Greig, P.D., Elwyn, D.H., Askanazi, J. and Kinney, J.M. (1987) Parenteral nutrition in septic patients: effect of increasing nitrogen intake. *Am. J. Clin. Nutr.*, **46**, 1040–7.
26. Lee, H.A. (1988) The nutritional management of renal disease, in *Nutrition in the Clinical Management of Disease* (eds J.W.T. Dickerson and H.A. Lee), Edward Arnold, London, pp. 263–79.
27. Abel, R.M., Beck, C.H., Abbott, W.M. *et al.* (1973) Improved survival from acute renal failure after treatment with intravenous essential amino acids and glucose. *N. Engl. J. Med.*, **288**, 696–9.

28. Leonard, C.D., Luke, R.G. and Siegel, R.R. (1975) Parenteral essential amino acids in acute renal failure. *Urology*, **6**, 154–7.
29. Blackburn, G.L., Etter, G. and MacKenzie, W. (1978) Criteria for choosing amino acid therapy in acute renal failure. *Am. J. Clin. Nutr.*, **31**, 1841–5.
30. Feinstein, E.I., Heals, M., Kaffler, A. *et al.* (1983) Total parenteral nutrition with high or low nitrogen intakes in patients with acute renal failure. *Kidney Int.*, **26**, S319–24.
31. McMurray, S.D. *et al.* (1978) Prevailing patterns and predicatory variables in patients with acute tubular necrosis. *Arch. Intern. Med.*, **139**, 950–4.
32. Borst, J.G.G. (1948) Protein catabolism in uraemia. Effects of protein free diet, infections and blood transfusions. *Lancet*, **i**, 825–8.
33. Bull, G.M., Joekes, J.M. and Lowe, K.G. (1949) Conservative management of anuric anaemia. *Lancet*, **ii**, 229–31.
34. Ang, S.D., Leski, M.J. and Stein, T.P. (1983) The effect of increasing total parenteral nutrition on protein metabolism. *J. Parenter. Enter. Nutr.*, **7**, 525–9.
35. Schizgal, H.M. and Furse, R.H. (1980) Protein and caloric requirements with total parenteral nutrition. *Ann. Surg.*, **192**, 562–8.
36. Wolfe, R.R., Goodenough, R.D., Burke, J.F. and Wolfe, M.H. (1983) Protein dynamics in stress, in *Amino Acids: Metabolism and Medical Applications* (eds G.L. Blackburn, J.P. Grant and V.R. Young), John Wright, Boston.
37. Rainsford, D.J. (1987) Trends in management of acute renal failure, in *Renal Failure: Current Approaches*, (eds H.A. Lee and S.W. Parker), Duphar Medical Laboratories, Southampton, pp. 26–30.
38. Varcoe, A.R., Halliday, D., Carson, E.R. *et al.* (1975) Efficiency of the utilisation of urea nitrogen for albumin synthesis by chronically uraemic and normal man. *Clin. Sci. Molec. Med.*, **44**, 379–86.
39. Mitch, W.E., Leitman, P. and Walser, M. (1977) Effect of oral neomycin and kanamycin in chronic uraemic subjects. *Kidney Int.*, **11**, 122–7.
40. Buse, M.G. and Reid, S. (1975) Leucine: a possible regulator of protein turnover in muscle. *J. Clin. Invest.*, **65**, 1250–61.
41. Goldberg, A.L. and Tischler, M.E. (1981) Regulatory effects of leucine on carbohydrate and protein metabolism, in *Metabolism and Clinical Infections of Branched Chain Amino and Keto Acids* (Developments in Biochemistry Series) (eds M.M. Walser and J.R. Williamson), Vol. 18, pp. 205–16.
42. Sapir, D.G. and Walser, M. (1977) Nitrogen sparing induced early in starvation by infusion of branched chain keto acids. *Metabolism*, **26**, 302–8.
43. Mitch, W.E., Walser, M. and Sapir, D.G. (1981) Nitrogen sparing induced by leucine compared with that induced by its keto analogue alpha-ketoisocaproate in fasting obese man. *J. Clin. Invest.*, **67**, 553–62.
44. Proietti, R., Pelosi, G., Santori, R. *et al.* (1983) Nutrition in acute renal failure. *Resuscitation*, **10**, 159–66.
45. Brissac, C., Saint-Aubert, B., Joyeux, A. *et al.* (1981) Alpha-ketoacids in acute renal insufficiency in the dog, in *Metabolism and Clinical Implications of Branched-chain Amino Acids and Keto Acids* (eds M. Walser and J.R. Williamson), Elsevier, North Holland, pp. 599–604.
46. Furst, P., Alber, S. and Stehle, P. (1989) Evidence for a nutritional need for glutamine (Gln) in catabolic patients. *Kidney Int.*, **32**, 216–21.
47. Wilmore, D.W. (1977) Energy requirements for maximum nitrogen retention, in Proceeding of Symposium on Amino Acid Metabolism, Houston, Texas, (eds H.L. Green, M.A. Halliday and H.N. Munro), American Medical Association, Chicago, pp. 47–57.

48. Roulet, M., Detsky, A.S., Marliss, E.B. *et al.* (1983) A controlled trial of the effect of parenteral nutritional support on patients with respiratory failure and sepsis. *Clin. Nutr.*, **2**, 97–105.
49. Woolfson, A.M.M., Heatley, R.V. and Allison, S.P. (1979) Insulin to inhibit protein catabolism after injury. *N. Engl. J. Med.*, **300**, 14–7.
50. Askanazi, J., Carpentier, Y.A., Elwyn, D.H. *et al.* (1980) Influence of total parenteral nutrition in fuel utilisation in injury and sepsis. *Ann. Surg.*, **191**, 40–6.
51. Clark, A.S. and Mitch, W.E. (1983) Muscle protein turnover and glucose uptake in acute uraemic rats. Effects of insulin and the duration of renal insufficiency. *J. Clin. Invest.*, **72**, 836–45.
52. Mondon, C.E., Dolkas, C.B. and Reaven, G.M. (1978) The site of insulin resistance in acute uraemia. *Diabetes*, **27**, 571–6.
53. Jackson, J.M., Talbot, S.T. and Lee, H.A. (1995) Plasma non-esterified fatty acid response to dialysate acetate concentration during haemodialysis in humans. *Clin. Chim. Acta*, **239**, 81–9.
54. Kleinknecht, D., Jungers, P., Chanard, J. *et al.* (1972) Uraemic and non-uraemic complications in acute renal failure: evaluation of early and frequent dialysis on prognosis. *Kidney Int.*, **1**, 190–6.
55. Conger, J.D. (1975) A controlled evaluation of prophylactic dialysis in post traumatic acute renal failure. *J. Trauma*, **15**, 1056–63.
56. Baek, S.M., Makaboli, G.G., Bryan-Brown, C.W. *et al.* (1975) The influence of parenteral nutrition on the course of acute renal failure. *Surg. Gynaecol. Obstet.*, **141**, 405–8.
57. Pelosi, G., Proietti, R., Arcangeli, A. *et al.* (1981) Total parenteral nutrition infusate. An approach to its optimal composition in post-traumatic acute renal failure. *Resuscitation*, **9**, 45–51.
58. Shear, L. (1967) Internal redistribution of tissue protein synthesis in uraemia. *J. Clin. Invest.*, **48**, 1252–6.
59. Lee, H.A. (1984) Total parenteral nutrition (TPN) in chronic renal failure patients, in *Surgery in Chronic Renal Failure* (eds F.W. Eigler and H.D. Jakubowski), G. Thieme Verlag, Stuttgart, pp. 19–23.

# 14

# Paediatric aspects

*M.E. McGraw*

The disease spectrum seen within paediatric nephrology differs from that seen in adult nephrology as do many aspects of treatment. It is not possible to cover all aspects of renal disease in children within this chapter, which will aim to concentrate upon those conditions which are common in childhood or in which the management is significantly different from that in adults.

## 14.1 URINARY TRACT INFECTION

The most common problem encountered by any paediatric nephrologist is that of urinary tract infection (UTI). The risk of developing a urinary tract infection between one month and eleven years of age is approximately 0.7% for boys and 2.8% for girls. The frequency in neonates is 0.14% [1]. Female preponderance for urinary tract infection is seen at all ages beyond the neonatal period.

Features at presentation are also influenced by age. The neonate often has bacteraemia and presents with the clinical symptoms of sepsis. The infant may present with non-specific symptoms associated with a febrile illness including vomiting, diarrhoea, meningism and failure to thrive. It is only in the toddler and older children that a urinary tract infection is likely to present with classical urinary tract symptoms.

The diagnosis of UTI requires a high index of suspicion together with an appropriate urine collection for culture. Kass' criterion for the diagnosis of urinary tract infection (of $>10^5$ organisms/ml in a clean-voided urine) however, needs to be modified for use in children. Urine bags are still widely used for the collection of urine from babies even

*Renal Disease.* Edited by G. Venkat Raman. Published in 1998 by Chapman & Hall, London. ISBN 0 412 45700 8.

though bacterial contamination may occur in around 50%. Clean voided urines also have a high contamination rate due to labial and preputial contamination and therefore this and bag specimens may only be useful in excluding the diagnosis of UTI, rather than to make the diagnosis. A variety of other methods have been suggested to improve diagnostic accuracy. Pyuria often accompanies bacteruria but its presence is not diagnostic and there are other causes of pyuria. Pyuria may be absent in up to 50% of patients with significant bacteruria, particularly in neonates.

The best available method for the accurate diagnosis of urinary tract infection in infancy remains the culture of urine obtained by suprapubic aspiration. In infants and young children the bladder is an abdominal organ and percutaneous suprapubic aspiration of urine is a safe and easy method of obtaining a reliable urine specimen. Under these circumstances no organisms should be found although skin contamination may produce up to $10^3$ organisms/ml of Gram positive cocci.

Leucocyte esterase and nitrite dipsticks in combination have excellent negative predictive value and may provide a suitable screening test [2]. However in children with complex renal problems, when infection with non-nitrite-producing organisms such as *Pseudomonas* and group B streptococcus is a real possibility, then urine microscopy and culture is mandatory.

### 14.1.1 Treatment and prevention

*Treatment of the acute infection*

Eighty to ninety per cent of first-time urinary tract infections are caused by coliforms, the majority of which are sensitive to the commonly used antibiotics. In neonates, infection with *Klebsiella* species, often resistant to amoxycillin, is common and in boys a third of infections are caused by *Proteus* species, usually resistant to nitrofurantoin. Although the final choice of antibiotic is made upon the sensitivities of the organism, treatment often needs to be commenced before this information is available. Commonly used agents include co-trimoxazole, nitrofurantoin, amoxycillin and cephalosporins. Oral treatment is usually adequate, although in neonates and in children who are vomiting and those with clinical septicaemia, intravenous treatment with aminoglycosides, broad-spectrum penicillins or cephalosporins is required. In children with recurrent infections resistant organisms may emerge and drugs which have been used in the preceding months should be avoided. Treatment for five to seven days is adequate in most situations.

Single-dose treatment has been found to be effective but should be reserved for girls over two years of age with acute dysuric symptoms and no systemic features. In these circumstances the drugs used should be slowly excreted, such as co-trimoxazole, and not rapidly excreted drugs such as amoxycillin and short-acting cephalosporins [3].

### 14.1.2 Antibiotic prophylaxis

Prophylactic antibiotics are indicated in all children at high risk of developing renal scarring. Risk factors include underlying structural abnormality, including vesicoureteric reflux (VUR) and obstruction. Age is also an important risk factor with an increased risk of scarring throughout the first year of life, but declining to low rates after the age of seven years. Diagnostic imaging is therefore carried out in all children presenting with their first urinary tract infection, the extent of the investigation dependent on the age of the child.

A Working Party of the Royal College of Physicians [4] has recommended the following:

1. Children under one year: ultrasound, plain abdominal X-ray, micturating cystourethrogram and DMSA scan.
2. Children between one and seven years: ultrasound, plain abdominal X-ray and DMSA scan, with cystourethrography confined to children with abnormalities shown on these investigations, a clinical history suggestive of acute pyelonephritis, a family history of reflux nephropathy or recurrent infections.
3. Children over seven years: ultrasound and plain abdominal X-ray.

In those in whom vesicoureteric reflux is demonstrated long-term treatment with prophylactic antibiotics, such as trimethoprim 2 mg/kg/day (or co-trimoxazole), should be continued. Long-term follow-up studies have shown no benefit of operative management [5] and that the incidence of new scar formation declines steeply after the age of seven years. Therefore current recommendations would be to continue prophylaxis until seven years of age or until the reflux has disappeared.

### 14.1.3 Antenatal ultrasonography

Routine antenatal ultrasonography now often includes examination of the fetal renal tract. The estimated incidence of fetal uropathy varies widely from 0.14% to 0.65% [6, 7]. Neonates shown to have antenatal hydronephrosis should be commenced on prophylactic antibiotics from birth, pending full postnatal investigation of the urinary tract. It is not yet known whether this will influence the natural history of conditions such as reflux nephropathy. One study of infants presenting with urinary tract infection demonstrated that 46% of urinary tract malformations were detected antenatally in a population where just over 50% of pregnancies were screened [8]. However, even in patients who had been investigated antenatally potentially recognizable lesions had been missed. Therefore the role of prenatal diagnosis has yet to be evaluated.

## 14.2 NEPHROTIC SYNDROME

Nephrotic syndrome is the most common clinical form of glomerulopathy, with an incidence of 2–3/100 000 population per annum. Over 60% of children will present under the age of five years with a 2:1 male preponderance. Presentation is with oedema, initially periorbital extending to pedal oedema and ascites. Diagnosis is confirmed by the finding of heavy proteinuria (greater than 50 mg/kg/24 h or >40 mg/hour/$m^2$ or a protein/creatinine ratio on an early morning urine >200 mg/mmol) and a low serum albumin (less than 25 g/l).

Eighty per cent of children will have minimal change nephropathy (MCN) and a renal biopsy is not indicated at presentation. However, the proportion of children with this diagnosis decreases with age, with only 55% of children between the ages of eight and 16 years showing minimal change histology [9]. However, children with other histologies may also respond to corticosteroids and therefore, even in older children, a renal biopsy is rarely indicated before a trial of steroids. The exception would be in those children with evidence of impaired renal function and an active urinary sediment, with the possibility of a more serious disorder such as membranoproliferative glomerulonephritis (MPGN). An abnormally low serum complement is highly suggestive of MPGN, though 25% of patients with this disease may have a normal serum complement.

In order to address this the International Study for Kidney Disease in Childhood (ISKDC) performed multivariate analyses and derived an equation based on various clinical and laboratory criteria, which can discriminate between MPGN and other forms of glomerular diseases [9].

### 14.2.1 Treatment and prevention

*Corticosteroids*

The British Association for Paediatric Nephrology (BAPN) has produced a consensus statement on the management of steroid responsive nephrotic syndrome [10]. A series of levels of treatment are recommended, commencing with steroid therapy and progressing to other agents if a frequently relapsing course develops. At present high-dose steroids (60 mg/$m^2$/day, maximum 80 mg/day) are accepted for the induction of remission, and once remission is induced the dose is reduced to 40 mg/m$^2$ on alternate days for the next few weeks. Remission of MCN has also been reported following intravenous pulse methylprednisolone [11] and lower doses of prednisolone 30 mg/m$^2$/day [12].

Studies looking at the total duration of steroids in relation to long-term outcome have suggested that shorter courses of steroids are associated with an increased rate of relapse [13]. On BAPN regimen the relapse rate is up to 95%. If the daily steroids are continued for four weeks the relapse rate falls to 75%. If the daily steroids are continued for six weeks followed by six weeks alternate-day steroids the relapse rate falls to 50%. Although the side effects need to be balanced against the response rates, the use of longer courses of steroids requires further evaluation.

Twenty-four per cent of children will become frequent relapsers (two relapses within six months of initial therapy or four relapses within a twelve-month period). Many of these cases can be satisfactorily maintained on alternate-day steroid therapy, 35 mg/m$^2$ on alternate days [14]. For such steroid-dependent children it is helpful to assess the steroid threshold, i.e. the lowest dose at which relapses can be prevented. The maintenance dose to prevent relapse should therefore be just above this. If doses above 35 mg/m$^2$ on alternate days are required to maintain remission, then alternate therapies should be considered.

### *Cyclophosphamide*

This is a well-established drug for the prevention of relapse in steroid-responsive nephrotic syndrome. Fifty per cent of children treated with cyclophosphamide relapsed compared to 90% treated with steroids alone [8]. An eight-week course of cyclophosphamide at 3 mg/kg/day resulted in 75% of cases remaining in remission for one year and 50% for five years [15]. Gonadal toxicity is related to total dosage. Total doses of less than 300 mg/kg in boys treated for less than 112 days have been shown to be associated with normal sperm counts in adulthood [16].

In children failing to respond to the initial eight-week course of steroids, despite varying histology, 56% have been shown to become protein-free after cyclophosphamide [17].

### *Chlorambucil and nitrogen mustard*

Although less frequently used, both chlorambucil 0.2 mg/kg/day for eight weeks and nitrogen mustard 0.1 mg/kg for four days have been shown to be effective. There are concerns regarding the long-term toxicity of chlorambucil, although nitrogen mustard may be less toxic than cyclophosphamide.

*Levamisole*

Levamisole, an immunostimulant originally developed as an anthelmintic, has been shown in a prospective randomized controlled trial to be superior to placebo in maintaining remission in frequently relapsing steroid-sensitive and dependent nephrotic syndrome [18]. At a dose of 2.5 mg/kg on alternate days 45% of patients receiving levamisole remained in remission and off steroids at 16 weeks. Although the optimum dose, frequency, and duration of treatment have not been established, longer courses of therapy would seem justified in patients with steroid toxicity.

*Cyclosporin A*

Cyclosporin A is effective in steroid-responsive nephrotic syndrome and early studies suggested that 80% of children would remain in remission with a cessation of steroids [19]. A British study following the BAPN guidelines however suggested that 72% of children on cyclosporin A had a relapse, 40% in the first year, and that 40% required, in addition, maintenance steroids [20].

Studies on the response to cyclosporin A in steroid-resistant nephrotic syndrome are conflicting but there is a suggestion that cyclosporin A will reduce the proteinuria and slow progression to end stage renal disease [21] although the risk of developing nephrotoxicity appears to be higher in steroid-resistant patients [19].

## 14.3 HYPERTENSION

Blood pressure in children rises with age and its variability is greater than in adults. Indices of body mass are major determinants of blood pressure in childhood although it is also influenced by the interaction of other genetic and environmental factors. 'Tracking' of blood pressure, which is the maintenance of rank order within the distribution over time, is present in childhood but its predictive power is low. Although epidemiological studies have suggested that the origins of adult hypertension may begin in childhood or even fetal life, in individuals the predictive value of childhood blood pressure readings is less certain.

The prevalence of hypertension is between 1 and 3%. It may be defined as a blood pressure greater than the 95th centile for age [22] or height [23] confirmed on at least three readings [24]. The blood pressure should be obtained using the largest cuff that can comfortably be applied to the arm so that the inflatable part of the cuff, the bladder, should cover at least two thirds of the circumference of the upper arm and the lower edge should not touch the stethoscope applied to the cubital artery. A minimum of four cuffs is necessary to cover the school-age population: bladder sizes 4 × 13 cm, 8 × 18 cm, 12 × 24 cm, 14 × 33 cm. The appearance of the first Korotkoff sound should be taken to indicate the systolic blood pressure measurement and the complete disappearance, Korotkoff 5, for the diastolic pressure.

### 14.3.1 Clinical features

Many children with hypertension are asymptomatic. In infancy symptoms include failure to thrive, irritability, heart failure and respiratory distress. In older children symptoms include poor growth, headache, vomiting, visual symptoms, facial palsy, polyuria and epistaxis. Important features to note include growth, delayed pulses and blood pressure differences between upper and lower limbs, palpable abdominal masses, a renal bruit (over the epigastrium), the presence of skin lesions of neurofibromatosis and retinal changes.

The recommendations for the investigation of hypertension in children [24] depend on the persistence and degree of hypertension. Mild hypertension will require no more than a careful family history, drug history and routine urinalysis and renal biochemistry. Mild to moderate hypertension, i.e. blood pressure consistently above the 95th centile with no evidence of end organ damage, will require full blood count, urinalysis, renal biochemistry including calcium, 24-hour urinary vanillyl mandelic acid, peripheral renin and aldosterone, together with renal imaging (renal ultrasound and DMSA scan), and cardiac assessment with ECG and chest X-ray.

Severe hypertension will need all of the above investigations and, depending on the results, more invasive procedures, such as renal arteriogram, and computed tomography. If catecholamines are high, an isotope-labelled *meta*-iodobenzylguanidine (MIBG) scan would be indicated.

The most common causes of childhood hypertension are renin mediated, and include renovascular disease, renal parenchymal disease (reflux nephropathy and chronic pyelonephritis, glomerulonephritis, polycystic kidneys) or renal tumours. In infants coarctation of the aorta is the most common cause. Endocrine causes, including phaeochromocytoma, neuroblastoma, congenital adrenal hyperplasia, Conn's and Cushing's syndromes, are rare.

### 14.3.2 Treatment and prevention

Non-pharmacological intervention should be considered first particularly in those with primary or mild hypertension. This should include weight reduction, dietary sodium restriction, and life style changes with

**Table 14.1** Hypertensive crisis treatment dosage

| Drug | Dose |
|---|---|
| Labetolol | 1–3 mg/kg/h IV |
| Nitroprusside | 0.5–8 μg/kg/min IV |
| Diazoxide | 2–10 mg/kg/IV bolus |
| Hydralazine | 0.1–0.2 mg/kg/IV |
| Nifedipine | 0.25 mg/kg sublingual |

emphasis on dynamic rather than static exercise, although most children tend to be reasonably active.

*Hypertensive crisis*

Severe symptomatic hypertension should be treated with parenteral antihypertensives with the aim of lowering the blood pressure immediately but slowly. Extreme caution should be observed so as to avoid a precipitous fall in blood pressure, which could lead to cerebral infarction. The drugs of choice are labetolol and nitroprusside, although diazoxide and hydralazine may be used as second-line drugs. If intravenous (IV) access is difficult, sublingual nifedipine has been found to be effective. The dosages are given in Table 14.1.

*Standard antihypertensive treatment*

Most children can be effectively managed with a beta-blocker with or without a vasodilator and/or a diuretic. As most children will have some form of renin-dependent hypertension, angiotensin-converting enzyme (ACE) inhibitors are increasingly being used as first-line treatment. The dosages are given in Table 14.2.

**Table 14.2** Standard antihypertensive treatment dosages

| Drug | Dose (mg/kg/day) |
|---|---|
| Propranolol | 1–6 |
| Atenolol | 1–2 |
| Nifedipine | 0.25–1 |
| Hydralazine | 1–4 |
| Prazosin | 0.05–0.4 |
| Minoxidil | 0.1–1 |
| Chlorthiazide | 10–40 |
| Captopril | 0.5–4 |

*Screening*

The recent working party of the British Hypertension Society [25] did not recommend the routine screening of the paediatric population for blood pressure. Whilst screening may seem prudent in those with a family history, interpretation of results is often difficult. However, it is recommended that the blood pressure is measured in all children presenting to clinicians when ill and in those with diseases known to be associated with hypertension, including any form of renal, urological or cardiovascular disease, meningomyelocoele, diabetes mellitus and neurofibromatosis.

## 14.4 ACUTE RENAL FAILURE

Acute renal failure results from a sudden deterioration in renal function resulting in an accumulation of nitrogenous wastes and associated fluid and electrolyte imbalance. In children a urine output of 300 ml/m$^2$/24 h (or 0.5 ml/kg/h in infants) is required to excrete the daily solute output.

The pathogenesis includes pre-renal causes due to volume depletion, impaired cardiac output or hypoalbuminaemic states. Renal causes include acute glomerulonephritis, acute interstitial nephritis and acute vascular causes such as renal vein thrombosis, vasculitis and haemolytic uraemic syndrome. Post-renal causes are mainly congenital, the major causes of which would be posterior urethral valves and bilateral hydronephrosis due to either pelvi-ureteric junction obstruction or vesicoureteric junction obstruction. Obstruction due to nephrolithiasis may present at any age.

The presentation will depend on the cause, although important features in the history will include the presence of any known underlying illness, diarrhoea and vomiting, poor urinary stream and exposure to drugs.

### 14.4.1 Treatment and prevention

*Fluids and circulation*

Volume depletion with a low blood pressure, low central venous pressure and a wide peripheral core temperature gap requires resuscitation with either volume expanders, e.g. isotonic saline or plasma 20 ml/kg. If the low blood pressure persists despite adequate volume, an inotrope may be indicated. Dopamine 2 μg/kg/min improves renal perfusion but doses of 5–10 μg/kg/min may be required to elevate systemic blood pressure. If poor peripheral perfusion remains, i.e. a wide peripheral core temperature gap, despite an adequate circulating volume and perfusion pressure, a vasodilator such as hydralazine (0.2 mg/kg) may reverse the peripheral vasoconstriction.

Volume overload with hypertension, raised central venous pressure and oedema may be treated with a diuretic such as frusemide, 1–5 mg/kg intravenously. If there is no response, dialysis is indicated. Maintenance fluids should be calculated as insensible losses together with continuing losses. Insensible losses may be calculated as 300 ml/m$^2$/24 h with increases of 13% per °C rise in temperature.

### *Electrolyte disturbances*

#### *Hyperkalaemia*

Ten per cent calcium gluconate 0.5 ml/kg over 5–10 min antagonizes the effect of hyperkalaemia on cells and is useful for the prevention or treatment of cardiac dysrhythmias.

Sodium bicarbonate (8.5%, 1–2 mmol/kg) may lower serum potassium, particularly in the presence of acidosis.

0.5 g/kg/h glucose with insulin 0.1 U/kg/h intravenously acts rapidly (within one hour) to lower serum potassium.

Salbutamol intravenously (4 $\mu$g/kg in 10 ml water over 10 min) or by nebulizer (2.5 mg $<$ 25 kg body weight or 5 mg $>$ 25 kg body weight) has recently tended to become first-line treatment.

Calcium resonium 1 g/kg/day in divided doses, orally or rectally, acts more slowly.

#### *Hyponatraemia*

Hyponatraemia may be associated with neurological disturbances and convulsions particularly with values less than 120 mmol/l. This is often due to fluid overload and therefore treatment should be aimed at fluid removal. However excess losses, particularly gastrointestinal, are associated with true sodium deficits which should be replaced. Sodium deficit may be calculated as follows:

$$\text{Deficit in mmol} = (140 - \text{serum sodium}) \times 0.6 \times \text{body weight in kg.}$$

Half the deficit should be replaced in the first 24 hours and the situation reviewed.

#### *Hypocalcaemia*

Symptomatic patients may be given a bolus of 10% calcium gluconate 0.5 ml/kg intravenously over 5–10 min. Slower correction may be achieved by an infusion of 10% calcium gluconate, 0.1 mmol calcium/kg body weight/h. The dose should be adjusted by frequent blood monitoring at least six hourly.

*Hypomagnesaemia*

Magnesium sulphate (50%, 0.1 ml/kg) intramuscularly is usually effective.

*Acidosis*

Sodium bicarbonate (2 mmol/kg) is given intravenously as immediate treatment. The total deficit may be calculated as follows:

$$(24 - \text{the actual bicarbonate}) \times 0.6 \times \text{body weight in kg}$$

Half this amount may be given as an infusion over 4–6 hours, and the acid–base status rechecked. Sodium bicarbonate needs to be given with caution particularly in neonates and infants as it may cause sodium, and thus fluid, overload.

*Convulsions*

Convulsions may be due to electrolyte disturbances, uraemia, hypertension, or the underlying disease. Many anticonvulsants tend to accumulate in renal failure. The safest emergency treatment is diazepam 0.25 mg/kg intravenously.

*Diet*

Adequate nutrition is essential to compensate for catabolism and the child should receive at least the estimated average requirement (EAR) for energy for chronological age. Calories are best provided as a combination of fat and carbohydrate often using glucose polymers and fat emulsions. The protein, phosphate and electrolyte content of complete feeds often need to be analysed carefully as many are unsuitable for use in renal failure.

### 14.4.2 Dialysis

Indications for dialysis include uncontrollable fluid overload/hypertension, uncontrollable acidosis, symptomatic electrolyte disturbances not controlled by the above measures, symptomatic uraemia, presence of a dialysable toxin, or anuria even if the above are not present. Obstruction must always be considered and excluded. Peritoneal dialysis is the preferred option, except in those in whom it is contraindicated, e.g. following abdominal surgery, although it is often possible to institute this treatment in uncomplicated abdominal surgery within 24 to 48 hours. There are a variety of peritoneal catheters available for dialysis.

Trocar catheters were first developed in the 1960s, and were the first type of catheter to be used in children. They are still used today, although they tend to have been replaced by more recently developed models. They consist of a rigid polyethylene catheter which has a fixed distal curve with side holes. The metal introducer is placed inside the catheter and both are introduced together percutaneously directly through the anterior abdominal wall. In neonates a standard neonatal chest drain may be used. The major disadvantages of this type of catheter are risk of intra-abdominal trauma and leakage.

The use of a Seldinger technique to insert peritoneal dialysis catheters was first described in 1984 [26] and is safer than the trocar technique. Problems encountered with this type of dialysis are poor drainage and catheter blockage. Catheters therefore frequently need to be changed. This is relatively easy using the Seldinger technique, reinserting a new catheter in the same site as the previous one.

Tenckhoff catheters made of flexible silicone rubber were first introduced for chronic dialysis, but recently they have been used for acute dialysis and the results compared with the trocar catheter [27]. A technique has been described for inserting the Tenckhoff catheter percutaneously through a hollow plastic sheath using a Seldinger technique [28]. There would appear to be fewer complications with this technique when performed by an experienced operator.

To initiate dialysis the patient should be sedated and the chosen catheter inserted under local anaesthetic using strict aseptic technique. The abdomen should be filled with normal saline or dialysate fluid until it feels firm (20–50 ml/kg), although this may not be necessary if the child has ascites) using a small intravenous cannula; this both aids the insertion of the cannula and helps prevent perforation of an intra-abdominal viscus. If using a Seldinger technique it is important to use a cannula of sufficient diameter to enable the guide wire to be threaded through it.

Standard commercially available dialysis solutions are used with potassium added according to the serum potassium. A standard regimen would be 25–30 ml/kg/cycle hourly with 10 min fill, 30 min dwell and 20 min drainage. Smaller cycle volumes may be needed in patients with respiratory or cardiac compromise. Glucose strength is chosen according to the ultrafiltration required. It is customary to start with the lower tonicity solutions with dialysate glucose of 1.5 g/100 ml, which should give ultrafiltration rates of approximately 10% of the dialysate volume. If higher ultrafiltration rates are required then higher tonicity solutions should be used.

Haemodialysis requires adequate vascular access which is often difficult in children and is the major limitation of this technique. Access may be achieved by either an arteriovenous shunt or an indwelling venous catheter. The Scribner arteriovenous shunt has been in use since 1960 with commercially available paediatric shunts and vessel tips. In small children the distal vessels are usually too small to allow the placement of the shunt and therefore proximal vessels are more often used. However, the newer intravenous cannulae suitable for dialysis have almost entirely replaced the arteriovenous shunt.

A variety of single and double lumen dialysis cannulae which may be inserted percutaneously using the Seldinger technique are now commercially available. Even small children, under 10 kg, may be dialysed using these cannulae. The choice of dialyser and lines should be governed by the patient's size so that the maximum extracorporeal blood volume does not exceed 10% of the patient's blood volume, calculated as 80 ml/kg. In children <10 kg it is preferable to prime the lines with transfused blood. Blood flow rates will depend on the efficacy of the vascular access. Maximum flow rates may be calculated as follows:

100 ml/min in children <10 kg
100 + 2.5 × body weight in kg in ml/min for children 10–40 kg

Urea clearances should not exceed 3–4 ml/min. Ultrafiltration should be carefully and continuously monitored and should not exceed 5% of the patient's body weight. In acute renal failure short daily dialyses are often better tolerated than longer dialysis procedures. In sick, acidotic children bicarbonate dialysis is preferred.

### *Haemofiltration*

Due to the technical advances which have led to the production of haemofilters suitable for use in children, continuous (arteriovenous or venovenous) haemofiltration, a convection based extracorporeal treatment, has become an effective and often preferred form of renal replacement therapy in acute renal failure in children, including neonates [29]. It is most suitable when peritoneal dialysis cannot be performed and when the circulation is too unstable to tolerate conventional haemodialysis. It has the advantage of being a continuous procedure which results in minimum haemodynamic disturbance, yielding excellent ultrafiltration rates and requiring only small extracorporeal volumes. The disadvantage is the need for continuous anticoagulation.

Arterial and venous access is required using standard intravascular catheters. A minimum of a 20 g arterial line is required together with the largest intravenous catheter that it is technically possible to insert (at least as big as arterial line.) In practice a central venous line is often preferred. The choice of filter is often governed by the priming volumes, with the small filters suitable for use in neonates having priming volumes of 2–6 ml.

Blood from the arterial line is driven by the patient's own cardiac output through the haemofilter and returned to the patient through the venous line. Ultrafiltrate forming across the membrane is collected into its own drainage chamber. Heparin is administered by a continuous infusion into a connector on the arterial side of the haemofilter. Suitable anticoagulation is provided by a bolus dose of heparin 5–10 U/kg/h followed by a continuous infusion of heparin 4 U/kg/h with prostacyclin 6 ng/kg/min aiming for whole blood clotting times of 30 min. Commercially available electrolyte solutions replace electrolytes lost in the ultrafiltrate. These can be combined with hyperalimentation fluids to provide nutrition.

If arterial access is difficult, a modified technique of continuous venous haemofiltration can be used. Venous access is most easily provided by the standard double lumen catheters used for haemodialysis. A blood pump as used in haemodialysis is required in the exit venous line, and therefore this technique requires more careful monitoring and training of staff.

A further modification of both of these techniques is continuous haemodiafiltration. The extracorporeal circuit is similar to that used in standard haemofiltration with the addition of dialysate infused countercurrent to the blood flow. At dialysis flow rates of 15 ml/kg/h there may be a two-fold increase in urea clearance. This technique has been used to treat both acute renal failure and electrolyte disturbances such as hypernatraemia [30].

#### *Drugs*

The altered physiology of renal failure affects the metabolism of most pharmacological agents and therefore modification of drug dosages becomes necessary with renal failure. Since peritoneal and haemodialysis also alter drug clearance, prescribing in renal failure should be undertaken with great care and always with reference to data on the influence of renal failure and dialysis on the drug's metabolism [31].

## 14.5 HAEMOLYTIC URAEMIC SYNDROME

The haemolytic uraemic syndromes (HUS) comprise a heterogeneous group of disorders in which microangiopathic haemolytic anaemia, thrombocytopenia and acute renal failure occur together (including an overlap with thrombotic thrombocytopenic purpura in adults). They are a major cause of acute renal failure in childhood responsible for around 150 to 200 cases per annum in the UK and can be classified into two categories, the epidemic and sporadic forms.

The epidemic form occurs most commonly in the summer months, affects younger children and is associated with a prodromal illness usually of bloody diarrhoea. The majority of these cases are associated with infections, the commonest aetiologic agent being the verocytotoxin producing *E. coli*. A variety of other bacteria, viruses and rickettsia have also been described in association with the syndrome. Shigella infection is an important cause in the developing world. The prognosis in this group is excellent and 85% can be expected to make a full recovery.

The sporadic form is much rarer and accounts for only 5% of the total number of cases. There is no seasonal incidence nor a prodromal illness. This group includes those rare relapsing and familial cases. Seventy per cent of this group progress to chronic renal failure.

### 14.5.1 Pathogenesis

A wide variety of pathogenetic mechanisms have been postulated. These are described below.

*Cytotoxins*

The association of a verocytotoxin producing *E. coli* with the epidemic form of HUS was first described in 1983. Up to 75% of these *E. coli* are of serotype 0157:H7. Screening for this organism is most often performed using the non-fermentation of sorbitol. However, the wider availability of gene probes for the rapid identification of verocytotoxin producing organisms, augmented by the development of serological techniques, may increase the identification rate.

Two toxins have been identified and, because of their similarity to the toxin produced by *Shigella dysenteriae*, are often called shiga-like toxins 1 and 2. The toxins consist of a biologically active subunit A linked to B subunits, which bind specific receptors. Once attached to the cell surface, subunit A enters the cell and inhibits protein synthesis by inactivating 60s ribosomal subunits, leading to cell death.

Glomerular endothelium is the main site of injury in HUS, and verocytotoxin has been shown to be cytopathic to cultured endothelial cells. Other observations have suggested that neutrophils may also have an important role in the pathogenesis. A high neutrophil count, $>20 \times 10^9$, is associated with an adverse prognosis [32]. Neutrophils from patients with HUS have also been shown to have increased adhesion to endothelium and are able to induce endothelial injury *in vitro*. It is postulated that these activated neutrophils degranulate onto endothelium, causing damage by local release of proteases such as elastase, which has been found to be elevated in patients with HUS.

*von Willebrand factor multimers*

Verocytotoxin also causes the release of von Willebrand factor (factor VIII-related antigen) which mediates platelet adhesion to subendothelium and promotes the formation of platelet thrombi. Raised factor VIII-related antigens, together with an abnormal multimer pattern, have been described in HUS [33]. These abnormalities return to normal on recovery but have been shown to persist in patients with recurrent episodes or in patients with progressive disease.

*Prostacyclin*

Prostacyclin is produced by normal endothelial cells and is a powerful inhibitor of platelet aggregation. Its precise role in the pathogenesis of HUS remains controversial. Endothelial cells in patients with HUS may be incapable of producing prostacyclin. Plasma from some patients with HUS has reduced capacity to support prostacyclin production by normal endothelial tissue [34]. That this may be corrected by plasma infusions led to the hypothesis of a prostacyclin deficiency, but the fact that other patients responded only to plasma exchange led to the alternative hypothesis of the presence of a prostacyclin inhibitor in the plasma of patients with HUS. An inhibitor has been identified in some patients and preliminary characterization suggests it may be an abnormal lipid peroxidase. Excessively rapid degradation of prostacyclin has also been noted in some patients. All these data have been obtained from a variety of patients with both epidemic and sporadic cases of HUS together with some patients with thrombotic thrombocytopenic purpura (TTP). However it is most often those patients with the non-epidemic forms of the disease in whom these abnormalities are demonstrable.

*Neuraminidase*

Neuraminidase is an enzyme produced by a number of microorganisms, although in many it is cell-bound and not released. It removes sialic acid from erythrocytes, platelets and glomeruli exposing the hidden Thomsen–Friedenreich antigen (T-cryptantigen). Anti-T, an IgM antibody present in most adult plasma, can then react with this exposed antigen leading to all the clinical manifestations of HUS. This phenomenon has been described in association with influenza, parainfluenza, *Clostridium perfringens*, *Bacteroides fragilis* and most commonly *Streptococcus pneumoniae* infections [35].

### 14.5.2 Prevention and treatment

Many children with haemolytic uraemic syndrome can be successfully managed with supportive therapy and careful attention to fluid balance without the need for dialysis. A prospective study of HUS showed that 57% of children received dialysis [36]. However, it is essential to establish the diagnosis as soon as possible because much morbidity can be induced by inappropriate rehydration in patients with compromised renal function. Therefore, the diagnosis should be suspected in any child with acute bloody diarrhoea, and biochemistry, haematology and fluid balance should be monitored appropriately. Children with deteriorating renal function, oligoanuria or poor prognostic features should be referred early to a paediatric nephrology centre. Poor prognostic features would include older children without a diarrhoeal prodrome, evidence of non-renal involvement including encephalopathy or cardiomyopathy, or those children with a high neutrophil count of $>20 \times 10^9/l$. Treatments other than careful supportive therapy together with dialysis should be reserved for those children with the more severe disease who would be predicted to have a poorer outcome. A wide variety of treatments have been used in HUS but none have been shown to have unequivocal benefit. These have included anticoagulants, antiplatelet agents and fibrinolytic activators. Current attention has focused on the following modalities.

### *Plasma*

The findings that prostacyclin production is reduced in some patients with HUS and that in others a platelet-aggregating factor inhibited by normal plasma is present, have led to the theory that plasma infusions may ameliorate the clinical course of HUS. In a randomized trial in 32 children with HUS Rizzoni [37] failed to demonstrate a significant benefit of plasma infusion. However, a French multicentre prospective trial in 79 patients [38] using a similar regimen of 10 ml/kg/day for seven days concluded that plasma infusions were beneficial as determined by a decreased incidence of cortical necrosis, lower creatinine at three months and lower incidence of proteinuria at six months in the treated group compared to controls. Both of these trials are disadvantaged by the inclusion of children with epidemic HUS (who could be expected to have a good prognosis) as well as those with sporadic HUS (who would be expected to have a poorer prognosis). The benefits of plasma need to be weighed against the disadvantages. Such disadvantages would include the risk of volume overload, the transmission of blood-borne viral diseases and the worsening haemolysis that may be seen in those patients with neuraminidase-associated HUS.

### *Plasma exchange*

In TTP, plasma exchange has been shown to be of benefit in both the acute illness and in patients with recurrent episodes. There is insufficient data on children with HUS. There are theoretical reasons why it may be beneficial and its use may be justified in the child with a deteriorating course, particularly with neurological involvement.

*Prostacyclin*

The observed abnormalities of prostacyclin metabolism seen in some patients with HUS have also led to the use of prostacyclin infusions. Early results were conflicting [39], but a recent pilot study aimed at patients with epidemic HUS and a high neutrophil count at presentation demonstrated an encouraging improvement in outcome [40].

### 14.5.3 Long-term outcome

The acute mortality of HUS is around 5%. The long-term consequences are less well documented and although the majority of survivors recover completely, a small proportion do develop a secondary decline in renal function. Evidence of hypertension or impaired glomerular filtration rate may be seen in 11 to 25%. A positive correlation between microalbuminuria and systolic blood pressure and a negative correlation between microalbuminuria and glomerular filtration rate [41] suggests that children with albuminuria should receive longer and closer follow up to identify occult nephropathy. A normal protein/creatinine ratio at one year appears to be a reliable discriminator between those with a favourable outcome and those with a poor outcome [42]. However, the full implications of the long-term sequelae of HUS are not yet clear. It has been demonstrated that patients who had apparently made a complete recovery presented abnormalities in their renal functional reserve, similar to those seen in children with a single kidney. Furthermore, the patients with HUS showed an increase in microalbuminuria after a protein load, which may imply a poorer long-term prognosis [43].

## 14.6 CHRONIC RENAL FAILURE

The precise incidence of severe chronic renal failure in childhood is not known. The European Dialysis Transplant Association (EDTA) register of children under 15 years of age accepted for renal replacement therapy suggests an incidence of between four and eight children per million child population per annum. [44].

The number of patients receiving treatment is increasing as the treatment criteria broaden and, in particular, younger children are now accepted for renal replacement therapy. The proportion of treated children below the age of six years has risen from 14 to 21% over the past decade, with a third of these being under the age of two years at the start of treatment [45].

The incidence of chronic renal failure is uncertain. Swedish data [46] noted a prevalence of preterminal renal failure (defined as glomerular filtration rate (GFR) of $<30\,ml/min/1.73\,m^2$) of 26.1 per million child population in 1985, having risen from 14.1 in 1978. These data excluded children under the age of six months.

A similar epidemiological study in France [47] found a prevalence of 34–43 per million children between 1975 and 1990. A UK study [48] also suggested a prevalence of at least 53 per million children but as all studies use different definitions of chronic renal failure direct comparisons are difficult.

The primary renal diseases also vary between countries although the main groups include malformations (30–50% including dysplasia, reflux and obstruction), hereditary disorders (16–20%), glomerulopathies (14–33%) and renal vascular diseases (5–10%).

### 14.6.1 Antenatal diagnosis

The increasing use of routine antenatal ultrasound has resulted in many congenital abnormalities of the urinary tract being detected *in utero*. The frequency of abnormalities is approximately one to two per thousand live births. This variability is related to the timing of the ultrasound and the selection of the obstetric population scanned. The lesions detected and their frequency are as follows [49]:

| | |
|---|---|
| pelviureteric junction obstruction | 31% |
| multicystic dysplastic kidney | 22% |
| vesicoureteric reflux | 13% |
| vesicoureteric junction obstruction | 11% |
| posterior urethral valves | 8% |
| megacystis megaureter | 4% |
| other | 5% |
| transient hydronephrosis | 6% |

These abnormalities and disorders, which may lead to chronic renal failure, can be detected and treated before there is significant functional decline or symptoms.

### 14.6.2 Clinical features

*Growth*

Growth failure is a major problem for children with chronic renal failure. The severity of the growth failure is related to the age at presentation, with 50% of children with renal failure during infancy having growth failure (>2 standard deviations below the mean height for age) in contrast to 10% of those with acquired disease after infancy [50]. Important factors contributing to the growth failure include uraemia, acidosis, salt depletion, renal osteodystrophy and energy malnutrition. Determination of renal function should be a routine investigation in a child presenting with unexplained growth failure.

### *Renal osteodystrophy*

The severity of the bone disease is related to age at onset, the nature of the underlying renal disease, and the severity and duration of renal dysfunction. It is more common with congenital and obstructive uropathies and rarely manifests clinically with a GFR above 20 ml/min/ $1.73\,m^2$.

### *Anaemia*

Anaemia secondary to a lack of erythropoietin is also a well-recognized complication of renal failure and may be the presenting feature.

### *Hypertension*

Renin-dependent hypertension is the most common form of hypertension in childhood and may be associated with renal failure. The presentation of renal failure may be with the symptoms of hypertension.

### *Neurological development*

Eighty per cent of postnatal brain growth takes place in the first year of life. Insult or injury at this critical phase of development may lead to irreversible damage. Early reports of the treatment of infants with chronic renal failure indicated a high incidence of developmental delay in children with chronic renal failure since infancy. The major contributing factors were thought to include the biochemical abnormalities associated with chronic renal failure, in particular hyperparathyroidism, malnutrition, aluminium neurotoxicity from the use of aluminium-containing phosphate binders and psychosocial factors including prolonged hospitalization. More recent studies from the same institutions as the previous reports [51, 52] have demonstrated a greatly improved developmental outcome with changes in clinical management. These have included early, aggressive treatment of chronic renal failure including nasogastric feeding, early dialysis, the avoidance of aluminium-containing phosphate binders, more meticulous outpatient management and psychosocial support. Furthermore, there are suggestions that successful renal transplantation accelerates development in young children with chronic renal failure [52].

### 14.6.3 Prevention

*Antenatal diagnosis*

The detection of a severe abnormality early in gestation may lead to termination of pregnancy or intrauterine intervention. The role of intrauterine intervention is not yet established. A study of 53 cases failed to demonstrate any definite improvement [53]. If the indication for intrauterine intervention is the preservation of renal function, then it is important to be able to assess antenatal renal function accurately. Although not uniformly accepted, prognostic indicators include urine volume and urinary electrolytes. Intrauterine intervention may also prevent oligohydramnios and subsequent pulmonary hypoplasia. In a study of 17 fetuses, 53% had amniotic fluid restored and no neonate with restored amniotic fluid had pulmonary hypoplasia [54].

Ultrasonographic findings may also identify conditions that may not be detected postnatally on clinical examination. Eighty-three per cent of live-born neonates with a prenatal diagnosis of urinary tract abnormalities had no physical findings on clinical examination with potentially treatable conditions involving a solitary kidney or both kidneys in 17% [55]. Early detection of these abnormalities together with appropriate surgical intervention or infection prophylaxis with antibiotics may alter the natural history of conditions that lead to renal failure. Further results from controlled long-term studies will be required.

*Dietary manipulation*

Over the last decade considerable attention has focused on dietary modifications to retard the progression of chronic renal failure. Of particular interest has been the role of restriction of dietary phosphate and protein. A meta-analysis of six controlled randomized trials [56] strongly supported the effectiveness of low-protein diets in delaying the onset of end stage renal disease. However none of these trials included children, and both the efficacy and safety of severe protein restriction in growing children require evaluation.

General recommendations for children with chronic renal failure suggest that children should have at least the estimated average requirement (EAR) for chronological age for calories although many will need additional calories to promote growth. Protein intake should be the reference nutrient intake (RNI) for protein for height and age. It is recommended that 50% of protein should be of high biological value and 8% of the calories should be derived from protein [57]. This is considerably lower than the diets of most children in the UK in which protein provides 15% of dietary energy. With energy supplementation of fat and carbohydrate, lower percentages of calories provided by protein are acceptable. Recommended intakes are:

- Infants: 1.5–2 g protein/kg/day<br>130–150 kcal/kg/day
- children between one and seven years: 1–1.5 g protein/kg/day<br>100–130 kcal/kg/day

Individual dietary and biochemical assessment will determine requirements as well as the stage of management. However, the following principles may act as guidelines. Many children, particularly infants, will not ingest this spontaneously and may require enteral feeding, either nasogastrically or via a gastrostomy. Phosphorus restriction naturally follows protein restriction although phosphate binders may still be required, particularly in more advanced chronic renal failure.

An important problem in the evaluation of protein restriction trials is the outcome measured, and in particular the use of creatinine as a measurement of GFR. Creatinine levels are related to muscle mass, which may be affected by protein restriction. Accepting these limitations, one study of ten children, using a diet of 1–1.2 g protein/kg/day together with amino acid supplementation, showed a rate of deterioration of renal function less than would have been expected on their previous diet of 2 g/kg/day. Moreover, height and weight velocities increased on the reduced protein regimen [58]. However, a one-year analysis of a multicentre randomized European trial on 105 patients using 1.1–0.8 g protein/kg/day according to age failed to show any change in glomerular filtration rate or height and weight velocity [59]. A three-year analysis of another prospective randomised trial of 56 children showed similar results [60]. Compliance with dietary manipulations in childhood is often poor and in the European study only 76% of children adhered to their dietary prescription. Further studies are needed before such treatments are recommended for widespread clinical use in children.

### 14.6.4 Management

The treatment of some complications of renal failure may in turn prevent further functional decline. Of particular importance is the treatment of hypertension, urinary tract infection and poorly functioning bladders with self-intermittent catheterization or cystoplasty to decrease intravesical pressure.

*Fluid and electrolyte therapy*

Many children with congenital renal diseases, in particular dysplasia, obstructive uropathy and nephronopthisis, have poor renal concentrating capacity with polyuria and salt loss. Since salt deficiency is an important cause of poor growth in these infants, salt supplementation is often necessary. Children with acquired diseases, in particular focal glomerulosclerosis and other forms of glomerulonephritis, may have salt and water retention and require salt restriction.

### *Renal osteodystrophy*

The pathogenesis of renal osteodystrophy (ROD) is due to a combination of factors, including phosphate retention, skeletal resistance to parathyroid hormone, the impairment of renal production of 1,25-dihydroxycholecalciferol and intestinal malabsorption of calcium leading to hypocalcaemia and secondary hyperparathyroidism.

Although ROD is rarely seen with GFR above $20\,\mathrm{ml/min/1.73\,m^2}$ introduction of vitamin D replacement at this level of GFR is recommended. The usual treatment would be with 1,25-dihydroxycholecalciferol (or alphacalcidol) at a starting dose of 10 ng/kg/day. This dose can be increased according to clinical and biochemical parameters up to dosages of 50 ng/kg/day.

Hyperphosphataemia, which usually occurs when the GFR falls to $20–30\,\mathrm{ml/min/1.73\,m^2}$, also plays an important role in the development and maintenance of secondary hyperparathyroidism. Initially dietary phosphate restriction may be sufficient to control hyperphosphataemia, although this can be difficult in young infants on a predominantly milk diet. With further loss of renal function phosphate binders become necessary and calcium carbonate is the binder of choice. Aluminium is best avoided in children because of concern regarding neurotoxic effects particularly on developmental progress.

### *Erythropoietin*

The production of human erythropoietin (EPO) by recombinant DNA techniques has made possible the treatment of the anaemia of chronic renal failure and significantly improves the quality of life for many patients. The use of EPO given intravenously [61] or subcutaneously [62] has been shown to be effective in raising the haematocrit of children with end stage renal failure. There are also trials of the use of EPO in predialysis patients [63] although these trials have not included children. Again, the efficacy is well demonstrated although there are concerns regarding safety. EPO may elevate blood pressure in both dialysis and predialysis patients. In animal models the administration of EPO may increase blood viscosity causing glomerular hypertension hyperfiltration with acceleration of functional renal decline. It is not known if this effect is independent or consequent upon changes in blood pressure. Further trials in children with preterminal renal failure are required to answer these questions.

*Growth hormone*

Short stature is a serious problem for children with chronic renal failure. Endogenous growth hormone (GH) secretion is normal as are serum levels of insulin-like growth factors I and II. However, exogenous GH has been shown to increase the height velocity in a number of conditions in which GH secretion is not impaired. GH increases the short-term growth velocity of prepubertal children with chronic renal failure. The effect on final height is not known and there is conflicting evidence from the trials of the effect of GH on bone age [64, 65]. This treatment is not without potential side effects. Of most concern is the possibility that GH may accelerate renal functional decline by increasing renal plasma flow and glomerular hyperfiltration. In view of this possibility, its use should be restricted to children who are below the third centile for height and in whom all other abnormalities such as hypertension, electrolyte and acid–base balance, renal osteodystrophy and nutritional deficiencies have been corrected.

### 14.6.5 Dialysis

Although renal replacement therapy is outside the scope of this chapter, a short discussion is included. There has been a dramatic growth in continuous ambulatory peritoneal dialysis (CAPD) over the last decade as the maintenance renal replacement therapy for children awaiting transplantation. First introduced in Canada in 1978, by 1989 68% of Canadian children with end stage renal failure were being treated by some form of peritoneal dialysis [66].

The contribution of CAPD towards the treatment of end stage renal failure in Europe is substantially less than in Canada but is increasing. It was used as the initial renal replacement therapy in only 8.5% of children reported to the EDTA registry in 1980 but by 1986 this had risen to 23.6% [67]. The UK has consistently treated more children with CAPD than other European countries and by 1992 74% of them were on some form of peritoneal dialysis [48]. Over this time there has also been a growth in the use of continuous cycling peritoneal dialysis (CCPD) and in Canada in 1989 57% of patients on peritoneal dialysis were on CCPD. Similar trends are being seen in the UK.

Peritoneal dialysis is the treatment of choice for infants and young children, although in older children the choice between peritoneal dialysis and haemodialysis will depend on patient preference, and geographical and practical considerations. CCPD produces better clearances and ultrafiltration than CAPD and is particularly suited to the needs of small infants in whom rapid peritoneal glucose absorption from the peritoneum favours shorter cycles and in whom dialysis often needs to be combined with enteral tube feeding. The increasing availability of automated cyclers capable of delivering exchange volumes as small as 50 to 100 ml has further facilitated this development. CCPD is also particularly useful in the anephric or oliguric patient in whom fluid balance control on CAPD may be difficult.

The major disadvantage is peritonitis and although CCPD involves fewer disconnections, its effect on peritonitis rates is variable. Some authors have noted no difference in peritonitis rates between CAPD and CCPD, although in one study of 83 patients peritonitis rates were found to be one episode per 12.9 months on CCPD compared to one per 8.1 months on CAPD [68]. The most common reason for discontinuation of peritoneal dialysis is transplantation, although peritonitis is the most common technical reason for failure, accounting for 50% of technical failures. Growth rates in children on peritoneal dialysis, even with early attention to diet, electrolyte disturbance and prevention of renal osteodystrophy, are below normal but are better than those on haemodialysis. Psychological rehabilitation and school attendance are also better on peritoneal dialysis in comparison to haemodialysis.

The major disadvantage of haemodialysis is the need to create vascular access. Arteriovenous fistulae may be technically difficult to create in small children and repeated needling can be distressing particularly to the younger child. An alternative technique is the insertion of an in-dwelling catheter, usually into a subclavian vein. With technological improvements in such catheters in many units this is the method of choice particularly for short and medium-term haemodialysis. The principles of haemodialysis are similar in adults and children; however due to the technical challenges presented by the smaller intravascular volumes of children, the potential haemodynamic instability, and the psychological issues, it is recommended that children be treated in units with paediatric expertise.

### 14.6.6 Transplantation

Renal transplantation is the best mode of renal replacement therapy for children and adolescents. At all ages paediatric renal transplant recipients have better survival than do dialysis patients of the same age. Moreover, successful transplantation confers a degree of physiological and psychological rehabilitation not seen with any form of dialysis.

Graft success rates reported from the North American Paediatric Renal Transplant Cooperative Study (NAPRTCS) were 89% at one year and 80% at three years for live donor grafts and 74% and 62%, respectively, for cadaver grafts [69]. Forty-three percent of these allografts were from live donors, 37% from a parent. Similar results for graft survival were reported to the EDTA [70], although a smaller proportion of children received live donor grafts. Overall, 20% of children received live donor grafts, although in Belgium the figure was similar to that seen in the USA, and in Sweden and Norway the rate was as high as 71%. More recent results from centres in the UK suggest 80% graft success at one year for cadaver grafts. Pre-emptive transplant was performed in 22% of children in the North American study compared to 11% in the EDTA report.

Analysis of the risk factors in paediatric transplantation from the American study based on a proportional hazards model has identified the following:

1. age of donor less than six years;
2. cold ischaemic time more than 24 hours;
3. age of recipient less than two years;
4. no known antilymphocyte preparation, e.g. ATG, ALG, OKT3;
5. previous transplantation;
6. no known HLA-DR matches.

There has been recent concern about the poor graft survival of organs from young donors. In a Canadian study [71] it was noted that the youngest recipients experienced better graft survival when they were matched with older donors. However, as recipient age increased donor age became progressively less important. The NAPRTCS also noted that kidneys from young donors were at increased risk of graft loss [72]. The ideal donor age was found to be 20–25 years with the probability of graft function at one year from donors of 0–5 years, 5–10 years and 10–15 years being 55, 67 and 79% respectively [73]. Cold storage time was found to have an added impact on graft survival with those grafts with cold storage times greater than 24 hours being one and a half times more likely to fail than grafts with shorter cold storage times for all donor ages.

The effect of recipient age is seen in the EDTA registry data [69] which reports graft survival rates of 65% at one year for children 0–5 years, 78% for 5–10 years and 76% for 10–15 years. These figures are similar to those found in the NAPRTCS. However, there is a tendency to use young donors in young recipients and when the data are statified for the donor age, the recipient age does not seem to influence graft outcome significantly. More encouraging results in the transplantation of young children have been reported by groups using live donor transplantation, with graft survival rates of 85–95% at one year in children less than two years of age [74, 75]. Poor graft survival in the young has been attributed to technical problems and graft thrombosis. The Canadian group observed that 44% of recipients under three years of age who received cadaveric grafts from donors less than four years of age lost their grafts as a result of thrombosis, ischaemia and technical problems. In contrast the Los Angeles group using live donors noted no graft losses due to technical failures or graft thromboses in children less than two years.

Overall, immunosuppressive regimens are similar to those used in adults, with increasing use of 'triple therapy' with prednisolone, cyclosporin and azathioprine. Young children metabolize cyclosporin more rapidly than do adolescents or adults and often require higher dosages to achieve satisfactory blood levels. Low-dose steroids allow optimal growth with improved growth rates on an alternate-day regimen. Reports of the use of immunosuppressive agent FK506 or Tacrolimus in children [76] are emerging and although the early results are encouraging, the results of prospective randomized trials comparing FK506 with cyclosporin A are awaited. There is a suggestion that infants may have a heightened immune response, and improved results with cadaveric transplantation have been reported using quadruple immunosuppressive therapy, with the addition of antithymocyte globulin to cyclosporin A, azathioprine and prednisolone, although these data are still preliminary [74, 75].

It has long been recognized that second and subsequent grafts are less successful than first grafts, and that previous transplantation is therefore a risk factor. More recently the importance of HLA matching has also been recognized and in the Collaborative Transplant Study the effect of matching for the HLA-B and HLA-DR was highly statistically significant with a stepwise decrease in graft survival rates noted as the number of HLA mismatches increased – graft survival of 74% at five years with no mismatches compared to 41% with four mismatches [77]. Again, this is highly influenced by donor age as the allocation policy tends to favour small kidneys to small children and this tends to impair HLA matching.

Some of the important long-term problems that may follow successful transplantation in childhood include hypertension, recurrence of the original disease, hyperlipidaemia and non-compliance. In NAPRTCS 72% of children were found to require antihypertensive therapy one month after transplantation although this fell to 53% at 30 months. Disease recurrence is higher than in adults and accounts for 7% of all graft failures; the most common recurrent disease is focal segmental glomerulosclerosis.

Post-transplant hyperlipidaemia is a common problem and in one survey [78] the mean serum cholesterol exceeded the 90th centile for all age groups at all times after transplantation. The long-term significance of this, particularly in association with hypertension on future cardiovascular health, is not established, but likely to be deleterious.

Finally, non-compliance with immunosuppression is a well-recognized problem particularly in adolescence. It is important to recognize those individuals who may be at high risk of such behaviour and intervene with early psychological support.

Delay in transplantation in children has considerable implications for growth. Children on dialysis grow less well than children transplanted and delay in transplantation can lead to a permanent loss of height. Growth rates post-transplantation are dependent on three factors: age at transplantation, steroid dosage and renal function. Accelerated growth rates are seen in children post-transplant up until adolescence (over 13 years) when deceleration in growth occurs. Gains in growth are most marked in children under the age of five years. Therefore, vigorous attempts should be made to transplant children as early as possible and certainly before they reach adolescence. The effect on neurological function is also a strong argument in favour of early transplantation. This issue has been addressed in the USA where the United Network for Organ Sharing has recently established a new method for expediting renal transplantation in children by adding extra points to increase the child's priority on the waiting list. The aim is to reduce the median waiting time to transplantation to six months for children up to five years and for older children, one year. The waiting time to transplantation in Europe, which is increasing annually, in 1988 was less than one year in 33%, 1–3 years in 39% and more than three years in 18%. A survey in the UK [68] in 1992 revealed that 58% were transplanted within one year, and a further 26% within two years; however, the number awaiting a transplant was some 50% more than the number transplanted.

Renal transplantation is a highly successful treatment option for children with end stage renal failure. To achieve the best results it is important to address the many unique differences in paediatric transplantation, many of which are related to the age and developmental stage of the recipient. Although transplantation of the very young remains controversial, with meticulous attention to detail and the avoidance of known risk factors for poor graft outcome, excellent results can be achieved even in this age group.

## REFERENCES

1. Winberg, J., Anderson, H.J. and Bergstrom, T. *et al.* (1974) Epidemiology of symptomatic urinary tract infection in childhood. *Acta Paediat. Scand.*, suppl. 252.
2. Woodward, M.N. and Griffiths, D.M. (1993) Use of dipsticks for routine analysis of urine from children with acute abdominal pain. *Br. Med. J.*, **306**, 1512–3.

3. Jodal, U. and Winberg, J. (1987) Management of children with unobstructed urinary tract infection. *Paediat. Nephrol.*, **1**, 647–56.
4. Working group of the research unit, Royal College of Physicians (1991) Guidelines for the management of acute urinary tract infection in childhood. *J. Roy. Coll. Phys.*, **25**, 36–42.
5. Birmingham Reflux Study Group (1987) Prospective trial of operative versus non operative treatment of severe vesico-ureteric reflux in children: five years observation. *Br. Med. J.*, **295**, 237–41.
6. Dudley, J.A., Fenton, T.H., Haworth, J.M. *et al.* (1997) The spectrum of antenatal hydronephrosis: clinical significance and applications. *Arch. Dis. Childh.*, **76**, F31–34.
7. Livera, L.N., Brookfield, D.S.K., Eggington, J.A. *et al.* (1989) Antenatal ultrasonography to detect fetal renal abnormalities: a prospective screening programme. *Br. Med. J.*, **298**, 1421–3.
8. Ring, E. and Zobel, G. (1988) Urinary infection and malformations of urinary tract in infancy. *Arch. Dis. Childh.*, **63**, 818–20.
9. International Study of Kidney Disease in Childhood (1978) Nephrotic syndrome in children: prediction of histopathology from clinical and laboratory characteristics at the time of diagnosis. *Kidney Int.*, **13**, 159–65.
10. British Association of Paediatric Nephrology and Research Unit, Royal College of Physicians (1994) Consensus statement on management and audit potential for steroid responsive nephrotic syndrome. *Arch. Dis. Childh.*, **70**, 151–7.
11. Imbasciati, E., Gusmano, R., Edefonti, A. *et al.* (1985) Controlled trial of methylprednisolone pulses and low dose oral prednisolone for the minimal change nephrotic syndrome. *Br. Med. J.*, **291**, 1305–8.
12. Choonara, I.A., Heney, D. and Meadow, S.R. (1989) Low dose prednisolone in nephrotic syndrome. *Arch. Dis. Childh.*, **64**, 610–21.
13. Arbeitsgemeinschaft fur Padiatrische Nephrologie (1988) Short versus standard prednisolone therapy for initial treatment of idiopathic nephrotic syndrome in children. *Lancet*, **i**, 380–3.
14. Arbeitsgemeinschaft für Pädiatrische Nephrologie (1970) Alternate day versus intermittent prednisolone in frequently relapsing nephrotic syndrome. *Lancet*, **i**, 401–3.
15. Barratt, T.M., Bercowscy, A., Osofsky, S.G. *et al.* (1973) A comparative trial of 2 weeks and 8 weeks cyclophosphamide in steroid sensitive relapsing nephrotic syndrome. *Arch. Dis. Childh.*, **48**, 286–90.
16. Watson, A.R., Rance, C.P. and Bain, J. (1985) Long term effects of cyclophosphamide on testicular function. *Br. Med. J.*, **291**, 1457–60.
17. International Study of Kidney Disease in Children (1974) Prospective controlled trial of cyclosphosphamide therapy in children with the nephrotic syndrome. *Lancet*, **ii**, 423–7.
18. British Association for Paediatric Nephrology (1991) Levamisole for corticosteroid-dependent nephrotic syndrome in childhood. *Lancet*, **337**, 1555–7.
19. Niaudet, P., Broyer, M. and Habib, R. (1991) Treatment of idiopathic nephrotic syndrome with cyclosporin A in children. *Clin. Nephrol.*, **35**, S31–36.
20. Hulton, S.A., Neuhaus, T.J., Dillon, M.J. and Barrat, T.M. (1994) Long term cyclosporin A treatment of minimal change nephrotic syndrome. *Paediat. Nephrol.*, **8**, 401–3.
21. Ingulli, E., Singh, A., Bagi, N. *et al.* (1995) Aggressive long term cyclosporin therapy in steroid resistant focal segmental glomerulosclerosis. *J. Am. Soc. Nephrol.*, **5**, 1820–5.

22. Report of the Second Task Force on Blood Pressure in Children (1987) *Pediatrics*, **79**, 1–25.
23. Andre, J.L., Deschamps, J.P. and Guegen, R. (1980) La tension artérielle chez l'enfant et l'adolescent. Valeurs rapportées à l'age et à la taille 17067 sujets. *Arch. Fr. Pediat.*, **37**, 477–82.
24. Recommendations for management of hypertension in children and adolescents (1987) *Pediat. Nephrol.*, **1**, 56–8.
25. de Swiet, M., Dillon, M.J., Littler, *et al.* (1989) Measurement of blood pressure in children. Recommendations of a working party of the British Hypertension Society. *Br. Med. J.*, **299**, 497.
26. Nakanashi, T., Yanase, M., Tanaka, Y. *et al.* (1984) New acute peritoneal dialysis technique: guide wire insertion and long term indwelling of peritoneal catheter. *Nephron*, **37**, 128–32.
27. Wong, S.N. and Geary, D.F. (1988) Comparison of temporary and permanent catheters for acute peritoneal dialysis. *Arch. Dis. Childh.*, **63**, 827–31.
28. Lewis, M.A. and Nycyk, J.A. (1992) Practical peritoneal dialysis – the Tenckhoff catheter in acute renal failure. *Pediat. Nephrol.*, **6**, 470–6.
29. Lieberman, K.V. (1987) Continuous arteriovenous haemofiltration in children. *Pediat. Nephrol.*, **1**, 330–8.
30. Moss, G.D., Primavesi, R.J., McGraw, M.E. and Chambers, T.L. (1990) Correction of hypernatraemia with continuous arteriovenous haemodiafiltration. *Arch. Dis. Childh.*, **65**, 628–30.
31. Trompeter, R.S. (1987) A review of drug prescribing in children with end-stage renal failure. *Pediat. Nephrol.*, **1**, 183–94.
32. Walters, M.D.S., Matthei, I.U., Kay, R. *et al.* (1989) The polymorphonuclear leucocyte count in childhood haemolytic uraemic syndrome. *Pediat. Nephrol.*, **3**, 130–4.
33. Rose, P.E., Enayat, S.M., Sunderland, R. *et al.* (1984) Abnormalities of factor VIII related protein multimers in the haemolytic uraemic syndrome. *Arch. Dis. Childh.*, **59**, 1135–40.
34. Remuzzi, G., Marchesi, D., Mecca, G. *et al.* (1978) Haemolytic uraemic syndrome: deficiency of plasma factor(s) regulating prostacyclin activity? *Lancet*, **ii**, 871–2.
35. McGraw, M.E., Lendon, M., Stevens, R. *et al.* (1989) Haemolytic uraemic syndrome and the Thomsen Friedenreich antigen. *Pediat. Nephrol.*, **3**, 135–9.
36. Milford, D.V., Taylor, C.M., Guttridge, B. *et al.* (1990) Haemolytic uraemic syndromes in the British Isles 1985–8: association with verocytotoxin producing *Eschericia coli*. Part 1: clinical and epidemiological aspects. *Arch. Dis. Childh.*, **65**, 716–21.
37. Rizzoni, G., Pavenello, L., Claris Appiani, A. *et al.* (1987) Treatment of children with haemolytic uraemic syndrome with plasma: a multicentre controlled trial. *Pediat. Nephrol.*, **1**, C14.
38. Loirat, C., Sonsino, E., Hinglais, N. *et al.* (1988) Treatment of childhood haemolytic uraemic syndrome with plasma. *Pediat. Nephrol.*, **2**, 279–85.
39. Defreyn, G., Proesmans, W., Machin, S.J. *et al.* (1982) Abnormal prostacyclin metabolism in hemolytic uraemic syndrome: equivocal effects of prostacyclin infusions. *Clin. Nephrol.*, **18**, 43–9.
40. Parida, S.K., Milford, D.V. and Taylor, C.M. (1991) Pilot study of Epoprostenol (PGI2) treatment in diarrhoea associated haemolytic uraemic syndrome. *Pediat. Nephrol.*, **5**, C31.
41. Fitzpatrick, M.M., Shah, V., Trompeter, R.S. *et al.* (1991) Long term outcome of childhood haemolytic uraemic syndrome. *Br. Med. J.*, **303**, 489–92.

42. Milford, D.V., White, R.H.R. and Taylor, C.M. (1991) Prognostic significance of proteinuria one year after onset of diarrhoea-associated hemolytic uremic syndrome. *J. Pediat.*, **118**, 191–4.
43. Perelstein, E.M., Grunfield, B.G., Simsolo, R.B. *et al.* (1991) Renal functional reserve compared in haemolytic uraemic syndrome and single kidney. *Arch. Dis. Childh.*, **65**, 728–31.
44. Broyer, M. (1986) Combined report on regular dialysis and transplantation in Europe XVI 1985. Proceedings of the European Dialysis Transplant Association–European Renal Association.
45. Rizzoni, G. (1989) Combined report on regular dialysis and transplantation in Europe XVI 1988. Proceedings of the European Dialysis Transplant Association–European Renal Association.
46. Esbjorner, E., Aronson, S., Berg, U. *et al.* (1990) Children with chronic renal failure in Sweden 1978–1985. *Pediat. Nephrol.*, **4**, 249–52.
47. Delau, J., Andre, J.-L., Briancon, S. and Musse, J.P. (1994) Chronic renal failure in children and epidemiological survey in Lorraine (France) 1975–1990. *Paediat. Nephrol.*, **8**, 472–6.
48. Report of a Working Party of the British Association of Paediatric Nephrology (1995) The provision of services in the United Kingdom for children and adolescents with renal disease.
49. Watson, A.R. (1992) The management of antenatally detected urinary tract abnormalities. *Current Medical Literature Paediatrics*, **1**, 3–5.
50. Betts, P.R. and McGrath, G. (1974) Growth pattern and dietary intake of children with chronic renal failure. *Br. Med. J.*, **1**, 189–93.
51. Geary, D.F. and Haka-Ikse, K. (1989) Neurodevelopmental progress of young children with chronic renal disease. *Pediatrics*, **84**, 68–72.
52. Davis, I.D., Chang, P.N. and Nevins, T.E. (1990) Successful renal transplantation accelerates development in young uraemic children. *Pediatrics*, **86**, 594–600.
53. Elder, J.S., Duckett, J.W. and Snyder, H.M. (1987) Intervention for fetal obstructive uropathy: has it been effective? *Lancet*, **i**, 1007–10.
54. Crombleholme, T.M., Harrison, M.R., Golbus, M.S. *et al.* (1990) Fetal intervention in obstructive uropathy: prognostic indicators and efficacy of intervention. *Am. J. Obstet. Gynecol.*, **162**, 1239–44.
55. Thomas, D.F.M. and Gordon, A.C. (1989) Management of prenatally diagnosed uropathies. *Arch. Dis. Childh.*, **64**, 58–63.
56. Fouque, D., Laville, M., Boissel, J.P. *et al.* (1992) Controlled low protein diets in chronic renal insufficiency: meta-analysis. *Br. Med. J.*, **304**, 216–20.
57. Hellerstein, S., Holliday, M.A., Grupe, W.E. *et al.* (1987) Nutritional management of children with chronic renal failure. *Pediat. Nephrol.*, **1**, 195–211.
58. Jureidini, K.F., Hogg, R.J., van Renen, M.J. *et al.* (1990) Evaluation of long term aggressive dietary management of chronic renal failure in children. *Pediat. Nephrol.*, **4**, 1–10.
59. Wingen, A.M., Fabian-Bach, C. and Mehls, O. (1991) Low protein diets in children with chronic renal failure. *Pediat. Nephrol.*, **5**, 496–500.
60. Kist-van Holthe tot Echten, J.E., Nauta, J., Hop, W.C.J. *et al.* (1993) Protein restriction in chronic renal failure. *Arch. Dis. Childh.*, **68**, 371–5.
61. Offner, G., Hoyer, P.F., Latta, K. *et al.* (1990) One year's experience with recombinant erythropoietin in children undergoing continuous ambulatory or cycling peritoneal dialysis. *Pediat. Nephrol.*, **4**, 498–500.

62. Warady, B.A., Sabath, R.J., Smith, C.A. *et al.* (1991) Recombinant human erythropoietin therapy in paediatric patients receiving long term peritoneal dialysis. *Pediat. Nephrol.*, **5**, 718–23.
63. Stone, W.J., Graber, S.E., Krantz, S.B. *et al.* (1988) Treatment of the anaemia of perdialysis patients with recombinant human erythropoetin: a randomized, placebo-controlled trial. *Am. J. Med. Sci.*, **296**, 171–9.
64. Rees, L., Rigden, S.P., Ward, G. *et al.* (1990) Treatment of short stature in renal disease with recombinant human growth hormone. *Arch. Dis. Childh.*, **65**, 856–60.
65. Hokken-Koelga, A.C.S., Stinjnen, T., de Keizer-Schrama, S.M.P.F. *et al.* (1991) Placebo controlled, double blind, cross over trial of growth hormone in prepubertal children with chronic renal failure. *Lancet*, **338**, 585–90.
66. Alexander, S.R. and Honda, M. (1993) Continuous peritoneal dialysis for children: a decade of worldwide growth and development. *Kidney Int.*, **43**, suppl. 40, S65-S74.
67. Rizzoni, G., Broyer, M., Ehrich, J.H.H. *et al.* (1990) The use of continuous peritoneal dialysis in Europe for the treatment of children with end-stage renal failure: data from the EDTA registry. *Nephrol. Dial. Transplant.*, **5**, 985–90.
68. Levy, M., Balfe, J.W., Geary, D.F. *et al.* (1989) Clinical aspects of peritonitis during continuous and cycling peritoneal dialysis in children: a ten year experience. *Pediat. Nephrol.*, **3**, C221.
69. McEnery, P.T., Stablein, D.M., Arbus, G. *et al.* (1992) Renal transplantation in children. A report of the North American Pediatric Renal Transplant Cooperative Study. *N. Engl. J. Med.*, **326**, 1727–32.
70. Ehrich, J.H.H., Rizzoni, G., Brunner, F.P. *et al.* (1991) Combined report on regular dialysis and transplantation of children in Europe 1989. *Nephrol. Dial. Transplant.*, **6**, suppl. 1, 37–47.
71. Arbus, G.S., Rochon, J. and Thompson, D. (1991) Survival of cadaveric renal transplant grafts from young donors and in young recipients. *Pediat. Nephrol.*, **5**, 152–7.
72. Harmon, W.E., Alexander, S.R., Tejani, A. *et al.* (1992) The effect of donor age on graft survival in pediatric cadavert renal transplant recipients: a report of the North American Pediatric Renal Transplant Cooperative Study. *Transplantation*, **54**, 232–7.
73. Alexander, S.R., Arbus, G.S., Butt, K.H.M. *et al.* (1990) The 1989 report of the North American Renal Transplant Cooperative Study. *Pediat. Nephrol.*, **4**, 542–53.
74. Najarian, J.S., Frey, D.J. and Matas, A.J. (1990) Renal transplantation in infants. *Ann. Surg.*, **212**, 353–65.
75. Briscoe, D.M., Kim, M.S., Lillehei, C. *et al.* (1992) Outcome of renal transplantation in children less than two years. *Kidney Int.*, **42**, 657–62.
76. Scneck, F.X., Jordan, M.L., Jenson, W.B. *et al.* (1992) Pediatric renal transplantation under FK-506 immunosuppression. *J. Urol.*, **147**, 1585–7.
77. Opelz, G. (1991) The influence of blood transfusions and tissue matching on graft survival in children treated with cyclosporin. *Pediat. Nephrol.*, **5**, C16.
78. Ettenger, R.B., Rosenthal, J.T., Marik, J. *et al.* (1990) Cadaver renal transplantation in children: Results with long term cyclosporin immunosuppression. *Clin. Transplant.*, **4**, 329–39.

# 15

# Medical aspects of renal transplantation

*A. Wilkinson*

All of those involved in renal transplantation have had to accept that while transplantation will provide a welcome respite from dialysis, this reprieve does not come without a number of significant long-term complications. The management of these complications has often taken second place to a narrow focus on allograft survival as we have struggled to extend the life of the transplanted organ. Even though the mean survival of cadaveric kidney allografts has remained at about eight years [1], the number of people with functioning grafts has increased enormously as one-year allograft survival has improved and transplantation has become more widespread. These patients are at risk from a number of problems which, if not treated aggressively, will have a major impact on their lives, not only during the life of this allograft, but also during subsequent transplants and future years on dialysis. It is our role as transplant physicians to focus on preventing the toll these co-morbidities take on the quality of life of our patients [2, 3].

This chapter will discuss the most common problems affecting those transplant patients in whom the graft continues to function successfully over many years. It will conclude with a section on some of the causes of late graft loss and on current immunosuppression.

## 15.1 HYPERTENSION

The importance of treating high blood pressure in the general population is well recognized. Hypertension continues to complicate the lives

*Renal Disease.* Edited by G. Venkat Raman. Published in 1998 by Chapman & Hall, London. ISBN 0 412 45700 8.

of most dialysis patients. Unfortunately hypertension is very common after transplantation. Its prevalence was roughly 50% in the azathioprine era and is 75% in the cyclosporine era [4]. This increased prevalence is in part a consequence of the introduction of cyclosporine. It is also greater because we now transplant patients who were previously considered too old or high risk, and who are at higher risk of developing hypertension. Early post-transplant hypertension may normalize as graft function improves and the doses of immunosuppressive drugs are reduced. However many patients will continue to require treatment during long-term follow-up. A number of factors play a part in post-transplant hypertension.

### 15.1.1 Etiology of post-transplant hypertension

*Immunosuppressive medications*

In the early weeks and months following transplantation high doses of corticosteroids are associated with an increased risk of hypertension. The way in which corticosteroids increase the blood pressure is not entirely clear. Factors which are thought important include their mineralocorticoid activity with sodium and water retention, an increased plasma volume, inhibition of vasodilatation by prostaglandins and increased sodium–potassium ATPase activity. As time goes on the dose of corticosteroids is reduced to low maintenance doses which should no longer cause hypertension. Prior to the introduction of cyclosporin, when patients were maintained on azathioprine and corticosteroids, hypertension occurred in half of the patients. This hypertension was different from that now seen in patients receiving cyclosporine. It was not salt-sensitive, and more likely a result of one of the other factors discussed below, rather than the immunosuppression itself. It was more common when graft function was impaired.

The introduction of cyclosporine, a calcineurin inhibitor, added considerably to the problem of post-transplant hypertension. Cyclosporine treatment results in a salt-sensitive hypertension in transplant patients and also patients who are treated with this drug for other reasons. It can occur even when graft function is normal. The new calcineurin inhibitor, tacrolimus, appears to cause hypertension somewhat less frequently than cyclosporine. Cyclosporine can increase sympathetic activity and causes direct vasoconstriction. These are probably the most important factors in cyclosporine-induced hypertension, but sodium retention with volume expansion is also important. Although in humans peripheral renin levels are suppressed, it is possible that the local intra-renal levels of renin are increased and this may be another factor in this hypertensive response. There is no correlation between blood levels of cyclosporine and the degree of hypertension.

*Rejection*

Deterioration in graft function may result in hypertension. Acute rejection, when severe, is often associated with an increased blood pressure. This is most common when there is a vascular component to the hypertension as seen with hyperacute or acute vascular rejection. It is not so often a typical feature of acute cellular rejection, though the presence or absence of hypertension does not exclude possibility of acute rejection. Almost all patients with chronic graft loss will have a degree of hypertension. Chronic rejection or chronic graft vasculopathy is associated with arteriolar intimal hyperplasia and progressive ischemia and an increase in renin production. This hypertension usually responds to the use of angiotensin-converting enzyme inhibitors (ACEI).

*Renal artery stenosis*

Stenosis of the artery supplying the allograft kidney will cause hypertension analogous to native renal artery stenosis. Some reports suggest that significant narrowing of the artery, more than 70% of the lumen, may occur in as many as 12% of transplant patients [5]. This complication may be more common when living donors are used as this requires an end-to-end anastomosis of the recipient and donor arteries with a higher chance of transplant renal artery stenosis (TRAS) where they are joined. In most cadaveric donors the donor artery is on a patch of aorta and TRAS at the suture line is uncommon. Atherosclerosis of the recipient vessel is one possible cause of TRAS. This may also occur proximally at the level of the iliac vessels. When there is no narrowing of the renal artery by Doppler ultrasonography, it is important to exclude the possibility of iliac stenosis. Ischaemic injury of the endothelium at the time the kidney is acquired for transplantation, or endothelial damage during episodes of rejection may promote the development of an area of TRAS.

TRAS should be considered in hypertensive patients who develop a new audible bruit over the allograft. The presence of a bruit is not specific as turbulent flow can occur if the vessel is tortuous but not narrowed. For this reason it is important to document whether the bruit was always present, or has become louder or whether it is a new finding. TRAS is not always accompanied by hypertension and may only become apparent when there is a decline in graft function. Other signs of TRAS include polycythemia, changes in renal function which are unusually sensitive to small fluctuations in hydration, or intractable fluid retention in the absence of proteinuria. An abrupt decline in renal function after the introduction of ACEI strongly suggests the presence of renal artery stenosis.

The only definite way to confirm the presence of significant stenosis is to perform conventional or carbon dioxide angiography. In experienced hands Colorflow Doppler ultrasonography is a reliable screening test. Magnetic resonance angiography has also been used in some centers [6]. Renal artery narrowing should be corrected by percutaneous trans-luminal angioplasty. Success rates of 60–80% have been reported using this approach. As many as 30% of these cases will restenose. This rate of restenosis is reduced if a stent is placed at the site of narrowing [7]. There is a high rate of graft loss following surgical correction of renal artery stenosis as the approach is difficult and complicated by the extensive scar tissue which surrounds the vessel.

*Retained native kidneys*

In patients who are anephric post-transplant, hypertension is less common. The removal of the native kidneys should be considered pre-transplantation in patients whose elevated blood pressure is difficult to control. Removal of the native kidneys post-transplantation will frequently return blood pressure to normal and reduce vascular resistance in the allograft. There is an improvement in the glomerular filtration rate of the transplant kidney similar to that seen with successful ACEI treatment.

### 15.1.2 Treatment of post-transplant hypertension

Most of the usual antihypertensive drugs will successfully lower the blood pressure in these patients [8]. Diuretics and restriction of salt are not usually effective in treating this hypertension when used alone but are useful in conjunction with other antihypertensive drugs. Diuretics can aggravate glucose intolerance and the tendency to develop gout. They can contribute to the problems of hyperlipidemia. However many transplant patients will require diuretics to control fluid retention. Beta-blockers are effective provided that the usual cautions are taken in prescribing them. Their proven benefit in patients with coronary artery disease should be considered in patients who have concomitant ischemic heart disease. The alpha-blockers are all generally effective. They can cause incontinence in women, but are particularly useful in men with prostatic hypertrophy. Severe hypertension will usually respond to the introduction of minoxidil. This drug can markedly increase the tendency to develop hirsutism, already a side effect of cyclosporine. It can also result in significant fluid retention.

Long-acting calcium channel blockers (CCB) and ACEI are frequently recommended as first-line therapy for post-transplant hypertension. They have a number of beneficial effects on renal hemodynamics and do not have any significant metabolic side effects. Their long-term use may prolong the life of these allografts. CCB may ameliorate some of the effects of cyclosporine. They cause vasodilatation of the afferent glomerular arteriole, counteracting the constriction caused by cyclosporine. A study of the glomerular filtration rates of patients one year after transplantation maintained on calcium channel blockers showed that they were significantly greater, $57 \pm 3.3$ ml/min, compared to $38.7 \pm 3.8$ ml/min in controls [9, 10]. When using CCB it is important to remember that both diltiazem and verapamil reduce the metabolism of cyclosporine whereas the dihydropyridine derivatives have variable effects. Gingival hyperplasia which is common in cyclosporine-treated patients may be aggravated by the use of CCB, especially nifedipine. The most problematic side effects of this class of drugs are edema and headaches.

ACEI should be used with caution, and only when there is no suspicion or evidence of TRAS. They reduce proteinuria and have a natriuretic effect. Hyperkalemia can occur when these agents are used. Anemia has been reported as a complication of ACEI therapy. The early introduction of ACEI treatment, before allograft function is stable, may complicate the management of these patients. In some patients on cyclosporine the introduction of an agent which dilates the efferent arteriole may reduce the glomerular filtration rate sufficiently to produce a decline in kidney function which could be misinterpreted as an episode of rejection. This is an important reason for avoiding ACEI in the early stages following transplantation when relatively large doses of cyclosporine are used. In patients in whom there is chronic transplant vasculopathy the glomerular filtration rate may fall significantly if ACEI are introduced. This risk should be balanced against the benefit of using ACEI in patients with impaired renal function.

Hricik [11] has shown that steroid sparing protocols are useful in reducing the blood pressure in post-transplant hypertension. In this study the mean systolic blood pressure fell from $142 \pm 19$ to $135 \pm 18$ mm Hg ($P < 0.0001$), mean arterial pressure decreased from $106 \pm 13$ to $100 \pm 12$ mm Hg ($P < 0.0001$) and mean diastolic pressure from $87 \pm 11$ to $83 \pm 11$ mm Hg ($P < 0.004$). The sparing of corticosteroids also has beneficial effects on hyperlipidemia, glucose intolerance and many of the other long-term complications of transplantation. The introduction of a new immunosuppressive agent that would allow the removal of steroids from the post-transplant protocol would reduce the long-term morbidity considerably.

## 15.2 HYPERLIPIDEMIA, CORONARY ARTERY DISEASE AND ATHEROSCLEROSIS

Death from infection used to be the most important cause of mortality in transplant patients. As we have become better at diagnosing and treating these infections, vascular diseases and hyperlipidemia are becoming more serious problems. By the start of the second year after transplantation these diseases become the leading cause of death. The prevalence of cardiovascular disease is high in dialysis patients. In diabetic dialysis patients cardiovascular disease is increased 30 times when compared to patients not on dialysis. A number of studies have shown that there is a parallel increase in the frequency of coronary artery disease and hyperlipidemia in the years following transplantation. The reported incidence of hyperlipidemia varies from 22 to 70% [12–14].

The most significant risk factors for coronary disease are pretransplant hypertension and diabetes. Statistical analysis has shown that other important factors are age, gender, smoking, serum cholesterol and the cumulative dose of corticosteroids. While patients are on dialysis awaiting transplantation every effort should be made to minimize the risk factors for vascular disease. Hyperlipidemia should be treated aggressively to bring the total cholesterol and particularly the low-density lipoprotein levels down to the levels recommended for the prevention of the progression of vascular disease. This same approach must continue in the years after transplantation. It Is important to discuss changes in life style, stopping cigarette smoking, weight reduction and exercise at every opportunity.

### 15.2.1 Hyperlipidemia

Within three months of transplantation about half the patients have an elevated serum cholesterol, with or without hypertriglyceridemia [12, 14]. This elevation persists in studies of long-term transplant recipients with 15% having a cholesterol greater than 7.7 mmol/l (300 mg/dl) at two years. The levels of all forms of cholesterol are increased. Low-density lipoproteins (LDL) and the very low-density lipoproteins (VLDL) are usually the most affected. Though high-density lipoprotein (HDL) levels may be high, the HDL in this patient group may not be as protective as in the general population as it is unusually rich in cholesterol and triglycerides. Triglyceride levels are high in the first few months following transplantation, but thereafter tend to decline steadily for the next three years [12].

There are a number of factors in the etiology of this hyperlipidemia. In some studies, but not all, cyclosporine-treated patients have had elevated lipoprotein(a) levels suggesting that cyclosporine may elevate lipoprotein(a) levels [15–18]. An elevated lipoprotein(a) level is an independent risk factor for the development of coronary artery disease [12]. Cyclosporine is lipophilic and binds to LDL receptors. This may result in abnormal cholesterol synthesis. Cyclosporine, in addition, increases glucose intolerance and impairs bile acid synthesis by inhibition of 26-hydroxylase activity.

Corticosteroid therapy appears to be a very important factor in the development of post-transplant hyperlipidemia and peripheral insulin resistance. The cumulative steroid dose and the daily steroid dose both correlate with hypertriglyceridemia and hypercholesterolemia. There is evidence that this insulin resistance is caused by an increase in the activity of the enzymes acetyl coenzyme A carboxylase and free fatty acid synthetase. Corticosteroids can inhibit lipoprotein lipase, resulting in increased triglyceride levels and decreased HDL levels. A number of other factors which correlate with hyperlipidemia are diabetes mellitus, renal dysfunction, age, beta-blocker treatment, marked weight gain and diuretic use. As in other nephrotic states patients with heavy proteinuria may have very high serum cholesterol levels.

### *Treatment of hyperlipidemia*

#### *Non-pharmacological treatment*

It is an important aspect of both pre- and post-transplant patient education to emphasize the increased risk of vascular disease in renal replacement therapies and to discuss ways patients can involve themselves in reducing the risk. Patients should be encouraged to reduce their weight close to their ideal lean body mass. A renal dietitian is crucial, and regular discussions are never wasted. When these facilities are available patients should be encouraged to enter rehabilitation programs. One of the less emphasized benefits of the correction of anemia by erythropoietin is that this will allow patients to exercise more regularly and more vigorously. It is now standard care to provide erythropoietin to all anemic dialysis patients. Unfortunately some of the guidelines for the use of this hormone are so restrictive as to seriously compromise the potential benefits of its use. Post-transplantation exercise training is worthwhile for its effect on patients' sense of well-being and overall rehabilitation, but it is not yet proven that this will prevent the progression of pre-existing vascular disease. Nutritional counseling should be provided to encourage patients to adopt a fat-modified low-cholesterol diet [19, 20].

#### *Reduction in corticosteroid dose*

There are a number of potential benefits of reducing the overall exposure of patients to corticosteroids. Weight loss may be easier to achieve as the dose is reduced. Muscle strength is likely to increase which will make it more feasible to exercise regularly. An improvement in the cosmetic changes which corticosteroids cause may make patients feel better about themselves, which will improve their adherence to weight loss and exercise programs. One of the most emphasized benefits of steroid reduction and withdrawal is the potential impact on hypercholesterolemia. In patients who no longer take corticosteroids there is a significant reduction in total cholesterol and LDL. However HDL levels also fall and there is not yet conclusive data that this strategy will diminish post-transplant vascular morbidity.

*Pharmacological treatment of hyperlipidemia*

The National Cholesterol Education Program [21] guidelines for the treatment of non-transplant patients can be used to guide therapy in transplant patients. These guidelines emphasize the use of the cardiovascular risk profile. Transplant patients usually have a number of risk factors in addition to an elevated LDL cholesterol. The positive risk factors are age (45 in men and 55 in women); a family history of cardiovascular disease; smoking; hypertension; HDL cholesterol $<0.9\,\text{mmol/l}$ ($35\,\text{mg/dl}$) and diabetes mellitus. Treatment decisions should be based on a previous history of coronary heart disease, the LDL cholesterol level and a risk-factor analysis.

There are a number of studies in transplant patients of drug therapy to reduce lipid levels. Whereas almost all of the approved agents will reduce lipid levels, each is associated with a number of potential problems. The hydroxymethylglutaryl-coenzyme A reductase inhibitors (HMG-CoA RI) are probably the most well tolerated. They effectively lower lipid levels in transplant patients. Initial concern that there would be an unacceptably high incidence of myositis or rhabdomyolysis when these agents were used at the same time as cyclosporine has not been confirmed by their continued use. These early reports of elevated creatinine phosphokinase (CPK) levels and rhabdomyolysis were in patients treated with higher doses of lovastatin than are now recommended, and this drug has been largely supplanted by better and safer agents. This complication also occurred when lovastatin was used in combination with gemfibrozil or niacin, two drugs which raise the serum levels of HMG-CoA RI. Pravastatin and simvastatin have gained wide acceptance in heart and kidney transplant recipients. The most common serious side effect is hepatotoxicity, which is rare. When patients develop elevated transaminase levels HMG-CoA RI treatment should be discontinued. In patients who complain of muscle pain CPK levels must be measured.

If patients develop significant hypertriglyceridemia it is possible to add a fibric acid derivative. Extreme care must be taken to monitor

CPK levels. Cholestyramine and colestipol may bind both cyclosporine and tacrolimus, which will be eliminated in the stool. If either of these immunosuppressive drugs is used with cholestyramine it is important to recalibrate the dose of the calcineurin inhibitor to obtain adequate blood levels. Nicotinic acid is poorly tolerated because of flushing and gastric toxicity. Some of these symptoms may be alleviated by the addition of low-dose aspirin therapy. Nicotinic acid may also be hepatotoxic in some patients. Clofibrate and gemfibrozil, the fibric acid derivatives, have also been associated with myositis in cyclosporine-treated patients.

## 15.3 DISEASES OF THE BONE

### 15.3.1 Osteonecrosis

The incidence of osteonecrosis has diminished as a result of a number of factors, but still occurs in as many as 6–8% of patients in the first few years after transplantation. The prevalence is higher in patients who receive high doses of intravenous methyl prednisolone [22–24]. The most commonly affected bone is the femoral neck and head, but osteonecrosis may also affect other weight-bearing bones and the humeral head. It causes considerable pain and loss of mobility, and in many patients results in further surgery, such as total hip replacement. The introduction of cyclosporine, with lower maintenance corticosteroid doses and fewer courses of high-dose steroid therapy for the treatment of allograft rejection, has had a beneficial impact on this problem, as has better control of calcium and phosphorus levels in patients on dialysis.

This diagnosis should be considered in all patients who complain of either hip or knee pain. The pain is usually aggravated by weight bearing and by heat, and may be worse at night. Early in the course of the disease magnetic resonance imaging is the most sensitive procedure for diagnosis, but as the necrosis progresses changes will be apparent on routine radiographs of the bones. Radionuclide bone scans have a high false positive rate, but are occasionally useful in reaching a diagnosis. Although this condition is most frequently diagnosed after six months have elapsed after transplantation, the process often begins much earlier, and protocols which discontinue steroids in the first half year have not reduced the incidence of this complication.

### 15.3.2 Osteoporosis

Patients on dialysis may suffer from a number of disorders of the bone and frequently have a low bone mineral density (BMD). After transplantation much of the deleterious effect of immunosuppressive therapy appears to occur within the first four months [25, 26]. There is a correlation with a further fall in BMD over the succeeding two years and the cumulative steroid dose, which should therefore be kept to a minimum. Corticosteroids inhibit the absorption of calcium from the intestine and calcium supplementation is frequently required. They also impair bone remodeling by interfering with osteoblast activity. Diabetic patients and post-menopausal women are at increased risk. The loss of bone may be reduced by exercise, calcium supplementation and therapy with inhibitors of osteoclast activity such as the etidronates. Vitamin D supplementation may be useful in some patients.

Persistent 'tertiary' hyperparathyroidism may be present for many months after transplantation. When this results in significant hypercalcemia or progressive bone loss, parathyroidectomy may be necessary. Another strategy is to use intermittent doses of high-dose oral vitamin D therapy and to avoid phosphate supplementation.

### 15.3.3 Non-specific musculoskeletal pain

Bone and joint pain has been described in patients receiving cyclosporine. As this frequently affects the lower femur, it is often confused with arthritis of the knee. Studies have suggested that cyclosporine can cause ischemia of the distal femur. This often occurs at night and may respond to treatment with calcium channel blockers [27]. It is postulated that these agents reverse cyclosporine-induced vasoconstriction. During or following high-dose corticosteroid therapy, particularly when the dose is reduced rapidly, a few patients complain of joint pain and myalgias.

Corticosteroid therapy may result in a protracted proximal myopathy and it is important to recognize this complication and advise physical therapy and a reduction in steroid dose. It is another reason to encourage fitness training in patients waiting for transplantation.

## 15.4 DISORDERS OF CALCIUM, MAGNESIUM AND PHOSPHORUS

### 15.4.1 Phosphorus

Well-functioning allografts may yet allow persistent phosphaturia which sometimes can result in profound hypophosphatemia. When serum phosphate levels are significantly reduced there is an increased risk of rhabdomyolysis. One of the more important factors in this persistent renal phosphate leak is hyperparathyroidism. It is not unusual for the parathyroid hormone levels (PTH) to remain abnormally high for the first year after transplantation. As discussed above this may also play a role in post-transplant osteopenia. Other factors include the possibility of a PTH-independent renal phosphate leak and inhibition by corticosteroids of phosphate reabsorption in the proximal tubule of the nephron. It is common to encounter a mild reduction in serum phosphate levels in the first weeks and months after transplantation. This will usually respond to an increased dietary intake of dairy products and other phosphate-rich foods, or the prescription of phosphate supplements. The use of these may be limited by the development of hyperkalemia or diarrhea. Some studies have supported the use of vitamin D supplementation to suppress PTH secretion [28, 29].

### 15.4.2 Magnesium

Magnesium deficiency is common after transplantation. This too is the result of a renal tubular magnesium leak inappropriate for the degree of hypomagnesemia. This leak appears to result directly from an action of cyclosporine. A number of studies have shown a correlation between hypertension and hypomagnesemia, and low magnesium levels have also been correlated with the neurotoxicity of cyclosporine. Oral magnesium supplementation is usually sufficient to restore levels to normal.

### 15.4.3 Calcium

The most common derangement in calcium homeostasis is the development of post-transplant hypercalcemia. This occurs in about 10% of patients and is a consequence of persistent excessive secretion of PTH [30]. The degree of hypercalcemia is seldom sufficient to cause symptoms but occasionally may become high enough to cause a reduction in allograft function which can be confused with rejection. Hypercalcemia can lead to an alteration in mental function which may be confused with cyclosporine neurotoxicity. Some patients respond to phosphate supplementation, and if the calcium is not already too high to risk a further elevation, vitamin D therapy may suppress PTH secretion sufficiently to lower the calcium level. This complication usually remits spontaneously with the involution of the enlarged parathyroid gland and only occasionally is parathyroidectomy required to correct this metabolic imbalance.

In the immediate postoperative period a profound and refractory hypocalcemia may occur in patients who have had a total parathyroidectomy pre-transplant. This mimics the 'hungry bone syndrome' in which even with continuous intravenous calcium supplementation it is difficult to correct the low calcium level. Tetanic spasms may occur in some patients. It is thought that the suppression of intestinal calcium reabsorption by corticosteroids and large urinary losses of calcium are both involved in maintaining the low calcium concentration. High doses of vitamin D and intravenous calcium infusions will be required to correct this deficit.

## 15.5 DISORDERS OF THE BLOOD

### 15.5.1 Erythrocytosis

This relatively common problem affects about 20% of patients at some time in the first two years after transplantation. It is more common when the native kidneys remain in place, even if the patient was anemic when on dialysis. It is also seen more commonly in patients on cyclosporine [31] and in males who also have high blood pressure. The pathophysiology of this complication appears to involve an abnormal feedback regulation of erythropoietin production, with an abnormally high set point for continued red cell production [32]. As discussed in Section 15.1 this complication may be associated with renal artery stenosis.

The polycythemia frequently results in the usual symptoms of this condition: headaches, hypertension, reduced cerebral blood flow and an increase in thromboembolic complications. Treatment of this condition used to require regular phlebotomy to reduce the elevated hematocrit. Once renal artery stenosis and secondary causes of erythrocytosis have been excluded it is now usual to treat this complication with an ACEI, such as lisinopril or enalapril [32, 33]. This class of drugs corrects the erythrocytosis to within the normal range, only rarely resulting in the development of anemia. This, and the fact that native nephrectomy may result in a correction of the elevated hematocrit suggests that poor blood flow to the native kidneys, aggravated by treatment with cyclosporine, may be a factor in the etiology of the condition. The cough which some patients develop on ACEI may respond to treatment with ipratropium bromide aerosolized inhalers. If the cough persists, or if patients are hypotensive on even low doses of ACEI, treatment can be tried with theophylline which antagonizes the regulation of erythropoietin production by adenosine.

## 15.6 MALIGNANCY

There are two important post-transplant malignant conditions of which physicians should be aware. The first usually occurs quite early after transplantation and the second many years after the start of immunosuppression. For both conditions it appears that the overall degree of immunosuppression is more important in their genesis than any single agent. The common cancers of breast, prostate, lung, colon and rectum do not occur any more frequently after transplantation. It is however very important not to transplant patients who have already developed tumors until they have been fully treated and have had a disease-free interval from two to five years depending on the site and extent of the tumor.

The tumor which usually occurs early after transplantation is termed 'post-transplant lymphoproliferative disease' (PTLD) and that which occurs late is carcinoma of the skin [34, 35].

### 15.6.1 Post-transplant lymphoproliferative disease

With the introduction of cyclosporine and other new agents into immunosuppressive protocols there has been an increase in the number of patients who develop either polyclonal or monoclonal proliferation of lymphocytes in a pattern akin to lymphomas. To differentiate these from true lymphomas they were called PTLD. They are usually confined to the allograft, but the more aggressive forms of this disorder may have spread more widely by the time a diagnosis is reached. It has become clear that this proliferative disorder is associated with the degree of overall immunosuppression [36]. They are for example more common with aggressive multidrug regimens or when antibody preparations such as OKT3 or antithymocyte globulin, which deplete lymphocytes, are used [37]. These tumors are also closely associated with active infection with the Epstein–Barr virus (EBV). Consequently seronegative recipients of organs from donors who were seropositive for EBV are at greatest risk. These tumors are of B cell origin and are classified as non-Hodgkin's lymphomas. Where there is spread beyond the allograft the disease is usually extranodal. These tumors, particularly when they are polyclonal, may respond to a reduction or discontinuation of the immunosuppression [35]. Prophylactic antiviral therapy with agents active against herpes viruses may have decreased their frequency, and when they occur in spite of this they may respond to more aggressive treatment with antiviral therapy.

The mortality rate is much higher, by as much as 50 times, than for lymphomas in the general population. The course may be rapid, with death within weeks of diagnosis in the more virulent monoclonal form of PTLD. It is thought that the role of the EBV is linked to its ability to infect, transform and immortalize B lymphocytes. Genomic EBV material can be found in most PTLD. It is believed that most PTLD would progress through a polyclonal form to a malignant monoclonal B cell lymphoma if not diagnosed early and immunosuppression reduced or withdrawn. Successful treatment is more likely at the polyclonal stage.

There is no specific way in which this complication can be prevented.

It is not practical to try to avoid the transplantation of kidneys from EBV seropositive donors into seronegative recipients. Antiviral prophylaxis with acyclovir against cytomegalovirus (CMV) may have had an impact on the frequency of this complication, as may the awareness of the risks of over-immunosuppression [38].

### 15.6.2 Skin cancer

In those geographic areas where skin cancers are already common, such as Australia, their incidence in renal transplant patients increases from 8% at one year to 17% at four years. Hardie calculates that by ten years the incidence will be 44%, 20 times greater than the annual incidence in a comparable general population [39]. Squamous cell carcinomas are more common than basal cell carcinomas, a reversal of the usual relationship. Multiple tumors are often already present at the time of first diagnosis, and these tumors are more aggressive and metastasize more frequently. In the Australian reports mortality from these cancers was increased ten-fold, and squamous carcinomas caused the death of 4% of patients with skin cancer [39]. By comparison 20% of malignant melanomas and 44% of other cancers were fatal.

It was initially thought that the antimetabolite azathioprine was the primary agent responsible for these tumors. Many patients were switched from that agent to cyclosporine, but it is now clear that patients who have never received azathioprine and were immunosuppressed from the start with cyclosporine are just as likely to develop these tumors, and that as for PTLD it is the overall degree of immunosuppression which is important. The increased incidence of skin cancers is a result of genetic background, immune responsiveness and environmental factors. Exposure to sunlight is a major risk factor and all patients from the time renal disease is first diagnosed, and through their years on dialysis, and after transplantation, must be warned repeatedly of the dangers of overexposure to the sun. In high-risk areas patients must be referred to a dermatology clinic on a regular basis for detection of early tumors.

Malignant melanomas are about twice as common in transplant patients as in the general population. Malignant and dysplastic lesions of the lips are particularly common in smokers who are also overexposed to the sun.

## 15.7 DISEASES OF THE LIVER

One of the most difficult areas to discuss with potential transplant recipients is their potential risk for accelerated liver disease if they have evidence of chronic hepatitis B or C infection [30]. Many of these patients feel extremely well and it is hard to persuade them that their safest course may be to stay on dialysis. I will not discuss the use of donors who are hepatitis C antibody positive, except to warn that even recipients who themselves have evidence of previous hepatitis C infection may develop worsening hepatitis if reinfected at the time of transplantation [40–42]. In patients with hepatitis, antilymphocyte antibody preparations should be used with great care as they may lead to reactivation of the virus.

### 15.7.1 Hepatitis C

This is becoming the most common viral cause of acute hepatitis in dialysis patients. The ability to screen blood for the evidence of previous hepatitis C infection (HCV) has reduced the rate of new infection [43–45]. In patients who are already infected the disease may progress without either symptoms or biochemical evidence of liver disease. The silent nature of this disease has meant that many patients received transplants when they already had significant chronic hepatitis, or even cirrhosis. In these patients from 30 to 70% develop worsening cirrhosis by the end of five to six years. Some transplant centers advise against the transplantation of any patient with positive HCV serology. Our strategy at UCLA is to perform a liver biopsy on all patients shown to have active viral replication. Unless the liver is normal or only mildly inflamed we advise against transplantation. There are studies which suggest that there is no difference in the long-term course of the infection, and its impact on hepatic function, between patients who remain on dialysis and those who are transplanted [46]. The data are still confusing and each center will have to devise its own algorithm until the evidence becomes clearer. There is no definitive treatment for HCV. Alpha-interferon may control the disease for the duration of treatment but does not appear to provide a long-term cure. Both mixed cryoglobulinemia and membranoproliferative nephritis occur with increased frequency in patients infected with HCV and these glomerulopathies may occur in the allograft. Some new antiviral agents are under investigation and may reduce the impact of chronic viral hepatitis.

A new dilemma facing renal transplant programs is that of patients with end stage liver disease from HCV infection who may also require a kidney transplant. The decision is less complicated at the time of a first liver allograft, but where the kidney failure occurs in the recipients of liver transplants who have recurrent aggressive HCV infection and failure of the liver allograft, the wisdom of offering these patients a combined kidney and liver transplant is less clear. It is likely that these patients will again develop recurrent HCV infection.

### 15.7.2 Hepatitis B

We recommend against kidney transplantation in patients infected with the hepatitis B virus (HBV), who remain surface antigen (HBsAg) positive with no evidence of conversion. We base this on data that suggest that carriers will progress more rapidly to cirrhosis when immunosuppressed. This is particularly true if the histological pattern is one of chronic active hepatitis where liver disease mortality increases to 45 to 60% [47]. If a liver biopsy shows chronic persistent hepatitis the post-transplant course is more benign and some would transplant this group of HBsAg positive patients. Whereas the progression to end stage liver disease in those positive for HBsAg is about 6% in the general population, in some studies of transplant patients as many as 80% of patients developed chronic active hepatitis or cirrhosis [30]. The presence of HBeAg, HBV DNA, or HBV DNA polymerase in the serum is a better predictor of active viral replication and these patients should remain on dialysis.

Corticosteroids may enhance viral replication via a steroid-responsive enhancer sequence. These HBsAg-positive patients are also at increased risk for the development of hepatomas. There is no definitive treatment for HBV infection although here too a number of new antiviral agents are showing some promise in the reduction of recurrence rates in patients who are immunosuppressed following orthotopic liver transplantation. These agents may gain a place in renal transplantation in the future.

## 15.8 PROGRESSIVE GRAFT FAILURE

The introduction of cyclosporine has significantly increased the one-year survival of renal allografts as compared to steroids and azathioprine by some 20%. However the subsequent rate of decline in function, and the rate of late graft loss over the next 10 years has not changed appreciably. The median life of renal allografts remains about eight years [1].

The loss of allografts after the period when acute rejection is the predominant problem, is a result of many different factors [48–50]:

1. 'chronic rejection' (or chronic allograft nephropathy) despite adherence to immunosuppression (24 to 67%);
2. chronic rejection in patients who admit failing to adhere to the recommended long-term treatment (2 to 28%);
3. death with a functioning allograft (22 to 48%);
4. recurrent disease (2 to 9%); and
5. other causes (2 to 13%), including loss from vascular stenosis and obstruction.

### 15.8.1 Chronic allograft nephropathy

The histological changes in the renal allograft which are known as 'chronic rejection' result from both immune and non-immune damage. For this reason that term is being replaced by the terms chronic allograft (or graft) nephropathy, vasculopathy or glomerulopathy. It is now understood that many factors interact to produce this slow decline in transplant function. Even before the allograft is placed in the recipient events occur, during organ retrieval and preservation, which have an impact on long-term graft survival [51, 52]. Table 15.1 lists possible factors which cause immune and non-immune damage to the transplanted kidney.

Unfortunately, there is currently no treatment which prevents the progression of chronic allograft nephropathy when this is caused by alloantigen-dependent factors. However every effort should be made to minimize the impact of non-immune factors. Here the treatments used should be similar to the strategies used to slow the progression of chronic renal failure in native kidneys [53, 54]. The use of ACEI for the treatment of hypertension, or even in the absence of hypertension, may prolong graft life. When the diastolic blood pressure is greater than 90 mm Hg the decline in graft function is more rapid. The treatment of hyperlipidemia is important for the reasons discussed earlier in this chapter and also because the reduction in lipid levels may slow fibrosis. Separate studies of early intervention to lower cholesterol by the use of HMG-CoA RI in heart and kidney transplant patients showed that in addition to their demonstrated efficacy in lowering cholesterol levels, they reduced significantly the incidence of acute rejection in the first six

**Table 15.1** Chronic allograft nephropathy

| |
|---|
| Alloantigen-dependent mechanisms |
| Acute rejection |
| HLA matching |
| Preformed cytotoxic antibodies |
| Persistent immunologic injury |
| |
| Alloantigen-independent mechanisms |
| Cold ischemia time |
| Reperfusion injury |
| Inadequate functional renal mass (donor sclerosis, donor age, organ size, race) |
| Hypertension |
| Hyperlipidemia |
| Drug nephrotoxicity |
| Cytomegalovirus infection |

months and also the frequency with which it was necessary to use anti-lymphocite preparations to treat steroid resistant rejection [55, 56]. These studies used pravastatin, but there is reason to believe that all agents of this class may have a similar effect. It is also hoped that these agents and mycophenolate mofetil, a new, potent immunosuppressive agent, may slow the progression of chronic allograft nephropathy.

### 15.8.2 Factors affecting allograft survival

*Alloantigen-dependent factors*

The persistence of donor antigens on the endothelial surface of the allograft vasculature and the absence of true tolerance means that the immune response, modified by the degree of histocompatibility matching, preformed cytotoxic antibody levels and the success of immunosuppression, continues to play a role throughout the life of the allograft.

*Histocompatibility*

The earliest successful transplants were performed between identical twins in whom rejection did not occur. There is a definite benefit in terms of long-term graft survival if there is a two haplotype match between the donor and recipient, and both one and zero haplotype living related transplants have a significantly better prognosis than do even the best-matched cadaveric transplants. However, recent data show that living unrelated transplants have survival curves *not* that different from one and zero haplotype related transplants [57, 58]. This suggests very strongly that the very short ischemic time and the quality of the kidney at the time of transplantation are of crucial importance in determining long-term outcome. These data will certainly lead to renewed efforts to improve the preservation of kidneys to minimize ischemic and reperfusion injury. Matching of cadaveric transplants is however also important as zero-mismatched transplants have a median survival of 13 years compared to eight years for completely mismatched allografts [1, 59]. It is not possible to obtain well-matched transplants for more than a small percentage of patients using the current histocompatibility methods, given the relative shortage of cadaveric organs. Studies are under way to determine whether the use of an alternative system in which kidneys are matched according to portions of the histocompatibility antigen which are shared between groups of these antigens, rather than by use of the whole antigen, will result in improved survival of more allografts. This is called public epitope matching or permissive mismatching [60].

*Preformed cytotoxic antibodies*

The degree of prior sensitization as a result of blood transfusion or previous transplants is another factor which has an impact on acute rejection and on long-term allograft survival. The introduction of erythropoietin has meant that patients require fewer blood transfusions and the majority of patients waiting for their first transplant now have no preformed antibodies. This should reduce the frequency of severe early rejection and improve the survival of the initial transplant. Even where patients do return to dialysis and to the waiting list for a second transplant they are likely to show less evidence of presensitization as the levels of these antibodies tend to be lower when the allograft lasts for a longer time. In addition where these patients initially have high levels of preformed antibody, the fact that they are not receiving multiple blood transfusions means that the level of antibody falls with time. This improves their chance of obtaining a second transplant, and increases the likelihood that the second graft will also last for a longer time. It is important to reserve the use of blood transfusions only for emergencies in order to avoid increasing the production of preformed antibodies.

*Acute rejection episodes*

The impact of even one episode of acute rejection has been documented in a number of studies and by analysis of registry data [61, 62]. These data show that where there has been no acute rejection the half-life of all cadaveric allografts is about 13 years. When there is more than one episode of rejection the half-life is reduced to six years. The newly approved immunosuppressive agent, mycophenolate mofetil, reduces the incidence of rejection episodes in the first six months from about 45% to 22% [63], though long-term graft survival data are not yet available. Studies of tacrolimus (FK506), another recently introduced drug, suggest that this agent may reduce the severity of acute rejection episodes [64]. During episodes of rejection it appears that events are set in motion which persist after the episode has been successfully treated. Biopsies of allografts with chronic allograft nephropathy show persistent perivascular inflammation and arteriosclerosis. It is probable that there is persistent endothelial and subendothelial damage in the arterioles which results in the continued secretion of cytokines, growth factors and adhesion molecules which produce intimal hyperplasia, with an obliterative vasculopathy, glomerulosclerosis and interstitial fibrosis.

*Immunosuppression*

Both non-adherence to prescribed immunosuppression and the prescription of inadequate immunosuppression are factors which have had an effect on long-term graft function. The demonstration that cyclosporine at high doses caused significant fibrosis in kidney allografts, and in the kidneys of patients receiving heart and liver transplants, resulted in protocols in which the dose of cyclosporine was reduced progressively provided the serum creatinine stayed stable. However, a number of studies demonstrate that allografts last longer when the cyclosporine levels are maintained at higher (though not toxic) concentrations. The steroid withdrawal studies have also shown that for some patients the price paid for lowering or stopping prednisone may be earlier loss of the graft.

Optimum cyclosporine treatment should suppress rejection of the allograft while minimizing cyclosporine toxicity but unfortunately it is not always possible to achieve this [65]. As the focus shifts from one-year and five-year allograft survival rates to factors which are important in long-term graft survival we may find that early beneficial effects from higher cyclosporine levels are lost as a consequence of cyclosporine toxicity. On the other hand data from living donor transplants show that it is possible to maintain good graft function for many years in patients immunosuppressed with cyclosporine.

### *Alloantigen-independent factors*

In addition to events during the procurement and preservation of the kidney, other factors which have been shown to affect long-term graft function include arterial hypertension, hyperlipidemia, cyclosporine and tacrolimus nephrotoxicity, and possibly cytomegalovirus infection. There are also data which suggest that in circumstances where the number of functioning nephrons in the allograft is insufficient, either by virtue of a size mismatch between the donor and recipient, or as a result of damage to the kidney from the factors already discussed, the kidney is likely to have a shorter life span. This needs further study in view of conflicting results [66, 67].

### *Recurrent disease*

The disease which caused the patient's original kidney failure may not be known and this makes estimates of the frequency of recurrent disease difficult to interpret. Although transplantation has become more successful with a lower loss of grafts from acute and chronic rejection, it is still unusual for the allografts to fail as a result of recurrent disease [2, 68]. A number of diseases can however have an impact on the survival of the graft. Primary oxalosis is a rare cause that can result in kidney failure. The preferred treatment for this condition is now combined kidney and liver transplantation. The structure of the glomerular basement membrane is abnormal in patients with Alport's disease, lacking the 'Goodpasture' antigen. When these patients are given a normal kidney about 10% develop antiglomerular basement membrane disease. This can lead to rapid loss of the allograft, and this may be mistaken for severe rejection unless the correct diagnosis is made by renal biopsy and serological tests.

About 10% of patients will have the diagnosis of recurrent glomerulonephritis confirmed by kidney biopsy. This is not usually of consequence. However in patients with focal and segmental glomerular sclerosis, especially in young patients in whom the primary disease had a rapid course, the disease may reoccur with the rapid onset of heavy proteinuria. Treatment with plasmapheresis and high-dose cyclosporine may result in a significant reduction in proteinuria. This recurrence is usually seen early after transplantation, but may occur late in the course of the allograft's life.

In patients with type 1 membranoproliferative nephritis (MPGN) there is an approximately 20–30% risk of recurrence and in those patients in whom the disease recurs 40% will lose the allograft. In type II MPGN there is an 80% risk of recurrence but only 10–20% of these patients will lose the graft [68, 70].

## 15.9 CURRENT IMMUNOSUPPRESSIVE THERAPIES

The last decade has seen an increase in the number of options available for maintenance immunosuppression (Table 15.2). In addition to glucocorticosteroids there are now two main classes of immunosuppressive agent. The first are calcineurin inhibitors (cyclosporine and tacrolimus)

**Table 15.2** Maintenance immunosuppressives

| |
|---|
| Glucocorticosteroids |
| Anti-inflammatory |
| Inhibit the transcription of cytokines (IL-1, IL-6, IFN-gamma) |
| |
| Calcineurin inhibitors/immunophilin-binding (inhibit IL-2 transcription) |
| Cyclosporine |
| Tacrolimus |
| |
| Non-calcineurin inhibitors/immunophilin binding |
| Sirolimus (rapamycin) |
| |
| Purine synthesis inhibitors |
| Azathioprine – non-selective |
| Mycophenolic acid – lymphocyte selective |

and the second are inhibitors of purine synthesis (azathioprine and mycophenolic acid). The majority of patients transplanted in the USA are immunosuppressed with cyclosporine, corticosteroid and mycophenolate mofetil, whereas in UK and Europe, the majority are treated with cyclosporine, steroids and azathioprine. At present about two-thirds of all new transplant patients are treated with mycophenolate. The remaining third either receive azathioprine as the third agent or only steroid and cyclosporine. Previously patients in many centers were treated initially for the first 7–14 days with an antilymphocyte preparation (OKT3, ATC, or ALG) in 'induction protocols'. They are now changing from this blanket approach to using antilymphocyte induction protocols only for patients at higher risk for early rejection or when there is delayed graft function [71]. The key to good immunosuppressive protocols is that they should minimize non-immune toxicity and immunodeficient complications while achieving an adequate immunosuppressive effect. To this end combinations of a number of agents are generally used. The two immunosuppressive medications most recently approved for use are mycophenolate mofetil (MMF) and tacrolimus (FK506).

### 15.9.1 Cyclosporin A (CyA)

This drug has become the mainstay of immunosuppression, and is increasingly used in immunological diseases, both renal and extra-renal. Considerable knowledge has been gained of the drug's properties. Ironically, nephrotoxicity remains its major defect. Clinical use requires considerable expertise, in order to achieve the fine balance between under-immunosuppression and toxicity. The differentiation can be extremely difficult, even with the aid of blood level and histology. Some aspects of CyA have been covered in the previous section.

The current consensus is to achieve induction with CyA at a dose of 10 mg/kg/day or less, and then reduce maintenance dose to 3–6 mg/kg/day in order to achieve trough blood concentrations of 100–300 ng/ml. It is important to reconcile a number of confusing facts, namely, nephrotoxicity may occur at 'therapeutic' blood concentrations, both high levels (>400 ng/ml) and 'subtherapeutic' levels (<100 ng/ml) may be associated with completely normal function (and no evidence of either toxicity or rejection), and there are no cast-iron features on histology! The manufacturers have recently marketed a new microemulsified formulation of CyA (Neoral) and this is the only formulation available from that company in many countries. The absorption is more consistent and predictable. The drug will not be considered in any further detail, given the huge amount of published literature available.

### 15.9.2 Mycophenolate mofetil

Converted *in vivo* to mycophenolic acid, this drug is a non-competitive and reversible inhibitor of inosine monophosphate dehydrogenase (IMPDH). This enzymatic step is required for the production of nucleic acids. Mycophenolic acid causes inhibition of T and B lymphocyte function. It appears to be very effective in those at high risk of rejection. In three large studies using mycophenylate there was a significant reduction in first rejection episodes within the first six months and in those patients in whom rejection occurred, fewer required treatment with OKT3 for steroid resistance [63, 72]. The drug has an excellent safety record. The major side effects were diarrhea, esophagitis and gastritis. The incidence of leukopenia and opportunistic infections was similar in the study and control groups. This new agent has had a profound impact on early events and it is hoped that this will have an effect on long-term graft survival.

### 15.9.3 Tacrolimus

Tacrolimus is a macrolactam produced by an actinomycete. It suppresses the immune response in a manner similar to cyclosporine. It binds to cytoplasmic FK binding proteins which in turn associate with the calcium-dependent calcineurin/calmodulin complex to impair calcineurin's serine/threonine phosphatase activity. As a result cytokine gene expression is reduced. Tacrolimus has been used successfully in liver, kidney and other organ allograft recipients. Although overall graft survival was not greater in primary cadaveric renal transplants, the incidence of first rejection episodes was reduced from 32% for cyclosporine to 14% for tacrolimus [73]. It has also been used successfully in treating refractory rejection in patients previously on cyclosporine [74]. High dosage in early studies leading to toxicity have taught us to reduce the starting dose to 0.2–0.3 mg/kg/day, reducing to 0.1 mg/kg/day, so as to achieve a target range of whole blood concentration of 5–15 ng/ml [73]. Adverse events most commonly seen are neurological, gastrointestinal and hyperglycaemia/diabetes. Nephrotoxicity and hypertension are seen as with cyclosporine.

### 15.9.4 Newer immunosuppressive agents

The reviews by Morris [75], Suthanthiran [76], Danovitch [71] and First [77], deal thoroughly with the new agents currently in trials to assess their place in clinical transplantation. Amongst these, two agents which show particular promise are sirolimus (rapamycin) and a humanized monoclonal antibody against the IL2 receptor, Zenapax (Roche).

### 15.9.5 Sirolimus (Rapamycin)

This, like tacrolimus, is the product of an actinomycete. As well as having some antifungal activity this molecule also suppresses the immune response. It binds intracellularly to the cytoplasmic FK binding protein. The target of this complex is not yet known, but it is not calcineurin. Sirolimus prevents T lymphocytes from progressing from G1 to the S phase of the cell cycle. Sirolimus also directly inhibits B cell immunoglobulin production. The combination of sirolimus and cyclosporine appears to be particularly effective, whereas because they both compete for the same binding protein this drug cannot be used together with tacrolimus.

### 15.9.6 Humanized anti-tac antibody (Zenapax)

OKT3 (Orthoclone), which is very successful in preventing and treating acute rejection, is the only monoclonal antibody available for use in transplantation. The use of this agent is limited by its quite significant side effects and by the development of antimurine antibodies which neutralize its action. Recent studies of a humanized anti-IL2 receptor antibody (Ro24-7375), Zenapax, suggest that this new agent reduces rejection in the recipients of primary cadaveric transplants by about 50% in the first six months. The lack of an immune response by the recipients to this antibody means that it will be possible to re-use it to treat acute rejection, and in patients receiving new transplants who were treated with this antibody for the previous transplant. It does not induce the cytokine release which produces the most severe side effects in patients given OKT3 and is well tolerated. The long half-life of this agent means that it only had to be given every two weeks to maintain suppression of T lymphocytes over the first eight weeks after transplantation. Even with the use of this agent for two months there was no increase in infectious complications [78].

## REFERENCES

1. Ceka, J.M. and Terasaki, P.I. (1995) The UNOS Scientific Renal Transplant Registry, in *Clinical Transplants 1995* (eds) J.M. Cecka and P.I. Terasaki), UCLA Tissue Typing Laboratory, Los Angeles, pp. 1–18.
2. Wilkinson, A.H., Rosenthal, J.T. and Danovitch, G.M. (1994) Developments and dilemmas in renal transplantation. *Adv. Renal Replac. Ther.*, **1**, 32–48.
3. Danovitch, G.M. (1996) *Handbook of Kidney Transplantation*, 2nd edn, Little, Brown and Company, Boston.
4. Curtis, J.J. (1994) Hypertension following kidney transplantation. *Am. J. Kidney Dis.*, **23**, 471–5.
5. Sankari, B.R., Geisinger, M., Zelch, M. *et al.* (1996) Post-transplant renal

artery stenosis: impact of therapy on long-term kidney function and blood pressure control. *J. Urol.*, **155**, 1860–4.

6. Loubeyre, P., Cahen, R., Grozel, F. *et al.* (1996) Transplant renal artery stenosis. Evaluation of diagnosis with magnetic resonance angiography compared with color duplex sonography and arteriography. *Transplantation*, **62**, 446–50.
7. Newman-Sanders, A.P., Gedroyc, W.G., Al-Kutoubi, M.A. *et al.* (1995) The use of expandable metal stents in transplant renal artery stenosis. *Clin. Radiol.*, **50**, 245–50.
8. Curtis, J.J. (1993) Management of hypertension after transplantation. *Kidney Int.*, **43**, S45–S49.
9. Ruggenetti, P., Perico, N., Mosconi, L. *et al.* (1993) Calcium channel blockers protect transplant patients from cyclosporine-induced daily renal hypoperfusion. *Kidney Int.*, **43**, 706–11.
10. Van der Schaaf, M.R., Hené, R.J., Floor, M.D. *et al.* (1995) Hypertension after renal transplantation. *Hypertension*, **25**, 77–81.
11. Hricik, D.E., Dear, E., Lautman, J. *et al.* (1992) Variable effects of steroid withdrawal on blood pressure reduction in cyclosporine-treated renal transplant recipients. *Transplantation*, **53**, 1232–5.
12. Massy, Z.A. and Kasiske, B.L. (1996) Post-transplant hyperlipidemia: mechanisms and management. *J. Am. Soc. Nephrol.*, **7**, 971–7.
13. Lindholm, A., Albrechtsen, D., Frödin, L. *et al.* (1995) Ischemic heart disease – major cause of death and graft loss after renal transplantation in Scandinavia. *Transplantation*, **60**, 451–7.
14. Kasiske, B.L., Guijarro, C., Massy, Z.A. *et al.* (1996) Cardiovascular disease after renal transplantation. *J. Am. Soc. Nephrol.*, **7**, 158–65.
15. Bartens, W. and Wanner, C. (1994) Lipoprotein (a): new insights into an atherogenic lipoprotein. *Clin. Invest.*, **72**, 558–67.
16. Gault, M.D.H., Longerich, L.L., Purchase, L. *et al.* (1995) Comparison of Lp (a) concentrations and some potential effects in hemodialysis, CAPD, transplantation, and control groups, and review of the literature. *Nephron*, **70**, 155–70.
17. Heimann, P., Josephson, M.A., Fellner, S.K. *et al.* (1991) Elevated lipoprotein (a) levels in renal transplantation and hemodialysis patients. *Am. J. Nephrol.* **11**, 174–5.
18. Sugahara, S., Koyama, I., Yoshikawa, Y. *et al.* (1994) Lipid and lipoprotein (a) in renal transplant recipients. *Transplant. Proc.*, **26**, 2080–1.
19. Strejc, J. and Weil, S. (1996) Nutrition management of the renal transplant recipient. *Clinical Strategies, American Kidney Foundation Newsletter for Nephrology*, **III**, 5–14.
20. Weil, S.E. (1996) Nutrition in the kidney transplant recipient, in *Handbook of Kidney Transplantation*, 2nd edn (ed. G.M. Danovitch), Little, Brown and Company, Boston, pp. 321–35.
21. Expert Panel on Detection Evaluation and Treatment of High Blood Cholesterol in Adults (1993) Summary of the Second Report of the National Cholesterol Education Program (NCEP) (Adult Treatment Panel II), *J. Am. Med. Assoc,*, **269**, 3015–23.
22. Mulliken, B.D., Renfrew, D.L., Brand, R.A. *et al.* (1994) Prevalence of previously undetected osteonecrosis of the femoral head in renal transplant recipients. *Radiology*, **192**, 831–4.
23. Fryer, J.P., Granger, D.K., Leventhal, J.R. *et al.* (1994) Steroid-related complications in the cyclosporine era. *Clin. Transplant.*, **8**, 224–9.

24. Saisu, T., Sakamoto, K., Yamada, K. *et al.* (1996) High incidence of osteonecrosis of femoral head in patients receiving more than 2 g of intravenous methylprednisolone after renal transplantation. *Transplant. Proc.*, **28**, 1559–60.
25. Katz, I.A. and Epstein, S. (1992) Perspectives. Posttransplantation bone disease. *J. Bone Min. Res.*, **7**, 123–6.
26. Reid, I.R. (1993) Steroid osteoporosis. *Osteo. Int.*, **3**, 349–54.
27. Barbosa, L.M., Gauthier, V.J., Davis, C.L. (1995) Bone pain that responds to calcium channel blockers. A retrospective and prospective study of transplant recipients. *Transplantation*, **59**, 541–4.
28. Fournier, A., Moriniere, P.H., Oprisiu, R. *et al.* (1995) 1-alpha-Hydroxyvitamin D3 derivatives in the treatment of renal bone diseases: justification and optimal modalities of administration. *Nephron*, **71**, 254–83.
29. Shigematsu, T., Kawaguchi, Y., Unemura, S. *et al.* (1993) Suppression of secondary hyperparathyroidism in chronic dialysis patients by single oral weekly dose of 1, 25-dihydroxycholecalciferol. *Intern. Med.*, **32**, 695–701.
30. Meyer, M.M., Norman, D.J., Danovitch, G.M. (1996) Long-term post-transplant management and complications, in *Handbook of Kidney Transplantation*, 2nd edn, (ed. G.M. Danovitch), Little, Brown and Company, Boston, pp. 154–86.
31. Perazella, M.A. and Bia, M.J. (1993) Posttransplant erythrocytosis: case report and review of newer treatment modalities. *J. Am. Soc. Nephrol.*, **3**, 1653–9.
32. Danovitch, G.M., Jamgotchian, N.J., Eggena, P.H. *et al.* (1995) Angiotensin-converting enzyme inhibition in the treatment of renal transplant erythrocytosis: clinical experience and observation of mechanism. *Transplantation*, **60**, 132.
33. Gaston, R.S., Julian, G.A. and Curtis, J.J. (1994) Posttransplant erythrocytosis: an enigma revisited. *Am. J. Kidney Dis.*, **24**, 1–11.
34. Penn, I. (1993) The effect of immunosuppression on pre-existing cancers. *Transplantation*, **55**, 742–7.
35. Hanto, D.W. (1992) Polyclonal and monoclonal posttransplant lymphoproliferative diseases (LPD) *Clin. Transplant.*, **6**, 227–34.
36. Wilkinson, A.H., Smith, J.L., Hunsicker, L.G. *et al.* (1989) Increased frequency of posttransplant lymphomas in patients treated with cyclosporine, azathioprine, and prednisone. *Transplantation*, **47**, 293–6.
37. Canfield, C.W., Hudnall, S.D., Colonna, J.O. *et al.* (1992) Fulminant Epstein–Barr virus-associated post-transplant lymphoproliferative disorders following LKT3 therapy. *Clin. Transplant.*, **6**, 1–9.
38. Walker, R.C., (1995) pretransplant assessment of the risk for posttransplant lymphoproliferative disorder. *Transplant. Proc.*, **27**, suppl. 1, 41.
39. Bavinck, J.N.B., Hardie, D.T., Green, A. *et al.* (1996) The risk of skin cancer in renal transplant recipients in Queensland, Australia. *Transplantation*, **61**, 715–21.
40. Fishman, J.A., Rubin, R.H., Koziel, M.J. *et al.* (1996) Hepatitis C virus and organ transplantation. *Transplantation*, **62**, 147–54.
41. Rao, K.V. and Anderson, W.R. (1992) Liver disease after renal transplantation. *Am. J. Kidney Dis.*, **XIX**, 496–501.
42. Martin, P. and Friedman, L.S. (1993) Chronic viral hcpatitis and the management of chronic renal failure. *Kidney Int.*, **47**, 1231–41.
43. Tesi, R.J., Waller, K., Morgan, C.J. *et al.* (1994) Transmission of hepatitis C by kidney transplantation – the risks. *Transplantation*, **57**, 826–31.

44. Periera, B.J.G., Wright, T.L., Schmid, C.H. *et al.* (1995) The impact of pretransplantation hepatitis C infection on the outcome of renal transplantation. *Transplantation*, **60**, 799–805.
45. Periera, B.J.G., Milford, E.L., Kirkman, R.L. *et al.* (1991) Transmission of hepatitis C virus by organ transplantation. *N. Engl. J. Med.*, **325**, 454–60.
46. Simon, N., Courouсé, A.M., Lemarrec, N. *et al.* (1994) A twelve year natural history of hepatitis C virus infection in hemodialyzed patients. *Kidney Int.*, **46**, 504–11.
47. Rao, K.V., Kasiske, B.L. and Anderson, W.R. (1991) Variability in the morphological spectrum and clinical outcome of chronic liver disease in hepatitis B-positive and B-negative renal transplant recipients. *Transplantation*, **51**, 391–6.
48. Troppmann, C., Benedetti, E., Gruessner, R.W.G. *et al.* (1995) Retransplantation after renal allograft loss due to noncompliance. *Transplantation*, **59**, 467–71.
49. Hilbrands, L.B., Hoitsma, A.J., Koene, R.A.P. (1995) Medication compliance after renal transplantation. *Transplantation*, **60**, 914–20.
50. Ettenger, R.B. (1996) Kidney Transplantation in Children, in *Handbook of Kidney Transplantation*, 2nd edn (ed. G.M. Danovitch), Little, Brown and Company, Boston, pp. 270–96.
51. Najarian, J.S., Gillingham, K.J., Sutherland, D.E.R. *et al.* (1994) The impact of the quality of initial graft function on cadaver kidney transplants. *Transplantation*, **57**, 812–16.
52. Shoskes, D.A. and Halloran, P.F. (1996) Delayed graft function in renal transplantation: etiology, management and long-term significance. *J. Urol.*, **155**, 1831–40.
53. Maschio, G., Alberti, D., Janin, G. *et al.* (1996) Effect of the angiotensin-converting-enzyme inhibitor benazepril on the progression of chronic renal insufficiency. *N. Engl. J. Med.*, **334**, 939–45.
54. Katznelson, S. and Wilkinson, A. (1995) HMGCoA reductase inhibitors and omega-3 fatty acids as adjunctive agents in maintenance immunosuppression after solid organ transplantation. *Clin. Transplant.*, **9**, 1–4.
55. Kobashigawa, J.A., Katznelson, S., Laks, H. *et al.* (1995) Impact of pravastatin on outcome after cardiac transplantation. *N. Engl. J. Med.*, **333**, 621.
56. Katznelson, S., Wilkinson, A.H., Kobashigawa, J.A. *et al.* (1996) The effect of pravastatin on acute rejection after kidney transplantation – a pilot study. *Transplantation*, **61**, 1469–74.
57. Terasaki, P.J., Cecka, J.M., Gjertson, D.W. *et al.* (1995) High survival rates of kidney transplants from spousal and living unrelated donors. *N. Engl. J. Med.*, **333**, 333–6.
58. Sesso, R., Klag, M.J., Ancao, M.S. *et al.* (1992) Kidney transplantation from living unrelated donors. *Ann. Intern. Med.*, **117**, 983–9.
59. Terasaki, P.I., McClelland, J.D., Yuge, J. *et al.* (1995) in *Clinical Transplants 1995*, (eds J.M. Cecka and P.I. Terasaki), UCLA Tissue Typing Laboratory, Los Angeles, pp. 487–501.
60. Takemoto, S. (1995) Sensitization and crossmatch, in *Clinical Transplants 1995*, (eds J.M. Cecka and P.I. Terasaki), UCLA Tissue Typing Laboratory, Los Angeles, pp. 417–85.
61. Matas, A.J., Gillingham, K.J., Payne, W.D. *et al.* (1994) The impact of an acute rejection episode on long-term renal allograft survival (t1/2). *Transplantation*, **57**, 857–9.

62. Cecka, J.M. (1991) Early rejection: determining the fate of renal transplants. *Transplant. Proc.*, **23**, 1263.
63. Sollinger, H.W. for the US Renal Transplant Mychophenolate Mofetil Study Group (1995) Mycophenolate mofetil for the prevention of acute rejection in primary cadaveric renal allograft recipients. *Transplantation*, **60**, 225–32.
64. Gjertson, D.W., Cecka, M.J. and Terasaki, P.I. (1995) The relative effects of FK506 and cyclosporine on short- and long-term kidney graft survival. *Transplantation*, **60**, 1384–8.
65. Bennet, W.M., DeMattos, A., Meyer, M.M. *et al.* (1996) Chronic cyclosporine nephropathy: the Achilles' heel of immunosuppressive therapy. *Kidney Int.*, **50**, 1089–100.
66. Massy, Z.A., Guijarro, C., Widerkehr, M.R. *et al.* (1996) Chronic renal allograft rejection: immunologic and nonimmunologic risk factors. *Kidney Int.*, **49**, 518–24.
67. Gaston, R.S., Hudson, S.L., Julian, B.A. *et al.* (1996) Impact of donor/recipient size matching on outcomes in renal transplantation. *Transplantation*, **61**, 383–8.
68. Michielsen, P. (1995) Recurrence of the original disease. Does this influence renal graft failure? *Kidney Int.*, **48**, S-79 – S-84.
69. Cameron, J.S. (1982) Glomerulonephritis in renal transplants. *Transplantation*, **34**, 237–45.
70. Kasiske, B.L., Eleanor, L., Ramos *et al.* (1995) The evaluation of renal transplant candidates: practice guidelines. *J. Am. Soc. Nephrol.*, **6**, 1–34.
71. Danovitch, G.M. (1996) Immunosuppressive medications and protocols for kidney transplantation, in *Handbook of Kidney Transplantation*, 2nd edn (ed. G.M. Danovitch), Little, Brown and Company, Boston, pp. 55–94.
72. European Mycophenolate Mofetil Cooperative Study Group (1995) Placebo-controlled study of mycophenolate mofetil combined with cyclosporin and corticosteroids for prevention of acute rejection. *Lancet*, **345**, 1321–5.
73. Laskow, D.A., Vincenti, F., Neylan, J.F. *et al.* (1996) An open-label concentration-ranging trial of FK506 in primary kidney transplantation. *Transplantation*, **62**, 900–5.
74. Woodle, E.S., Thistlethwaite, J.R., Gordon, J.H. *et al.* (1996) A multicenter trial of FK506 (tacrolimus) therapy in refractory acute renal allograft rejection. *Transplantation*, **62**, 594–9.
75. Morris, R.E. (1996) Mechanisms of action of new immunosuppressive drugs. *Kidney Int.*, **49**, S-26 – S-38.
76. Suthanthiran, M., Morris, R.E. and Strom, T.B. (1996) Immunosuppressants: cellular and molecular mechanisms of action. *Am. J. Kidney Dis.*, **28**, 159–71.
77. First, R.M. (1992) Renal transplantation for the nephrologist: new immunosuppressive drugs. *Am. J. Kidney Dis.*, **XIX**, 3–9.
78. Renal Transplant Humanized Anti-Tac Antibody Study Group (1996) Humanized anti-tac antibody (Ro24-7375) for the prevention of acute rejection in primary cadaveric renal allograft recipients (submitted).

# 16

# Practical dietetic aspects in chronic renal failure

*M. Vennegoor*

The modification of dietary protein intake in the treatment of uraemia has been practised for at least 50 years, well before renal replacement therapy (RRT) became a regular form of treatment to control biochemistry and sustain the life of patients with chronic renal failure (CRF).

Dietary treatment plays a major role in the total management of patients with chronic renal failure. The accumulation of fluid and metabolic waste can, to a certain extent, be controlled by diet.

The National Institute of Health Consensus Statement on Morbidity and Mortality of Dialysis states that the nutritional health of a patient prior to dialysis is an important indication of outcome [1].

The use of a low-protein diet in the range of 0.7–0.8 g per kg ideal body weight (IBW) per day, requires sufficient energy to maintain the nitrogen balance. The nutritional components of any renal diet need to be adapted to the specific needs of each patient. Malnutrition must be detected and treated early. Severe weight loss and a steady decline in serum albumin levels in non-nephrotic patients are obvious clinical signs.

## 16.1 THE AIMS OF CONSERVATIVE DIETARY MANAGEMENT

1. To maintain an optimal nutritional status by ensuring sufficient protein and energy, and to provide important nutrients such as vitamins and minerals.

*Renal Disease.* Edited by G. Venkat Raman. Published in 1998 by Chapman & Hall, London. ISBN 0 412 45700 8.

2. To reduce or to control the accumulation of waste products as chronic renal disease progresses (such as urea from protein metabolism, creatinine from muscle turnover and the unmeasurable uraemic toxins) as well as phosphate, potassium, sodium and fluid. Dietary treatment should be reviewed regularly in line with the deterioration of renal function and regular follow-up is important to support the patient to achieve maximum compliance.
3. To prevent or to ameliorate symptoms of uraemia such as lack of appetite, nausea, vomiting and a general feeling of lethargy until the patient starts renal replacement therapy (RRT).
4. To help prevent the long-term effects of renal disease such as cardiovascular disease (CVD) by manipulating the intake, and the types of fat and carbohydrate as a source of energy, as long as this manoeuvre does not affect the quality of the diet.
5. To provide sufficient dietary freedom and enable the patient to lead a near normal life. This means that dietary flexibility must be incorporated and relatives or friends should be involved while educating the patient to promote maximum dietary compliance.

It is very difficult to determine at what stage in progressive renal failure dietary treatment should begin. At the very latest, dietary intervention should be recommended once uraemic symptoms start to appear.

The results of the multicentre trial on the modification of diet in renal disease (MDRD) show initially a slower decline in the progression of renal disease in the absence of severe proteinuria and hypertension. There appears no further advantage in using a very low-protein diet (VLPD) supplement with essential amino acids (EAA) or keto aminoacids (*KAA*) [2].

Furthermore, secondary results are in the process of being published. A meta-analysis which includes the MDRD study, indicates that a low-protein diet (LPD) reduces the risk of renal failure or renal death in patients with non-diabetic renal disease [3].

Controlling the patient's blood chemistry is important and most patients acknowledge an improved feeling of well-being once they have started a protein-restricted diet, and mild symptoms such as 'morning sickness' or a 'metallic taste' in their mouth, may disappear.

## 16.2 NEPHROTIC SYNDROME

The nephrotic syndrome is associated with heavy proteinuria. The major protein lost is albumin, but other important protein-bound nutrients are also lost, such as iron bound to transferrin, vitamin D bound to vitamin D-binding protein, copper and zinc [4]. Hypoalbuminaemia can lead to severe fluid retention which is difficult to treat

**Table 16.1** Management of the nephrotic syndrome

| |
|---|
| Treatment of hypertension |
| drug therapy |
| moderate salt restriction |
| treat obesity |
| |
| Moderate protein restriction |
| 0.8–1.0 g/kg IBW |
| adequate energy |
| |
| Treatment of hyperlipidaemia |
| manipulate fat intake |
| lipid lowering drugs |
| increase exercise |
| stop smoking |

by diuretic therapy and dietary sodium and/or fluid restriction alone.

The current practice is to normalize blood pressure (often with angiotensin-converting enzyme inhibitors), to normalize the amount of dietary protein to 1.0 g/kg/IBW/day and to modify the energy intake to 35 kcal/kg/IBW (Table 16.1).

Hyperlipidaemia is also present as part of the nephrotic syndrome, proportional to the degree of proteinuria. General advice to reduce the long-term risk of cardiovascular disease would include:

1. weight loss as necessary;
2. diet low in animal fat, low in cholesterol, high in mono/polyunsaturates;
3. lipid-lowering drugs;
4. increase exercise;
5. eliminate smoking.

The following nutrients are important and should be routinely considered/assessed in the dietary management of CRF (see also Appendix 16.A):

1. protein;
2. energy (carbohydrate and fat);
3. sodium and fluid;
4. potassium;
5. phosphorus;
6. other minerals, such as calcium, iron and zinc;
7. vitamins.

## 16.3 DIETARY PROTEIN

Protein is an important nutrient for repair and maintenance of tissue and for growth. There are two important aspects to consider when prescribing a protein-restricted diet:

1. the quantity of protein;
2. the quality of protein.

### 16.3.1 Quantity

The level of dietary protein should maintain the nitrogen balance and the nutritional status as previously discussed. The calculation should be based on the ideal or acceptable body weight (see reference tables) and not on actual body weight, taking the patient's residual renal function into consideration (Table 16.1).

The amount can be decreased as renal function declines. For instance if a patient consumes a high-protein diet a reduction to 1.0 g/kg/IBW daily may initially be sufficient and can be reduced at a later stage to 0.7–0.8 g/kg IBW. This is an acceptable degree of protein restriction for long-term use and is well within the limit advised by the World Health Organization.

### 16.3.2 Quality

It is equally important that the correct type of protein is prescribed, for similar reasons, especially when protein restriction is $<0.7$ g/kg IBW. The majority of proteins should be obtained from animal sources such as meat, fish, eggs and milk. These foods contain a higher percentage of essential amino acids. Ideally 60–70% should be high biological value (HBV) protein, containing a high proportion of essential amino acids. Vegetarian patients may not be able to achieve this goal, particularly those, such as Asian women, who follow strict vegetarian or vegan diets.

The protein requirement for a 70 kg person is

$$70 \times 0.7\text{–}0.8 = 49\text{–}56\ \text{g, or approximately 50 g of protein}$$

This works out as 3.5 g for each 5 kg in weight.

Quality: approximately 60–70% should be HBV protein:

$$0.65 \times 49\text{–}56 = 30\text{–}36\ \text{g, or approximately 35 g of HBV protein.}$$

The remainder can be obtained as low biological value (LBV) protein, from sources such as cereals and vegetables. One 'unit' contains 6 g HBV protein; thus 30 g = five exchanges.

The quality of any dietary advice must be excellent in order to prevent the main problem of long-term protein restriction, namely malnutrition, and also to alleviate boredom, leading to non-compliance. This can be achieved by using experienced dietitians and frequent follow-up sessions either at the clinic or by telephone.

## 16.4 THE EFFECT OF PROTEIN RESTRICTION

An improvement in well-being is first noticed with often a corresponding decrease in serum urea and creatinine levels. The initial fall in creatinine is due to a reduction in the consumption of muscle protein (i.e. meat or fish). If urea levels do not show an improvement, the following should be investigated.

1. Urinary urea excretion measurement, indicating the amount of dietary protcin intake [5].
2. The protein content of the diet may be too high.
3. The intake of energy (carbohydrate and fat) is too low and protein is used to supplement energy requirements.
4. Other extra-renal catabolic factors can lead to excess breakdown of protein, particularly if there is a concomitant inadequacy of energy intake. This may occur, for example, as a result of a serious infection or major surgery.
5. Steroid therapy, to treat immune disease or as an immunosuppressant after transplantation. Steroids are catabolic and will cause nitrogen to be released from cells with a corresponding increase of urea.

In most cases treatment can continue, after correcting any of the dietary and/or metabolic aspects.

## 16.5 ENERGY

The amount of energy required for maintenance is just as important as the quantity and quality of the protein itself. Insufficient energy will lead to protein catabolism, a negative nitrogen balance to protein–energy malnutrition and weight loss.

Too much energy leading to obesity is equally undesirable especially with replacement therapy in mind. Where obesity is a problem, a low-energy diet could be considered at an early stage to achieve weight loss, in preparation for RRT later on. It is extremely difficult to achieve weight loss on chronic ambulatory peritoneal dialysis (CAPD), because of the peritoneal glucose load from the dialysate, and after transplantation, when steroids act as appetite stimulants.

The minimum requirement is 30–35 kcal (126–150 KJ)/kg/IBW for patients within the optimum or acceptable weight range. To calculate the energy requirements for a 70 kg person (ideal weight);

$$70 \times 30\text{–}35\,\text{kcal}\ (126\text{–}150\,\text{KJ}) = 2100\text{–}2450\,\text{kcal}\ (8.8\text{–}10.5\,\text{MJ})$$

### 16.5.1 Carbohydrate (1 g equals 4 kcal/18 KJ)

Ideally 50% of the dietary energy should be obtained from carbohydrate, the majority from starch and fibre-containing foods, such as wholemeal bread, whole grain cereals, biscuits, potatoes, brown rice and pasta. There is a small amount in vegetables and fruit. These foods contain some protein and some types of fruit and vegetables are high in potassium.

### 16.5.2 Fat (1 g = 9 kcal/38 KJ)

Approximately 30–35% of the dietary energy intake should be obtained from fat. To achieve a satisfactory energy intake this needs to be increased for patients on more severe protein restriction (1 g protein = 4 kcal/18 KJ) (see Table 16.2). Fat is a concentrated form of energy, and it makes more food palatable and provides a feeling of satiety.

Hyperlipidaemia is a common feature of chronic renal failure. Lowering the amount and changing to polyunsaturated types of fat may help to reduce the risk of cardiovascular disease at a later stage. This manoeuvre should not affect the quality of the individual dietary advice.

**Table 16.2** Dietary management of CRF

| |
|---|
| Protein: 0.8–1.0 g/kg IBW (60–70% HBV, 40–30% LBV) |
| Energy: 35–30 kcal/kg IBW |
| Fat: 40% of energy-reduced saturated fatty acids (animal fat), increased polyunsaturated fatty acids and monounsaturated fatty acids |
| Carbohydrate: 50% of energy, high fibre, increased polysaccharides |
| Phosphorus: 800–1000 mg |
| Sodium: 80–120 mmol/day (higher in salt wasters) |
| Potassium: approx. 1.0 mmol/kg IBW |
| Minerals: calcium (Ca-containing phosphate binders), iron and folate |
| Vitamins: water soluble 'renal' formula |

## 16.6 PROTEIN EXCHANGES

### 16.6.1 Food containing HBV protein (cooked weight)

1 unit = approximately 6 g protein

Meat: 1 oz/25 g. All types – beef, pork, lamb, veal. Offal – liver, tongue or tripe
1 oz/25 g poultry – chicken, turkey, duck, goose or pigeon
1 oz/25 g game – hare, rabbit or venison
1 oz/25 g fish – all kinds of white and oily fish, and squid
1 oz/25 g shell fish (weighed without shells) – prawns, shrimps, scallops, clams, oysters, lobster or crab
2 oz/50 g mussels (weighed without shells)

Eggs*: 50 g (1 small)

Cheese*:
1 oz/25 g hard cheese, all types
2 oz/50 g cheese spread, Brie, Gorgonzola, Roquefort
1 oz/25 g cottage cheese, fromage frais, quark, boursin, monchou, fromage blanc
8 oz/200 g cream cheese, crême fraiche (minimum fat content 50%, mostly saturated fat!)

Milk and milk products:
6 oz/180 ml milk*
5 oz/150 ml yoghurt*
6 oz/180 g dairy ice cream*
6 oz/180 ml single or sour cream (fat content 20%)*

### 16.6.2 Foods containing (LBV) protein

1 unit = 2 g protein

Cereals: 1 oz/25 g bread – wholemeal, high-fibre white or rye (= 1 thin slice) or 1 croissant
3/4 oz/20 g crispbread (2), cream crackers (2), Matzo, water biscuits (2). (High-fibre varieties whenever available)
1 small Yorkshire pudding
1 scone
5 oz/150 g porridge (made with water) or Ready Brek
2 oz/50 g breakfast cereals or 1 Weetabix or 1 Shredded Wheat†
1 oz/30 g biscuits (3 small), 1 thin slice plain cake, 1 doughnut, 1 pancake, fruit crumble, fruit tart, fruit pie, sponge pudding†

---

* Foods with high phosphorus content.

† Exclude those containing chocolate, nuts or dried fruit if potassium content of diet needs to be reduced.

Potatoes and other staple foods (cooked weight):

6 oz/150 g potato, sweet potato, yam, dasheen, eddoes.
Green banana or plantain (not with a potassium-restricted diet)
2 oz/50 g pasta or noodles
4 oz/100 g rice
2 oz/50 g couscous
3 oz/75 g rice flour or rice cakes
1 oz/25 g chapati (1/2) or 1 puri or pitta (1/2)

## 16.7 CALCIUM, PHOSPHORUS, OTHER MINERALS AND VITAMINS

Calcium and phosphorus are the main mineral constituents of bone tissue. Both minerals are obtained from foods such as milk and its products, hard cheese being especially rich in both. The balance of calcium and phosphorus is carefully maintained in health and vitamin D plays a major role. This balance is disrupted as vital renal functions fail leading to impaired production of active vitamin D and excretion of inorganic phosphate.

Renal osteodystrophy (ROD) is a major long-term problem (Chapter 10) and hyperphosphataemia is one of its features. A high calcium–phosphorus product (Ca $\times$ P product $>$ 5.0 mmol/l) may lead to secondary soft tissue calcification, particularly affecting blood vessels.

Hyperphosphataemia starts to occur when renal function is reduced to 25% or less. This roughly equates to a serum creatinine level of 250 mol/l [6]. Hypocalcaemia develops progressively alongside and is due to a deficiency in 1,25-dihydroxy cholecalciferol (1,25-DHCC), the active metabolite of vitamin D, converted from 25-HCC in the kidney.

The recommended calcium intake for predialysis patients is 1000–1500 mg daily. A protein-restricted diet tends to be lower in calcium as well as phosphorus, as these tend to coexist.

Secondary hyperparathyroidism is a result of hypocalcaemia. The excess parathyroid hormone leads to calcium resorption from bone, in an attempt to restore serum calcium. ROD develops over many years but can be ameliorated by starting treatment early with vitamin D, phosphate binders and restriction of dietary phosphorus.

### 16.7.1 Dietary treatment of bone disease

1. Moderate dietary restriction of protein at an early stage. Foods with a high protein content also contain a lot of phosphorus.
2. Avoid foods with a high phosphorus content such as hard cheese, excessive amounts of milk, yoghurt.

3. Use phosphate-binding agents such as calcium carbonate. The phosphorus from food forms an insoluble salt with calcium from the binders and is eliminated.
4. Phosphate binders must be taken with food, main meals in particular, or with snacks containing phosphorus.
5. Aluminium-containing phosphate binders are seldom used. They are very potent products and can be used to improve hyperphosphataemia initially.

Sometimes, especially in conservative management, calcium supplements may be prescribed to supplement dietary deficiency and these should then be taken at bedtime or in between meals.

In summary, the following principles should be observed.

1. Restrict the dietary intake of phosphorus to 0.5 mmol (15 mg)/kg ideal body weight (IBW) (Table 16.2).
2. Individualize the prescription of phosphate binders.
3. Monitor aluminium levels at regular intervals if aluminium-containing binders are used.
4. Change partly to calcium carbonate, observing the same guidelines as above.
5. Monitor calcium levels and if hypercalcaemia occurs, lower the dose of calcium carbonate and combine with an aluminium-containing phosphate binder.

It has been suggested that an increased intake of fibre has a clinical benefit for renal patients, without adversely affecting serum potassium levels. Serum phosphate levels may rise by 0.25 mmol [7]. The improvement in bowel habit, however, enhances the quality of life in renal patients [8].

### 16.7.2 Foods with a high phosphorus content

All foods with a high protein content also contain a fair amount of phosphorus. However some of these foods are an essential part of the diet and should not be eliminated.

The following foods can be excluded without altering the nutritional quality of the diet.

Most types of cheese (see also those listed as a protein exchange, and see Appendix 16.B for listed cheeses with various phosphorus contents)
Milk powder, cocoa powder, chocolate (also high in potassium)

The following foods should be restricted to a minimum as part of the diet.

Milk and milk puddings, yoghurt, buttermilk, eggs (no more than one daily). These quantities may need to be adapted for vegetarian diets.

Meat and meat products, poultry and game – follow the daily allowance
High-fibre foods with a high phosphorus content (see daily recommended intake) such as bran, wholemeal flour, oatmeal, wholemeal bread, whole grain cereals such as All-Bran, Puffed Wheat, Ready Brek, Shredded Wheat, Weetabix
Crispbread containing rye, oatcakes
Pulses such as dried peas, dried beans and all dishes containing these foods
Nuts, seeds and all types of foods containing these, peanut butter, marzipan

The following foods should be avoided.

Fish with edible bones such as whitebait
Remove bones from canned fish, such as herrings, tuna and salmon
All types of fish paste
Shell fish (may be used occasionally)
Fish roes

### 16.7.3 Magnesium

Magnesium is retained with impaired kidney function. Magnesium may be taken in the form of antacids, and is also a potent phosphate binder. However gastrointestinal symptoms are frequent (diarrhoea).

### 16.7.4 Iron

A low-protein diet may be deficient in iron, depending on the degree of protein restriction. Iron deficiency is common in chronic renal failure. Even if a patient is receiving human recombinant erythropoetin (EPO), iron supplements are often essential to correct anaemia.

Abnormal ferritin levels will indicate iron deficiency. As a guide, for patients on haemo- or peritoneal dialysis, those with a serum ferritin level of $<100$ mg/ml or a transferrin saturation of $<20\%$, an oral supplement of 200–300 mg of an iron compound per day will be needed to restore iron status [9].

Avoid prescribing iron supplement with phosphate binders; these should be taken separately. Iron should be taken in combination with folate, pyridoxine, $B_{12}$ and vitamin C (Section 16.7.6). Hyperparathyroidism may blunt the response to EPO.

### 16.7.5 Zinc

Meat, fish, pulses and wheat products are rich in zinc. These foods are restricted with a low-protein diet and zinc deficiency may occur in patients on long-term dietary treatment. This should be treated with supplements if zinc deficiency has been established.

### 16.7.6 Vitamins

Chronic renal failure causes abnormalities in the effective levels of water soluble vitamins. This is due to abnormal patterns of vitamin absorption and excretion, interaction of metabolites and toxins and abnormal protein binding [10].

The ideal supplement should contain all vitamins of the B group, including folic acid, and vitamin C in a moderate dose. The intake of vitamin C will be reduced once hyperkalaemia prevents the intake of sufficient fresh vegetables and fruit. Too much vitamin C can however eventually lead to oxalosis.

Supplementation of vitamin A is contraindicated. The vitamin A metabolites are less well excreted in chronic renal failure and accumulate over time. Generic vitamin D should not be taken; the active forms should only be used under close medical supervision.

The following vitamins are recommended for patients with renal failure [10]:

1. pyridoxine HCl ($B_6$) 5 mg;
2. ascorbic acid (C) 100 mg;
3. folic acid 1 mg;
4. thiamine ($B_1$) 1.5 mg;
5. riboflavine ($B_2$) 1.7 mg;
6. niacinamide 20 mg;
7. pantothenic acid 10 mg;
8. vitamin $B_{12}$ 6 μg;
9. biotin 300 μg.

## 16.8 POTASSIUM

Progressive renal failure is often complicated by hyperkalaemia, a potassium level of $>6$ mmol/l. This is a potential life-threatening situation and is not associated with physical warning signs. Dietary and non-dietary causes for hyperkalaemia should be considered.

Examples of non-dietary hyperkalaemia include metabolic acidosis, increased catabolism, endocrine abnormalities, drugs such as angiotension-converting enzyme inhibitors, non-steroidal anti-inflammatory drugs and excessive exercise [11].

Most foods contain potassium, but it is predominantly found in vegetables and fruits, some varieties containing more than others. Staple foods such as potatoes, yam, sweet potatoes, green bananas and plantain contain a lot of potassium, but can still be included in a carefully potassium-restricted diet.

Potassium is also found in salt substitutes where the sodium component is replaced by potassium. Potassium-containing salts, such as dipotassium phosphate, are used as food additives but usually in small quantities.

Dietary potassium restriction may be initiated either to prevent or to treat hyperkalaemia, alongside correction of other reasons for hyperkalaemia. A dietary intake of no more than 60–70 mmol/day (1 mmol/kg/IBW) is appropriate to prevent or treat hyperkalaemia by dietary means (Table 16.2).

### 16.8.1 Potassium binders

Potassium binders such as calcium or sodium ion exchange resin (i.e. calcium or sodium resonium) may be used to control hyperkalaemia. Calcium or sodium ions are exchanged for potassium in the gut and the potassium salt is then eliminated. The calcium-based resin should be used in preference to the sodium-based product in order to avoid salt and fluid overload.

Calcium resonium is presented as a gritty textured powder, to be taken in measures of 15 g once, twice or thrice daily. It is best taken with a sweet soft drink to mask its taste. Avoid mixing the resin with high-potassium fruit juice or milk! It tends to produce major constipation if used long term, unless appropriate laxatives are prescribed (check potassium content of laxatives and bulking agents).

### 16.8.2 Potassium and high-fibre foods

General recommended guidelines for a renal diet include advice to increase the intake of cereal products with a high-fibre content. These contain potassium and some of it is variably absorbed. The overall effect of a high-fibre diet on the serum potassium level is not significant at 0.3 mmol/l [12].

*Foods with a high potassium content*

These foods should be *excluded* if potassium restriction is required. Some of the foods below may be integrated into a renal diet as necessary.

1. Snacks
   *Bombay mix*, curry snacks, peanuts and raisins, potato crisps, potato hoops, tortilla chips, Twiglets, vegetable samosas

2. Sweets
   Chocolate, plain or milk, and all sweets containing chocolate or cocoa
   Liquorice Allsorts, toffees, fudge and all other sweets containing nuts, chocolate and dried fruit

3. Drinks
   Herb tea brewed for a long period of time
   Coffee in excess of 1 cup per day (either instant or fresh)
   Milk powder and drinks containing milk powder such as Ovaltine, Horlicks, Complan, Build up, drinking chocolate, milk shakes, Nutrament, cocoa powder
   Fruit juices unless exchanged for fruit: tomato juice, carrot juice, vegetable juice, cane sugar juice, pomegranate juice, guava, mango and lychee juice
   Strong ale (i.e. Guinness)
   Coffee Mate in excess

4. Fruit (see also fruit exchange list)
   Always avoid avocados, bananas, fresh black or red currants
   Dried fruit such as dried apples, dried apricots, dried banana chips, currants, dates, dried figs, prunes, raisins and sultanas.

5. Nuts
   All types of nuts including peanut butter and marzipan
   All types of seeds such as sesame seeds
   Chocolate and nut spread

6. Vegetables
   Ackee, Jerusalem artichokes, beetroot (only as part of a salad), mushrooms in excess, spinach, celeriac, squash, parsnips, grilled or fried tomatoes, fried onions in excess, potato waffles, plantain, green bananas
   Dried vegetables and pulses such as red kidney beans, broad beans, butter beans, black eyed beans, dried peas, chick peas, lentils
   Vegetables which can be eaten instead of potatoes: yam, sweet potato, couscous, parsnips

7. Cereals
   All Bran, Bran Flakes, Oat Bran Flakes, Fruit and Fibre, Oat and Wheat Bran, Raisin Wheats, Shredded Sultana Bran
   Malt bread, currant bread

8. Cakes and biscuits
   Fruit cake, mince pies, Christmas cake, ginger nuts
   Biscuits, buns, cakes or pastries containing nuts, chocolate, dried fruit

9. Pudding and desserts
   Bread pudding and Christmas pudding
   Chocolate ices, frozen ice cream desserts, chocolate mousse and other desserts containing chocolate

10. Meat substitutes
    Soya bean products, vegetarian meat substitutes, bean milk, convenience foods containing soya bean products, unless part of a vegetarian or vegan diet in which case small amounts may be allowed

11. Condiments and miscellaneous
    Sauces such as tomato ketchup, tomato chutney, tomato puree, tomato sauce (in small quantities)
    Meat and yeast extracts (dried or paste)
    Mineral salt and salt substitutes containing potassium chloride.
    Black treacle, molasses, apple syrup (in small quantities)

*Foods with a low potassium content*

1. Sweets
   Sugar, glucose, jam, marmalade, honey
   Glucose and glucose polymer powder or liquid
   Boiled sweets, barley sugars, peppermints, plain fudge, butterscotch, toffee and Turkish delight, fondant sweets, jelly babies, fruit gum, sherbets, chewing gum

2. Drinks
   Tea black or with milk from allowance or with a little coffee creamer
   Tonic, Seven Up, Coca Cola, Pepsi Cola, lemonade, Lucozade, soda water, mineral water, dry ginger ale, ginger beer, American ginger ale, bitter lemon, sparkling orange and other soft drinks with a low juice content
   Fruit squash with a low natural juice content
   Spirits (in small quantities): whisky, gin, vodka, brandy, rum and liqueurs (these can be mixed with any of the above soft drinks)

3. Fruit
   Crystallized or glacé fruit
   Olives

4. Vegetables
   Bean sprouts, bamboo shoots, water chestnuts
5. Cereal
   Rice, noodles, pasta, wild rice
   Bread, bread products
   Cream crackers, Crispbake, water biscuits
   Corn Flakes, Rice Krispies
   Plain cake, pastry and biscuits
   Arrowroot, flour, cornflour, custard powder
   Gelatine and yeast for baking
6. Fat (see advice on the use of these products)
   Butter, margarine, low-fat spreads, oil, olive oil
   French dressing, mayonnaise, salad cream
   Double cream, crême fraiche, cream cheese
7. Condiments
   Spices such as allspice, cinnamon, ginger powder, mustard powder, nutmeg, pepper
   Essences: almond, vanilla
   Vinegar, Worcester sauce
   Dried herbs or spices in moderation, such as basil, bayleaf, caraway seeds, chilli powder, cloves, coriander, curry powder, dill, mint, oregano, paprika, parsley, sage, tarragon, thyme, turmeric
   Garlic, lemon juice, Tabasco
   Piccalilli, horseradish, chutney and sweet pickles
   Fresh herbs: use sparingly, such as basil, bayleaf, coriander, dill, oregano, mint, tarragon, thyme

### 16.8.3 Leaching

Potassium can be removed from vegetables and fruit by the process of leaching (boiling in plenty of water). For example, the potassium content of potatoes can be reduced effectively by the double cooking method and slicing the potatoes. This results in a loss of approximately 70% of the potassium [13]. Potatoes need to be peeled, thinly sliced and brought to the boil in twice their volume of water. Drain, add fresh water and bring to the boil again, cook for 20 minutes or until 'ready'. There is no need for presoaking.

Sweet potatoes and yam can be treated similarly.

*Vegetables*

1. Peel and cut in small pieces.
2. Boil in plenty of water to remove the potassium.
3. Drain the vegetables well, then measure the portion.

4. Do not use a microwave oven, pressure cooker or steamer to cook vegetables as the potassium does not leach sufficiently. Avoid stir frying vegetables unless preboiled.
5. A microwave oven may be used to reheat food.
6. Canned vegetables contain more salt.

### 16.8.4 Potassium exchanges

Potassium exchanges can be used to encourage variety. Most fruits and vegetables contain potassium in varying quantities. Each exchange unit contains approximately 5 mmol (200 mg) potassium. Quantities are based on fresh or boiled vegetables or on fresh, stewed or canned fruit.

1. Potatoes (1 portion contains 10 mmol potassium)
   6 oz/150 g potatoes may be replaced by:
   - 6 oz/150 g new potatoes, peeled
   - 3 oz/75 g baked potato in skin
   - 3 oz/75 g new potatoes, boiled in skin
   - 3 oz/75 g roast potato
   - 2 oz/50 g chips
   - 6 oz/150 g risotto
   - 6 oz/150 g ravioli or spaghetti in tomato sauce
   - 6 oz/150 g yam, sweet potato, dasheen, eddoes, coco, boiled bread fruit
   - 6 oz/150 g rice and peas (without coconut)
   - 3 oz/75 g boiled green banana or plantain

2. Pulses (boiled weight, to be used instead of potatoes and use occasionally)
   6 oz/150 g soaked and boiled butter beans, haricot beans, black eyed beans, baked beans in tomato sauce, dried peas, split peas, chick peas
   4 oz/100 g lentils, boiled
   3 oz/75 g red kidney beans, boiled
   These are high in phosphorus

3. Vegetables (One unit (boiled and drained vegetables) contains approximately 5 mmol (200 mg) potassium)
   One unit equals 6 oz/150 g of

| | |
|---|---|
| Asparagus (6 medium spears) | Bean sprouts |
| Runner beans | Cauliflower |
| Bamboo shoots | Red or white cabbage |
| Carrots | Marrow |
| Globe artichoke | Peas |
| Chinese leaves | Spring greens |
| Pumpkin | Swedes |
| Onions, boiled, pickled or silverskin | |

One unit equals 4 oz/100 g of

Aubergine
Broccoli
Curly kale
Courgettes
Capsicum (red or green)
Sweetcorn
French beans
Celery
Mange tout
Leeks
Turnip

One unit equals 3 oz/75 g of

Brussels sprouts (6)
Fennel
Tomatoes (canned)
Okra (6 pods)
Mushrooms (boiled in water first)
Kohl rabi

4. Raw vegetables (one unit is 3 oz/75 g of salad vegetables)

Beetroot
Celery
Coleslaw
Cucumber
Mustard and cress
Radish
Tomato
Watercress
Red cabbage
Carrots
Chicory
Corn kernels
Lettuce
Peppers
Spring onions

5. Fruit

Canned, bottled, stewed or baked fruit in water contains less potassium than raw fruit. Drain the fruit before measuring a portion, as the juice also contains potassium and should be discarded.
One unit of fruit equals 6 oz/150 g of the following

**Fresh**

Apple (1)
Clementine (1)
Grapefruit ( small)
Mango ( small)
Melon varieties
Orange ( small)
Passion fruit (2)
Peach (1)
Pear (1)
Satsuma (1)
Tangerine (1)

**Canned**

Apples
Blackberries
Cranberries
Cherries
Fruit cocktail
Gooseberries
Grapefruit
Guava
Loganberries
Lychees
Mandarins
Mango
Paw paw
Peaches
Pears
Pineapple
Plums
Raspberries
Strawberries

One unit of fruit equals 4 oz/100 g of the following (canned or fresh)

Apricots (in syrup or juice only)
Blackberries (fresh or stewed)
Blackcurrants (stewed only)
Cherries (12)
Gooseberries (fresh or stewed)
Kumquats (6–8)
Lemon or lime
Loganberries (fresh)
Lychees (fresh)
Paw paw/papaya
Nectarine (1)
Pineapple
Pomegranate (2)
Plums
Raspberries (fresh)
Rhubarb (stewed or canned)
Sharon fruit (1)
Strawberries (6–8)

One unit of fruit equals 3 oz/75 g of the following (canned or fresh)

Damsons
Dates (5)
Figs (fresh) (1)
Greengages (fresh)
Kiwi (1)
Prunes (6)

## 16.9 SODIUM AND FLUID

Mild to moderate sodium (Na) and fluid retention occurs in most types of renal disease. Diuretics control this accumulation by increasing sodium excretion. A moderate salt-restricted diet (about 100 mmol Na/day), will help to prevent excessive accumulation of sodium.

In practice this means very simple advice:

1. use little salt in meal preparation;
2. avoid adding salt to food after preparation;
3. avoid excessive amounts of salty foods such as cured foods and convenience meals;
4. avoid monosodium glutamate, as used in Chinese and Asian meals.

Patients diagnosed as 'salt losers' need to add extra salt to their meals and/or salt supplements. One Slow Sodium tablet equals 10 mmol Na and two or three of these can be replaced by one cube of Oxo, which contains 25 mmol of sodium.

### 16.9.1 Foods with a high sodium (salt) content

These foods should be taken in moderation with a sodium-restricted diet.

1. Dairy products
   Salted butter, margarine, low-fat spreads. Use unsalted or salt-reduced alternatives instead
   All types of hard or soft cheeses (also high in phosphorus)

2. Meat and meat products
   Smoked and cured meats such as bacon, gammon, salt beef, corned beef, ham, tongue, brawn, black pudding, all types of sausages, paté
   Pies and quiches, sausage rolls
   Ready made meals, canned, frozen or purchased from take-away shops, such as beef burgers, fish and (salted) chips, curries, fried chicken pieces and others
3. Fish and shell fish
   All types of smoked or dried fish such as cod, haddock, kippers, bloaters, salmon, trout, mackerel
   Canned fish in tomato cause, oil or brine such as salmon, sardines, herrings, tuna, anchovy
   Shell fish such as crab, lobster, crayfish, prawns, scampi, shrimps, cockles
   Fish products such as fish fingers, fish cakes, fish paste, fish roes
4. Vegetables
   All types of canned vegetables, unless preserved without salt, such as sauerkraut, instant potato powders, salted potato crisps and other salted savoury snacks
5. Nuts
   Roasted and salted nuts, peanut butter
6. Miscellaneous
   Salt, mayonnaise, salad dressings, unless home made, bottled sauces, pickles
   Canned or packet soups or sauces
   Meat or yeast extracts and bouillon cubes, packet gravy, gravy cubes or powders
   All meals containing monosodium glutamate
7. Asian foods
   Poppadams, samosas, savoury snack, chutneys, pickles
8. Greek foods
   Taramasalata, canned vine leaves, houmous
9. Chinese foods
   Meat buns, salted eggs, Chinese luncheon meat, canned fish, dried fish, salted fish, dried shell fish or squid, soya sauce. These foods may form part of Chinese-style diet.

It may be impossible to eliminate all the above foods or meals. A low-sodium alternative may be utilized, but beware of substituting sodium chloride with potassium chloride, which is potentially more dangerous!

A compromise may be reached by allowing some salty foods for sandwiches at lunch, for instance, and to prepare meals at home without salt. Adding herbs and spices during meal preparation or thereafter compensates for the loss of salt.

## 16.10 THE RENAL DIABETIC DIET

Up to 30–40% of all patients with diabetes mellitus may develop end stage renal failure requiring RRT. The early detection of microalbuminuria, optimizing blood pressure control and frequent follow up, may help to prevent or delay progression to end stage renal failure.

Research has shown that a moderate reduction in dietary protein also plays an important role. It has been suggested that a moderate restriction of 0.8–1.0 g/kg IBW/day should be implemented at an early stage, once renal function starts to decline [14]. A further reduction may be necessary at a later stage as well as the restriction of sodium to control fluid retention and hypertension, potassium to control hyperkalaemia and phosphorus to control hyperphosphataemia.

The requirements for energy, calcium, iron, zinc and vitamins are similar to those for non-diabetic patients (Table 16.2).

### 16.1.1 Fibre

The intake of unrefined, complex carbohydrate with a natural high fibre content should be encouraged. This form of ingested carbohydrate is absorbed at a slower rate, preventing post-prandial hyperglycaemia peaks.

### 16.1.2 Hypoglycaemia

The requirements for glucose-lowering agents need to be reviewed at regular intervals to maintain optimal glycaemic control and patients should be encouraged to take a bedtime snack to prevent hypoglycaemia during the night or early hours of the morning.

### 16.1.3 Hyperkalaemia

Diabetic patients are more prone to hyperkalaemia due to extracellular pH changes (potassium shift from intracellular to extracellular fluid). This is due to poor glycaemic control.

### 16.1.4 Malnutrition

Hypoalbuminaemia is common as a result of proteinuria associated with diabetes. Uraemic symptoms mostly appear at an earlier stage, soon followed by dialysis.

### 16.1.5 besity

It will be in the patient's best interest to prevent obesity. A low-energy diet is contraindicated once the patient approaches the need for dialysis. Once dialysis has started, weight loss is difficult to achieve.

## 16.11 DIETARY MANAGEMENT OF RENAL REPLACEMENT THERAPY

During the predialysis period patients with end stage renal failure will be given information on haemodialysis (HD), peritoneal dialysis (PD) and transplantation (TLN). The initial mode of treatment may be changed, if and when the method fails, and any specific dietary requirements might then need to be adjusted. Current recommendations for dietary requirements for HD, PD, and TLN are shown in Table 16.3.

### 16.11.1 Protein requirements

During dialysis all water-soluble products, such as urea, creatinine, potassium, sodium and fluid, phosphates and other waste, are removed. During HD approximately 8–12 g amino acids are lost per treatment. The normal recommended intake of protein is 1.0 g/kg BW. A supplement of 0.1–0.2 g/kg is needed to cover these losses. Therefore the recommended intake of protein for HD patients totals 1.1–1.2 g/kg IBW/day.

During PD, a mean of 9 g albumin (Alb) is lost daily in addition to 5 g amino acids. About 2/3 of this protein is albumin. There may be a ten-fold difference in protein losses between patients, and this is dependent on the molecular weight of the protein, the permeability of the peritoneal membrane (transport characteristics), the composition of the dialysate, serum protein concentration, as well as clinical status [15].

During peritonitis, protein losses increase due to changes in the

**Table 16.3** Dietary recommendations for patients on renal replacement therapy

| | HD | PD | TLN |
|---|---|---|---|
| Protein (g/kg/day) | 1.0–1.2 | 1.1–1.3 | 1.0 |
| Energy (kcal/kg/day) | RDA | RDA-400 | RDA |
| Carbohydrates | 50% | 35% | 50% |
| Fat | 35% | 50% | 35% |
| Na (mmol/kg/day) | 1.0 | 1.5 | 1.0–1.5 |
| K (mmol/kg/day) | 1.0 | 1.2 | Free |
| P (mg) | 1000 | 1200 | Free |
| Vitamins | Renal | Renal | N/A |
| Phosphate binders | yes | yes | N/A |

permeability of the membrane. This should correct once the peritonitis has been treated. Nephrotic and diabetic patients suffer the greatest losses, as proteinuria continues until renal function ceases. The protein requirement for a patient with a good functioning transplant returns to normal: 1.0 g/kg IBW, to be reduced once again in the case of TLN failure.

### 16.11.2 Energy requirements

The energy requirement for HD and TLN can be adapted to the recommended values for age and activity. Patients on dialysis need 20–25 kcal/kg to lose weight and 45–50 kcal/kg to gain weight. The energy intake for subjects on PD may need to be adapted as dialysate glucose could provide 700 kcal of the total energy intake, depending on the strength of the solution. The recommended energy intake for a non-obese, well-nourished individual is likely to be of the order of 30 kcal/kg/day for PD and 35 kcal/kg/day for HD patients.

### 16.11.3 Sodium

Sodium intake should be restricted to control thirst, as well as prevent hypertension and fluid overload, with concomitant fluid restriction. Patients with a good urine output do not need generally to drastically reduce their salt intake. A restriction of 80–100 mmol per day is usually sufficient to control thirst and helps the patient to manage his/her fluid restriction.

Foods with a very high salt content should be avoided, little salt should be added to food during the cooking process and salt should not be added on top.

### 16.11.4 Potassium

The risk of hyperkalaemia is higher in anuric patients. The dietary intake of potassium should be reduced to 1.0 mmol/kg IBW/day for intermittent HD and to 1.2 mmol/kg/day for PD patients.

Most patients starting dialysis continue to produce some urine and this helps in the excretion of sodium and potassium. At this time it may be possible to relax the intake of sodium, fluid and potassium but urine output must be monitored regularly. Dietary restrictions should be introduced as the urine output diminishes.

### 16.11.5 Phosphorus

The recommended intake is approximately 1000 mg (33 mmol/day) for HD and 1200<mg (40 mmol/day) for PD, to prevent hyperphospha-

**Table 16.4** Dietary phosphorus intake versus treatment

| | Protein (g) | Phosphorus (mg (mol)) | Clearance |
|---|---|---|---|
| Predialysis | 0.8–1.0 | 800 (26) | Poor |
| HD | 1.0–1.2 | 1000 (32) | 24 mmol per week |
| PD | 1.1–1.3 | 1200 (34) | 70 mmol per week |
| Transplant | 1.0 | Free | Normal |

taemia. Dietary phosphorus restriction combined with phosphate binders and dialysis helps to prevent hyperphosphataemia.

Table 16.4 shows the dietary phosphorus intake versus modes of treatment. Phosphorus depends on protein intakc and the removal of phosphate depends of the mode of dialysis. With a daily dietary intake of 1000 mg (32 mmol) phosphorus, only 3 × 240 mg (8 mmol) phosphate is removed by thrice weekly HD (= 24 mmol). This is a net gain of 200 mmol/week.

With PD if the dietary intake is also 1000 mg (32 mmol) daily, only 300 mg (10 mmol) is removed (= 70 mmol). This is a net gain of 154 mmol/week. Thus the net gain of phosphate can only be controlled by using appropriate phosphate binders.

### 16.11.6 Vitamins

It is recommended that dialysis patients should supplement their water-soluble vitamin intake. See Section 16.7.6 for the recommended intake of vitamins for dialysis patients [10].

### 16.11.7 Fluid

The intake of fluid needs to be restricted as the urine output reduces. The interdialytic weight gain with HD should be kept to no more than 1.5–2.0 kg. A daily fluid allowance of 500 ml plus the volume of urine from the previous day is usually sufficient to prevent fluid overload.

The restriction of fluid is one of the most difficult aspects of the dialysis dietary regimen for the patient to adhere to, and up to 86% of patients may exceed the fluid weight guideline of 1.5 kg [16]. A multidisciplinary approach to this aspect of the general management is essential, as patients are often confused between flesh and fluid weight.

### 16.11.8 Some hints for fluid control

1. Avoid salt and highly salted foods.
2. Avoid meals prepared with monosodium glutamate, e.g. Chinese, Asian and other Far Eastern meals.
3. Measure the fluid allowance in a water jug. Divide the fluid allowance during the whole day, using small cups (150 ml each) instead of mugs (250 ml each). Drink only one cup at a time.
4. Ice cubes may be more thirst quenching, but each cubes equals about 30 ml fluid (2 tablespoons)
5. Rinse the mouth with water, gargle, but do not swallow.
6. Stimulate saliva production by sucking slices of lemon, sherbets or chewing gum.
7. Take medicines with the main meals unless contraindicated.
8. When going out save the allowance of fluid. This allows for an extra drink(s) when socializing.
9. A patient may be preoccupied with the desire for fluid. It is important to keep occupied with some form of activity.
10. A daily weight check will reveal the rate of fluid accumulation.

## 16.12 PRESCRIPTION DIALYSIS AND UREA KINETIC MODELLING

Urea kinetic modelling (UKM) is used to prescribe dialysis treatment using an established formula. UKM includes the calculation of the protein catabolic rate (PCR). Malnourished patients can be easily identified, alerting dietitians to spend time on those that are at risk [17].

### 16.12.1 Urea reduction rate (URR)

This is an alternative method of calculating dialysis adequacy.

URR = predialysis urea
– post-dialysis urea divided by the predialysis urea.

A urea reduction ratio of 50% equals a *Kt/V* of 0.8 and each additional 5% reduction equals an increase of the *Kt/V* by 0.2. Ideally the percentage should be 70–75% per HD treatment. This equals a *Kt/V* of 1.4 [18].

There are pros and cons to both methods of assessing the adequacy of dialysis. Table 16.5 gives a relationship between the two types of assessments compared to mortality rates, derived from a large database from the USA [19].

**Table 16.5** Relationship between the two assessments and the mortality rates [19]

| URR | *Kt/V* | Mortality |
|---|---|---|
| 50% | 0.82 | 25% |
| 60% | 1.05 | 22% |
| 70% | 1.40 | 17% |

## 16.13 MALNUTRITION

Malnutrition is recognized as a common and important problem amongst dialysis patients as it contributes to morbidity and mortality. Malnutrition is preventable and is linked to inadequate dialysis but may also be due to progressive worsening of renal function, with failure to adjust the dialysis prescription. It has been reported that, of patients on dialysis, approximately 47% on HD and 44% on PD were clinically malnourished [20].

Malnutrition must be corrected to avoid preventable morbidity and mortality. For instance each 10 g/l decrease in serum albumin concentration increases the likelihood of hospitalization, particularly in diabetics, where there is a ten-fold increase [21].

Consequences of malnutrition include:

1. delayed wound healing;
2. decreased resistance to infection;
3. electrolyte imbalance; and
4. prolonged hospitalization, increasing the cost of treatment.

There are several reasons for malnutrition in dialysis patients, and in any individual the cause is usually multifactorial.

1. Reduced dietary intake
   - Pre-existing malnutrition at the start of dialysis due to uraemia and unsupervised predialysis dietary restriction.
   - Inadequate dietary nutrient intake. Most patients consume less protein than is recommended. This may not always lead to a negative nitrogen balance in stable subjects when adequately supervised, for example with a protein intake of 0.7 g/kg IBW/day with a high energy consumption of 35–38 kcal/kg/day.
   - Conflicting dietary recommendations: increase in protein while reducing dietary phosphorus.
   - Financial constraints.
2. Reduced appetite
   - Inadequate dialysis, leading to uraemic anorexia.

- Suppression of appetite due to glucose absorption with PD, intra-abdominal compression, constipation and chronic depression.
- Coexisting gastrointestinal disease and co-morbidity such as cardiac failure and cancer.
- Prolonged hospitalization contributing to an inadequate nutritional intake.

3. Increased nutritional losses
   - Water-soluble nutrient losses, such as amino acid and vitamin losses during dialysis, albumin during PD.
   - Persistent proteinuria.
4. Altered metabolism
   - Protein degradation as a result of the dialysis process (HD).
   - Untreated acidosis contributes to protein catabolism.

### 16.13.1 Treatment of malnutrition

Intervention should start as soon as malnutrition is identified. This consists of dietary review and counselling by an experienced renal dietitian who will:

1. improve/increase the existing dietary prescription as required;
2. modify the consistency and composition of the meal, if chewing and/or swallowing are a problem;
3. gradually motivate the patient to improve his/her appetite if active depression is an underlying problem;
4. introduce nutritional support at an early stage;
5. monitor progress regularly.

## 16.14 NUTRITIONAL SUPPORT

There are a number of methods of supplemental feeding employed in clinical nephrology.

1. Oral or sip feeding is appropriate for patients who are able to eat and drink normally.
2. Nasogastric or gastrostomy feeding is necessary for patients who are unable or unwilling to eat or drink normally.
3. Oral and tube feeding can be combined, for instance tube feeding overnight, while the patient sleeps, and normal eating/drinking during the day.
4. Intraperitoneal nutrition (IPN) for those on PD.
5. Intradialysis parenteral nutrition (IDPN) during HD.
6. Total parenteral nutrition (TPN) for those who are unable to receive oral/sip or enteral methods of nutritional support.

**Table 16.6** Commercial nutritional products for sip or tube feeding

| Product (unit) | Energy (k/cal) | Protein (g) | K (mmol) | P (mg) |
|---|---|---|---|---|
| Nepro* (237 ml) | 475 | 17 | 6 | 171 |
| Suplena* (237 ml) | 475 | 7 | 7 | 173 |
| Ensure Plus* (200 ml) | 300 | 13 | 9 | 212 |
| Entera† (200 ml) | 300 | 11 | 9 | 103 |
| Protein Forte† (200 ml) | 200 | 20 | 8 | 200 |
| Fortisip‡ (200 ml) | 300 | 10 | 8 | 100 |
| Maxijul§ (200 ml) | 400 | – | – | – |

* Ross/Abbott Ltd
† Fresenius Ltd
‡ Cow and Gate Nutricia Ltd
§ Scientific Hospital Supplies Ltd

### 16.14.1 Nasogastric and sip feeding

Concentrated oral supplements could be used once malnutrition is diagnosed, and these should be prescribed as medicine. The insertion of a percutaneous enteral gastrostomy (PEG) feeding tube enables long-term feeding without the discomfort of a nasogastric feeding tube.

The manufacturers of nutritional support products have improved their range for oral consumption and of enteral tube feeding products. The high-protein and energy-dense products are best for the anuric patient requiring additional support, while those on PD would benefit from high-protein formulations. Low-volume enteral tube feeding regimes can be tailored to individual needs. These are highly viscous and need the assistance of a special feeding pump. Some formulations available are shown in Table 16.6.

### 16.14.2 Nutritional peritoneal dialysis

Recent studies indicate that using dialysate with a 1.1% amino acid concentration, providing 18 g amino acids in two litres of dialysate, improves the nutritional status of PD patients.

### 16.14.3 Intra-dialysis parenteral nutrition

Parenteral formulations containing approximately 10–12 g nitrogen (64–75 g protein) and 1000 kcal (mainly glucose), can be delivered during HD treatment. Glucose monitoring during the treatment is essential to prevent hyperglycaemia. The fluid balance can be adjusted accordingly.

It is a useful mode of nutritional support for patients for whom other forms of nutritional support have failed or are contraindicated.

### 16.14.4 Monitoring nutritional support

*Biochemistry*

Serum albumin is regarded as the easiest marker of malnutrition. However, it has a long half-life and should be assessed on a monthly basis. Patients with an acute or chronic illness may not show any improvement in serum albumin levels until recovery is taking place. Serum reactive protein (CRP), an acute-phase protein, rises with chronic inflammation, infection and tissue damage. When serum albumin levels are corrected for CRP they lose their significance as a nutritional marker. Serum albumin levels depend on fluid status, and will be lower in fluid-overloaded patients.

*Anthropometric measurements*

Weight loss of more than 10% in less than three months is a nutritional risk factor. If available, anthropometric measurements are useful in assessing lean body mass. The patient here acts as his/her own control, but fluid status can flaw the results. It is therefore necessary to perform these measurements after dialysis. Fistula arms should not be used to perform these measurements. There are limitations to anthropometry, such as observer error, instrument error and recording techniques. Other considerations include errors related to the patient's status and the interpretation of measurements. Anthropometry should therefore only be measured by well-trained personnel [22].

### 16.14.5 Quality standards for dialysis patients

Table 16.7 shows the recommended nutritional standards for dialysis patients. These are based on the publications of the American Health Care Finance Administration [23]. The British Renal Association and Royal College of Physicians have issued standards, which include nutritional guidelines to guarantee adequate treatment.

## 16.15 POST-TRANSPLANT NUTRITIONAL PROBLEMS

Some nutritional problems occurring after transplantation are related to immunosuppressive therapy. Side effects of steroids include protein hypercatabolism, obesity, hyperlipidaemia, glucose intolerance, hyperkalaemia and interference with the action of vitamin D. Obesity is a frequent problem. Post-transplantation dietary treatment should be taken into consideration.

**Table 16.7** Nutritional standards for patients on RRT

| | HD | PD |
|---|---|---|
| Albumin (g/l) | > 35 | > 35 |
| Urea (mmol/l) | < 30 | < 30 |
| K (mmol/l) | 3.5–6.5 | 3.5–6.5 |
| iP (mmol/l) | 1.1–1.9 | 1.1–1.9 |
| Ca (mmol/l) | 2.12–2.60 | 2.12–2.60 |
| UKM (*Kt/V*) | > 1.2 | 1.7 per week |
| URR | 65% | |

The immediate post-transplant recommended intake of protein ranges between 1.3 and 1.5 g/kg IBW/day, to a maintenance protein intake of 1 g/kg/day. The protein intake may need to be reduced with the onset of transplant failure [24]. Obesity is common with a successful transplant and is multifactorial:

1. appetite increase due to an increased feeling of well-being;
2. steroids stimulate appetite;
3. lack of exercise.

Obesity contributes to hypertension and hyperlipidaemia, and these in turn to accelerated atherosclerosis. It is important to maintain an ideal weight for height: an energy intake of 28–30 kcal/kg IBW/day. The patient should be made aware of the risks of obesity at an early stage.

The majority of transplanted patients develop hyperlipidaemia, with elevated serum triglycerides and cholesterol. This is in part due to steroids as well as cyclosporin therapy, and there is often associated glucose intolerance (insulin resistance). This can be treated by dietary manipulation of fat and carbohydrate intake, and by reducing the cholesterol intake to 300 mg per day.

### 16.15.1 Dietary treatment of hyperlipidaemia

Hyperlipidaemia is a common feature of the nephrotic syndrome, a functioning transplant and of PD. The latter is linked to continuous glucose absorption from the dialysate. It is important that the guidelines for healthy eating are incorporated whenever a renal patient is given dietary advice (Table 16.8).

## 16.16 DIETARY MANAGEMENT OF RENAL STONE DISEASE

Metabolic renal stone disease is a common disorder (see Chapter 8 for further details). The majority of stones are composed of calcium and oxalate. The formation of stones depends on:

**Table 16.8** Recommendations for healthy eating

| *Sources of energy:* | |
|---|---|
| Carbohydrate: | 50% of energy |
| | ↑ polysaccharides |
| | ↓ monosaccharides |
| | ↑ fibre |
| Fat: | 30–35% of energy |
| | ↓ saturated fatty acids |
| | ↑ mono- and |
| | ↑ polyunsaturated fatty acids |

1. the retention of the particles that promote crystal formation;
2. supersaturation of the urine with those minerals;
3. decrease of natural inhibitors that prevent precipitation of crystals.

Patients with multiple and recurring stone formation and those with abnormal urine chemistry would benefit from an assessment with the aim of correcting any dietary components contributing to stone formation. Working in hot conditions or living in a hot climate can cause dehydration if insufficient fluid is taken, thus contributing to stone formation. An excessive intake of calcium, oxalate, vitamin D, purines, fibre, protein and refined carbohydrate can increase the risk of idiopathic hypercalciuria.

### 16.16.1 Fluid requirement

It is very important that patients with a history of stone formation produce a dilute urine. An intake of 3 l/day is needed to produce 2–2.5 l urine. Additional fluid should be taken to compensate for losses such as perspiration and diarrhoea. The fluid should be taken *throughout* the day in divided quantities and at bedtime. Suitable drinks are water, weak coffee (black or with creamers or milk from the allowance), fruit squash, fruit juice, soft drinks (low calorie, if necessary).

### 16.16.2 Calcium

The recommended daily intake is 500–800 mg according to National recommended allowances and increases to 1200 mg for pregnant, lactating and postmenopausal women. A low-calcium diet is difficult to adhere to and may even contribute to secondary hyperoxaluria. It was an accepted wisdom to prescribe low-calcium diets, but there is little evidence to justify it now. A normal or moderately calcium-reduced diet (400–600 mg) may be prescribed. More importantly, a low-oxalate diet should be enforced.

*Foods with a high calcium content*

The following should not be taken in excess.

Milk and all foods made from milk, milk powder
Cheese, yoghurt, buttermilk, single or sour cream
Dairy ice cream
Manufactured foods and meals containing milk solids
Fish with small edible bones such as whitebait, herrings, tinned fish, such as pilchards, sardines, sprats, fish paste
Shell fish, mussels, cockles, oysters, scallops, shrimps, prawns, lobster
White bread, white fortified flour, digestive biscuits, scones, muesli
Broccoli, watercress, fruit gums and black treacle can be taken occasionally
Soya flour, soya added to food, i.e. to substitute for meat (Mince saver), bean curd, tofu (but soya milk is allowed)
Vitamin D supplements, cod liver oil or other types of fish oils.

*Foods with moderate calcium content*

The following may be taken freely.

Wholemeal bread and cereals, except muesli, All Bran, Weetabix, Shredded Wheat
Wholemeal flour, wholemeal or whole rye crispbreads
Brown pasta and brown rice
Milk should be reduced to half a pint (275 ml) or less daily
Yoghurts or buttermilk, evaporated or condensed milk, can replace the milk

The following may be taken in moderation.

Cream cheese with a high fat content, double cream, crême fraiche (these have a high energy and saturated fat content)
Margarine, butter, oil
Meat, poultry, fish, fruit and fruit juice, vegetables (except those with a high calcium content), potatoes
Wines and spirits, but in appropriate quantities!

### 16.16.3 Oxalate

The dietary intake of oxalate affects urinary oxalate excretion, even in small quantities. Urinary levels do not always indicate a high intake and it is therefore important to be aware of the stone composition, if at all possible. Sustained by hyperoxaluria may be due to:

1. excessive oxalate intake;
2. excessive absorption from the gut; or
3. excessive synthesis as a result of a metabolic disorder.

It is important to reduce the intake of oxalate-rich foods whether or not a low-calcium diet is prescribed. A low-oxalate diet should contain no more than 60–70 mg oxalate daily (1 mg/kg/day)

*Foods with a high oxalate content*

Tea, not more than 3–4 cups/1–2 mugs of weak tea per day
Rhubarb, beetroot, parsley, spinach, strawberries
Chocolate and cocoa
All types of nuts, peanut butter, marzipan
All foods containing cocoa, chocolate and/or nuts

### 16.16.4 Other dietary factors

Gastrointestinal calcium absorption may be increased when plasma levels of 1,25-dihydroxycholecalciferol or parathyroid hormone are raised. (Patients may take multi-vitamin supplements, containing vitamin D or cod liver oil.) Withdrawal of such supplements is important. A diet low in phosphorus, phytate (fibre) or fat may also contribute to an increased calcium absorption as the calcium remains unbound in the gut. A reduced sodium intake (100 mmol/day) also reduces the quantity of calcium excreted in the urine. A high-sodium diet may result in a high urinary calcium by promoting its excretion.

A high-protein diet normally increases calcium, oxalate and uric acid excretion and patients with recurrent renal stone formation may benefit from a normalized intake of protein (1 g/kg IBW/day), emphasizing a reduction in the consumption of meat and fish. This simple advice will automatically include a reduced intake of uric acid and purine, which further contribute to hypercalciuria. Other important components are the urinary pH and citrate levels.

### 16.16.5 Gout and uric acid stone formation

Despite the fact that drug therapy has replaced dietary restrictions (reducing or eliminating foods with a high purine content), it may still be advisable to include some advice if hyperuricaemia is refractory. Purine is found in plenty in offal and some types of fish.

Principal source of purine are:

| **Meat sources** | **Fish sources** |
|---|---|
| liver | anchovies |
| heart | crab |
| kidney | fish roes |
| sweetbreads | herring |
| meat extracts (Oxo) | mackerel |
| | sardines |
| | shrimps |
| | sprats |
| | whitebait |

## 16.17 DIETARY COMPLIANCE (LOW-PROTEIN DIET)

Prescribing any type of diet deprives the patients of the freedom to choose. A renal diet prior to or whilst on dialysis involves the manipulation of dietary nutrients and sources of energy. It is not surprising that the protein-restricted diet was unpopular for a long time. Protein–energy malnutrition was a frequent problem and it delayed rehabilitation once dialysis was started. More recently the importance of regular follow-up has been recognized and this has improved the quality of treatment, which includes regular dietary reviews. The results of the MDRD feasibility study have also shown how dietary compliance can be improved by frequent monitoring and patient self-management.

Initially protein restriction should be adapted to current eating habits. Thereafter, the protein intake can be lowered gradually to the required level. It is suggested that protein gram counting, instead of using protein exchanges, might also improve compliance [25]. A positive working relationship with the patient is obviously vital for success. This should be based on a mutual understanding. The rationale for any dietary restriction should be explained to each patient individually, if possible in the presence of a member of the family or a close friend. Renal patients require support from their family, friends and colleagues at work.

### 16.17.1 Socialii ng

Dietary restrictions should not prevent a patient from socializing. A sensible choice can be made irrespective of whether a meal is taken in a restaurant, a snackbar, the canteen at work or at a picnic.

1. Avoid dishes on the menu with ingredients containing a lot of protein, potassium, salt or phosphorus.
2. Avoid the addition of salt to the meal after preparation.

3. Make a sensible choice from a menu by choosing grills, salads etc.
4. Control portion size. Omit the protein portion of one meal and take a double quantity when eating out.

It is, furthermore, important not to expect an immediate response to complicated dietary interventions which have a major impact on the patient's freedom. Frequent follow-up, by telephone if necessary, is one obvious solution. Finally, all those involved in the care of renal patients need to provide as much support and understanding as possible to achieve maximum compliance.

**cknowle dgement**

Advice has been obtained from Ms Alison Anderton, SRD, formerly Senior Renal Dietitian, The Middlesex and St Peter's Hospital, London, UK, and Ms Barbara Wendland, RPDt, Mount Sinai Hospital, Toronto, Canada.

## APPENDIX 16.A DIETARY MANAGEMENT OF CHRONIC RENAL FAILURE

### Dietary components for conser atie management of CRF

Protein: 0.7–0.8 g per kg IBW/day (60–70% HBV protein)

Energy: 35–30 kcal/210–126 kJ/kg IBW/day
carbohydrate: 50% of total energy; use mainly polysaccharides if possible
fat: approximately 35% of total energy, unsaturated fats if possible

Sodium: 1–2 mmol/kg IBW/day; adapt to individual requirements (e.g. if salt-wasting)

Fluid: adapt to individual needs – a high sodium/fluid intake may be required with salt-losing nephropathy

Potassium: 1 mmol/kg IBW, initiate as soon as hyperkalaemia occurs, also investigate non-dietary causes of hyperkalaemia [11]

Phosphorus: 0.5 mmol (15 mg)/kg IBW/day, use phosphate binders as required

Calcium: 500–1000 mg (12–25 mmol) daily or as required to maintain serum calcium levels (in conjunction with vitamin D)

Iron: 10 mg for adult males and 12 mg for females

Vitamins: see Section 16.7.6

**Example of a days diet (for a 70 kg person moderately actie not oe rweight)**

Protein: 50–55 g; 30–35 g HBV and 20 g LBV
Energy: 2500–2100 kcal/10.5–8.8 MJ
Carbohydrate: 280–330 g
Fat: 90 g
Sodium: 70 mmol (1600 mg)
Potassium: 70 mmol (2730 mg)
Phosphorus: 23 mmol (700 mg)

Supplements of iron, vitamin $B_{12}$ and zinc, if deficient. Water-soluble vitamins.

**Example of a days menu**

Breakfast
2 slices (wholemeal) bread or 2 LBV protein exchanges
Unsaturated margarine, slightly salted
1 egg or 1 oz/25 g cheese (= 1 slice) or 1 small carton yoghurt
Jam, honey, marmalade

Lunch
2 oz/50 g meat or 2 HBV protein exchanges
2 slices (wholemeal) bread or 2 LBV protein exchanges
Unsaturated margarine
1 vegetable exchange unit (with potassium restriction)
1 fruit exchange unit (with potassium restriction)

Evening meal
2 oz/50 g meat or 2 HBV protein exchanges
6 oz/150 g potatoes
Unsaturated margarine or oil for cooking
1 vegetable exchange unit (with potassium restriction)
1 fruit exchange unit (with potassium restriction)

Daily
1/3 pint (180 ml) milk or yoghurt
2 oz/50 g unsaturated margarine or oil
4 biscuits (wholemeal and plain) or 2 LBV exchanges
6 slices (wholemeal) bread
8 biscuits (wholemeal) or alternative 4 LBV protein exchanges

## APPENDIX 16.B PHOSPHORUS CONTENT OF SOME TYPES OF CHEESE

The phosphorus content of cheese depends on its maturity and fat content. 'Young' cheeses and those with a high fat content contain less phosphorus and protein than mature cheese with a reduced fat content.

**Low phosphorus cheese (<25 mg/100 g)**

| | Protein (g) | Phosphorus (mg) |
|---|---|---|
| Cottage, plain or with herbs | 13 | 160 |
| Cream cheese | 3 | 100 |
| Fromage frais, plain | 7 | 110 |
| Full fat soft cheese | 9 | 130 |
| Goat's milk soft cheese | 13 | 210 |
| Quark | 15 | 200 |
| Ricotta | 9 | 170 |
| White stilton | 20 | 260 |

**Medium phosphorus cheese (<400 mg/100 g)**

| | Protein (g) | Phosphorus (mg) |
|---|---|---|
| Brie | 19 | 390 |
| Camembert | 21 | 316 |
| Cheshire | 27 | 400 |
| Feta | 16 | 280 |
| Danish blue | 20 | 370 |
| Lancashire | 23 | 400 |
| Roquefort | 20 | 400 |
| Stilton | 23 | 310 |

**High phosphorus cheese (>400 mg/100 g)**

| | Protein (g) | Phosphorus (mg) |
|---|---|---|
| Cheddar (average maturity) | 25 | 500 |
| Cheese spread | 16 | 800 |
| Edam | 26 | 530 |
| Emmenthaler | 27 | 590 |
| Gouda | 24 | 490 |
| Gruyere | 27 | 616 |
| Processed cheese | 21 | 800 |
| Mozzarella | 25 | 420 |

## REFERENCES


1. National Institute of Health (1993). Morbidity and mortality of dialysis. National Institute of Health Consensus Statement. Volume 11, Number 2, US Department of Health and Human Services, Public Health Service, Office of Medical Application of Research.
2. Klahr, S., Levey, A.S., Beck, G.J. *et al.* (1994) The effects of dietary protein restriction and blood-pressure control on the progression of chronic renal disease. *N. Engl. . Med.*, **330**, 877–84.
3. Levey, A.S., Beck, G.J., Caggiula, A.W. *et al.* (1995) Trends towards a beneficial effect of a low protein diet during additional follow-up in the modification of diet in renal disease study. European Dialysis and Transplant Association–European Renal Association (EDTA–ERA) abstracts, p. 985.
4. Kaysen, G.A. (1992) Nutritional management of nephrotic syndrome. . *Renal Nutr.*, **2**, 50–8.
5. Maroni, B.J. (1994) Nutrition in the pre-dialysis patient. *Dial. Transplant.*, **23**, 76–94.
6. Sakhaee, K. (1992) Management of Renal Osteodystrophy. *Semin. Nephrol.*, **12**, 101–8.
7. McKenzie, S.I. and Henderson, I.S. (1986) The effect of increased dietary fibre intake on regular haemodialysis patients. *Aspects Renal Care*, **1**, 172–7.
8. Pender, F.T. (1989) The effect of increasing the dietary fibre content of diets of patients with chronic renal failure treated by haemodialysis at home. . *um. Nutr. Dietetics*, **2**, 423–7.
9. Makoff, R. (1992) The importance and use of iron supplementation in uremia. *Nephrol. News Issues*, June, 14–9.
10. Makoff, R. (1991) Water-soluble vitamin status in patients with renal disease treated with hemodialysis of peritoneal dialysis. . *Renal Nutr.*, **1**, 56–73.
11. Bansal, V. (1992) Potassium metabolism in renal failure: nondietary rationale for hyperkalemia. . *Renal Nutr.*, **2**, suppl. 1, 8–12.
12. Pender, F.T. (1989) The effect of increasing the dietary fibre content of diets of patients with chronic renal failure treated by haemodialysis at home. . *um. Nutr. Dietetics*, **2**, 423–7.
13. Bower, J.A. (1989) Cooking for restricted potassium diets in dietary treatment of renal patients. . *um. Nutr. Dietetics*, **2**, 31–8.
14. Stenvinkel, P. (1993) Factors influencing the development and progression of diabetic nephropathy. *EDTNA ERCA ournal* , **I** , 2–4.
15. Kopple, J.D. and Blumenkrantz, M.J. (1983) Nutritional requirements for patients undergoing continuous ambulatory peritoneal dialysis. *Kidney Int.*, **24** (S 16) 295–302.
16. Halverson, N.A., Wilkens, K.G. and Worthington-Roberts, B. (1993) Interdialytic fluid gains in diabetic patients receiving hemodialysis treatment. . *Renal Nutr.*, **3**, 23–9.
17. Goldstein, D.J. and Frederico, C.B. (1987) The effect of urea kinetic modeling on the nutrition management of hemodialysis patients. . *Am. Dietetic Assoc.*, **87**, 474–9.
18. Lowrie, E.G. and Lew, N. (1991) The urea reduction ratio (URR): a simple method for evaluating hemodialysis treatment. *Contem. Dial. Nephrol.*, February, 11–20.
19. Boag, J.T. (1994) Basic truths in optimal hemodialysis. *Dial. Transplant.*, **23** 636–42.

20. Marckman, P. (1988) Nutritional status of patients on hemodialysis and peritoneal dialysis. *Clin. Nephrol.*, **29**, 75–8.
21. Spiegel, D.M., Anderson, M., Campbell, U. *et al.* (1993) Serum albumin: a marker for morbidity in peritoneal dialysis patients. *Am. . Kidney Dis.*, **21**, 26–30.
22. Nelson, E.E. (1991) Anthropometry in the nutritional assessment of adults with end-stage renal disease. . *Renal Nutr.*, **1**, 162–72.
23. Medford, S. (1992) Medical review criteria – HCFA. . *Renal Nutr.* **2**, 77–8.
24. Pagenkemper, J.J. and Foulks, C.J. (1991) Nutritional management of the adult renal transplant patient. . *Renal Nutr.* **1**, 119–24.
25. Snetselaar, L. (1994) Planning and implementing a reduced-protein diet. *Renal Nutr.*, **4**, 86–7.

## FURTHER READING

Blackwell, T.B. (ed.) (1993) *Manual of Dietetic Practice*, Blackwell Scientific Publications, Oxford

Holland, B., Unwin, I.D. and Buss, D.H. (1989) *McCance and iddowsons The Composition of Food*, 4th edn, Milk products and eggs, 4th suppl., Royal Society of Chemistry and Ministry of Agriculture, Fisheries and Food.

Holland, B., Welch, A.A., Unwin, I.D. *et al.* (1991) *McCance and iddowsons The Composition of Food*, 5th edn, Royal Society of Chemistry and Ministry of Agriculture, Fisheries and Food.

Smith, C.L. (1992) Dietary factors in calcium nephrolithiasis. . *Renal Nutr.*, **2**, 146–53.

Wendland, B. (1991) Nutritional management of patients with kidney stones, *Nephrol. News Issues*, October, 32–43.

# Index

Page numbers in *italic* refer to figures and page numbers in **bold** refer to tables